Praise for
JJ VIRGIN'S SUGAR IMPACT DIET COOKBOOK

"JJ Virgin has done it again with her *Sugar Impact Diet Cookbook*. Her delicious, nutritious recipes are guaranteed to be a huge hit!"

—Mark Hyman, MD, #1 *New York Times* bestselling author of *The Blood Sugar Solution*

"This cookbook makes it easier than ever to throw together a fabulous, fat-burning meal that is sure to please the whole family."

—Haylie Pomroy, #1 *New York Times* bestselling author of *The Fast Metabolism Diet*

"Sugar sucks! JJ Virgin's Sugar Impact Diet helps you avoid sugar without experiencing cravings. It's totally worth it!"

—Dave Asprey, *New York Times* bestselling author and creator of Bulletproof Coffee

"In *JJ Virgin's Sugar Impact Diet Cookbook*, the brilliant JJ Virgin shows you how to ditch hidden sugars, eat delicious food, and lose weight. If you buy one book this year make sure it's this one!"

—Rocco DiSpirito, celebrity chef and #1 *New York Times* bestselling author

"Good food is the foundation of brain health. This revolutionary cookbook makes it easier to lose weight and feel mentally healthier and sharper, while enjoying delicious meals."

—Daniel Amen, MD, *New York Times* bestselling author of *Change Your Brain, Change Your Life* and founder of Amen Clinics

"A groundbreaking new cookbook that will help you lose weight without feeling deprived or giving up your favorite foods."

—Sara Gottfried, MD, *New York Times* bestselling author of *The Hormone Cure*

"JJ helps you crush your sugar cravings without deprivation. If you've gone cold turkey and suffered, you're going to love these recipes."

—Alan Christianson, NMD, *New York Times* bestselling author of *The Adrenal Reset Diet* and founder of Integrative Health Care

"Pizza and pudding for fat loss? Yes, it's possible! JJ Virgin shows you how in this delicious new cookbook."

—Frank Lipman, author of *The New Health Rules*

JJ VIRGIN'S
SUGAR IMPACT
DIET COOKBOOK

Also by JJ Virgin

JJ Virgin's Sugar Impact Diet
The Virgin Diet Cookbook
The Virgin Diet
Six Weeks to Sleeveless and Sexy

JJ VIRGIN'S SUGAR IMPACT DIET COOKBOOK

150 Low-Sugar Recipes to
Help You Lose Up to
10 Pounds in Just 2 Weeks

JJ Virgin, CNS, CHFS

New York Times bestselling author of
JJ Virgin's Sugar Impact Diet

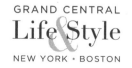

GRAND CENTRAL
Life & Style
NEW YORK • BOSTON

Copyright © 2015 by JJ Virgin

Photographs copyright © 2015 by Jonathan Heindemause

Grand Central Life & Style
Hachette Book Group
1290 Avenue of the Americas
New York, NY 10104

www.GrandCentralLifeandStyle.com

Printed in the United States of America

RRD-C

First Edition: May 2015

10 9 8 7 6 5 4 3 2 1

Grand Central Life & Style is an imprint of Grand Central Publishing.

The Grand Central Life & Style name and logo are trademarks of Hachette Book Group, Inc.

The Hachette Speakers Bureau provides a wide range of authors for speaking events. To find out more, go to www.HachetteSpeakersBureau.com or call (866) 376-6591.

The publisher is not responsible for websites (or their content) that are not owned by the publisher.

Library of Congress Cataloging-in-Publication Data

Virgin, JJ
    JJ Virgin's sugar impact diet cookbook : 150 low-sugar recipes to help you lose up to 10 pounds in just 2 weeks / JJ Virgin, CNS, CHFS ; *New York Times* bestselling author of JJ Virgin's Sugar Impact Diet.
        pages cm
    title: Sugar impact diet cookbook
    Includes bibliographical references and index.
    ISBN 978-1-4555-7787-3 (hardback)—ISBN 978-1-4555-7786-6 (ebook)   1. Sugar-free diet—Recipes.   2. Reducing diets—Recipes.   3. Weight loss.   I. Virgin, JJ. JJ Virgin's sugar impact diet. II. Title.   III. Title: Sugar impact diet cookbook.
    RM237.85V568 2015
    641.5'63837—dc23
                                                                                            2014049849

There is such power in knowing it's never too late to become your best self.
The secret is simply to decide to act. Please don't rob the world of the gift of you!

CONTENTS

PART III

THE SUGAR IMPACT DIET MEAL PLANS 205

JJ VIRGIN'S
SUGAR IMPACT
DIET COOKBOOK

DROP 7 SUGARS, LOSE 10 POUNDS, JUST 2 WEEKS

Think about sugar's place in all our happy memories, from birthday cakes to Halloween candy to after-school treats. Maybe there were sundaes with your grandparents or big boxes of candy at the movies with your friends. Boy, have times changed! It's hard to feel the same way about sugar now, but its hold over us is just as strong as it ever was.

Sugar is everywhere! It's nearly impossible to avoid, even though we know it's bad for us. But what if I told you I could give you a simple way to change the way you look at sugar and an easy plan to reduce it in your diet without feeling like you're being deprived? You'd jump at the chance, right? Cutting back on sugar is the secret to fast fat loss, breaking weight loss plateaus, reducing inflammation, balancing hormones, and improving mood and sleep more than any other change to diet or lifestyle. And it's not as hard as you think!

NOT ALL SUGARS ARE CREATED EQUAL

The key is understanding this one thing: not all sugar is created equal! It's the *impact* of sugar that matters. Sugar Impact (SI) is the very reason I've declared sugar—especially hidden sugars, which I'll describe in this book—Public Enemy #1. The high Sugar Impact of the 7 foods I'm going to share with you is the single biggest culprit when it comes to hijacking your weight and health.

High-impact sugars create dramatic spikes in your blood sugar and insulin response, and take aim at your weight, your skin, and your insides. Low-impact sugars are the key to a nice, steady stream of energy that fuels your body and eliminates the daily siege of sugar spikes and crashes.

I've helped hundreds of thousands of people overcome the vise grip of sugar, and I can help you, too. I can promise you amazing results if you follow the recipes and meal plans in this book. The revolutionary program I've created is a game changer. It's an easy to follow, step-by-step process that weans you off the foods with the highest and most damaging sugars—those with the highest Sugar Impact—so that you can lose weight, drop fat, and improve your health fast, all while satisfying your sweet tooth, and without the trauma of withdrawal or deprivation. By making simple sugar swaps for just 2 weeks, you'll heal your body and transform your life *forever*.

FROM YOUR GENES TO YOUR JEANS

Our love affair with sugar begins in the womb. We're genetically hardwired to want food that's sweet; every cell in our body needs the sugar glucose to function. So we can't—and shouldn't—cut it out entirely. But the line between what we want and what we need has become so blurred that our sugar consumption has gotten out of control. The average American eats more than 22 teaspoons a day. A day!

That's a far cry from how our ancestors ate. They gorged on fruit when it was ripe, and honey if they were lucky, to store energy. It wasn't often, and that was as sweet as it got. But when high-fructose corn syrup was introduced in the 1970s, our food got sweeter, which only increased our desire for sugar. It also happened to be the beginning of the war on fat, and when fat came out of food, so did the taste. Sugar was poured back in to compensate, and because high-fructose corn syrup was cheap, it was used in just about everything. Suddenly, eating low fat meant eating high sugar—and we were all being dosed with it.

By 2000, the average American was consuming a jaw-dropping 150 pounds of sugar a year (up from 5 pounds in 1900), with about 61 of those pounds coming from high-fructose corn syrup.

Even though we don't eat as much straight table sugar as we used to, we still don't always know how much sugar we're consuming. We're increasing the amount we eat by about 1% every year, which is faster than the world's population is growing. Many people come to me when they're at their wits' end—they've already cut out sweets, they use "healthy" substitutes like honey or maple syrup as sweeteners, they add fruit to their whole-grain cereal. They power through the day with low-calorie snack bars and live on salads and diet sodas. Of course, no one can live like that for long, and when they veer off course they beat themselves up for their lack of willpower. And after all that, they're still fighting weight gain, fatigue, cravings, mood swings, health issues like joint pain and insulin resistance, and maybe even diabetes. No wonder they're frustrated!

RESET YOUR SWEET TOOTH—IN JUST 2 WEEKS!

If you're eating healthy but you just can't drop that stubborn weight (maybe you're even gaining weight), here's your answer. The problem is that many diets people think of as healthy are loaded with *hidden* sugars. Sneaky sugars hide in surprising places—including foods you think are safe: whole foods, diet foods, fruit, enhanced waters, dressings . . . even sugar substitutes. Even when you're hypervigilant, it's hard to know all the places they take cover or how to avoid them. All told, there are more than 50 names for sugar!

But whether you're on the Sugar Impact Diet or you're just getting started, this cookbook is your low–Sugar Impact road map for easy, fun, delicious recipes that deliver benefits to your weight and health faster than you thought possible.

The recipes in this book make going low Sugar Impact so simple! They eliminate high–Sugar Impact foods for you and still serve up delicious, straightforward meals that are fun to make and eliminate your cravings.

You may have trouble picking your favorite out of the 150 scrumptious recipes, but rest assured, you'll never feel that you're missing anything or being deprived. These recipes help you enjoy taking control of your Sugar Impact, and just to be sure, they leave plenty of room for you to swap foods to your heart's content.

Plus, if you've ever been on a diet and felt paralyzed wondering whether you can do the program if you have diabetes or insulin resistance, or as a vegetarian or paleo dieter, the answer is—yes! I've created meal plans for all those scenarios and more and included them in this cookbook. In addition to the meal plan for the basic Sugar Impact Diet, I've given you 3-week meal plans for managing your blood sugar, gastrointestinal healing, and for vegetarians and vegans, as well as Paleo followers.

You'll be amazed at how easy it is to keep the weight off no matter where you are or what your eating style is.

People who've followed the Sugar Impact Diet had amazing results—most lost 10 pounds in just 2 weeks! And they feel better than they have in years—symptoms we're all told to believe are the normal signs of aging, like bloating, exhaustion, and joint pain, simply disappeared.

You can see results like this, too! You'll be surprised at how easy it is. I'll show you how to eliminate the hidden sugars holding your health and your waistline hostage from these 7 food groups:

Grains
Roots
Packaged Fruit
Low- and No-Fat Dairy and Diet Foods
Sugary Drinks
Sauces, Dressings, and Condiments
Sweeteners and Added Sugar

Dropping your Sugar Impact in these 7 categories resets and retrains your taste buds. You'll key back into the subtle sweetness of nature's treats and set yourself up to join my clients in losing up to 10 pounds in just 2 weeks—which is great news, since studies show that when you lose weight fast, you keep it off.

THE SUGAR IMPACT DIET BLUEPRINT

The strategic, step-by-step approach of the Sugar Impact Diet ensures your success by moving you through the program at your own speed, in tune with how your body responds to the changes in your diet. You have to know where you are when you start. Then you'll gently remove high-impact sugars, shift from being a sugar burner to a fat burner, and emerge on the other side, ready to chart your maintenance path forward.

Simply put, the journey to low–Sugar Impact freedom is guided by the 4Ts—Test,

Taper, Transition, Transformed! In just 2 weeks, you'll drop up to 10 pounds and no longer wonder what it feels like to be bursting with energy and feeling better than ever.

Cycle 1: TAPER

- Take the Sneaky Sugar Inventory to identify how much sugar you are actually eating.
- Take the Sugar Impact Quiz to identify the impact sugar is having on you.
- Trade your high-SI foods for medium-SI foods.
- Take your starting weight and measurements.
- Start the day with a Sugar Impact Shake.
- Focus on following the portions of the Sugar Impact Plate and eating by the Sugar Impact Clock.

Cycle 2: TRANSITION

- Trade your medium-SI foods for low-SI foods and avoid any low-SI foods that are asterisked (i.e., most fruit).
- Hide or toss the medium- and high-SI foods.
- Start the day with a Sugar Impact Shake.
- Take the Sugar Impact Quiz weekly.
- Take your weight and measurements weekly.
- Check in with the Sugar Impact Quiz at the 2-week mark to determine if you should stay in Cycle 2 or shift into Cycle 3.

Cycle 3: TRANSFORMED!

- Swap 3 or 4 low-SI servings for medium-SI servings; 1 or 2 of these servings should be from fruit.
- Have one high-SI serving at the end of the week.
- Weigh, measure, and retest at the end of the week. Decide if you can stay in Cycle 3 or need to return to Cycle 2.
- Once a year, repeat Cycles 1 and 2 to ensure you're retaining your sugar sensitivity and to bust any plateaus. You should also do Cycles 1 and 2 again if you "fall off the wagon."

At first, your success on the Sugar Impact Diet will be about how much weight you lose, but that's just the beginning. In time you'll see the gift it delivers in helping you stay at your goal weight forever. Most programs yank the sugar and then leave you without a path forward—and you usually end up right back where you started.

When you complete this program, Cycle 3 will be your guide to staying sugar sensitive for life. I still encourage you to redo Cycles 1 and 2 once a year, especially if you want to push yourself toward a new goal, but whether or not you do, you'll have 150 simple, delicious recipes to help you chart your course. They put you in complete control of your weight, energy, and health—whether you're eating at home or out, you're paleo or vegetarian, you're feeding a family on a budget or dealing with personal conditions like leaky gut or insulin resistance.

This book is organized to make the best use of your precious time—and to help you easily customize the Sugar Impact Diet for your lifestyle.

Part I is an explanation of Sugar Impact and what lowering it will mean to your weight, your health, and your life. Part II gets right to the good stuff with all the tasty recipes, and the meal plans in Part III make living your low–Sugar Impact life a no-brainer—just follow them as they're laid out and watch all the benefits of lower Sugar Impact come your way.

You're about to enter completely new weight loss territory. Be prepared for how quickly the changes come—and how empowering it will be to break free from the stranglehold of sugar in just 2 weeks!

PART I

UNDERSTANDING SUGAR IMPACT

1

NOT ALL SUGAR IS CREATED EQUAL

Starting a new diet is a little like waking up on Christmas morning—all the promise and wonder is so exciting! Well, here it is, the Sugar Impact Diet, just waiting to be unwrapped. And its present to you is that it's going to change your life in just 2 weeks! Once you see how easy it is to drop high–Sugar Impact foods and the huge benefits it has for you in your life, you'll never look back. Fast fat loss awaits—most people lose 10 pounds in just 2 weeks—but so does a more youthful-looking, energetic you. You can kiss your cravings good-bye, along with the brain fog, achy joints, and other oppressive symptoms that have made you feel old, sick, and tired before your time. And best of all, in your new low–Sugar Impact life, you'll be arming yourself against—or even reversing—serious diseases connected to obesity and high blood sugar, like insulin resistance and diabetes.

BURN, BABY, BURN

The secret sauce of fast fat loss is this: the Sugar Impact Diet is going to take you from being a sugar burner, which is what you are now, to a fat burner. Sugar burners begin burning the fuel in their food as soon as it hits their mouth, and they have to keep shoveling more fuel in the furnace to keep it lit, so to speak. So your body currently depends on a steady supply of carbs for energy—because you're in a vicious cycle where you'll crash without them. Even worse, your metabolism never dips into your fat reserves for energy because it doesn't have to and chronically elevated blood sugar and insulin levels prevent fat burning. To lose weight, you've got to start burning fat and stop burning sugar—and lowering your Sugar Impact is the key.

You'll have all of the support you need on your journey to becoming a fat burner. Simple swaps, delicious recipes, and easy-to-follow meal plans will be your road map— follow them, and your extra pounds will be in your rearview mirror so fast you won't even know what hit you! You'll not only lose weight fast, ditch your cravings, and be bursting with energy, you'll have fun along the way!

NO MORE COUNTING CALORIES

Another thing that sets the Sugar Impact Diet apart is that there will be no counting calories. In fact, I forbid it. Let me hear you say it—yay! Just as all sugar is not created equal, a calorie is not a calorie. I want you to start looking at food as the information it is. Every time you choose something to eat, it has consequences, for better or worse. It's going to send your body a message, and the payoff is either that you're being nourished or you're not. As you might imagine, your body responds a little differently to a hot fudge sundae than it does to a lean, organic chicken breast. But why?

WHY SUGAR IS PUBLIC ENEMY #1

All foods raise blood sugar, but high–Sugar Impact carbohydrates and sugary foods make your blood sugar go *way* up. Your pancreas produces the hormone insulin to get glucose, one of the sugars you eat, out of your bloodstream and shuttle it to your cells to use for energy—glucose is our fuel. What your cells can't use, your liver and muscles can store in the form of glycogen to be used for energy later.

But insulin also makes it easier for your body to store fat. Ack! Plus, it can lead to much bigger problems like insulin resistance and diabetes.

In addition to glucose, one of the other most common sugars in our food is fructose, the primary sugar in fruit. Fructose is also found in less natural "foods" like sugary drinks and packaged snacks in the form of high-fructose corn syrup. Fructose is metabolized differently than other sugars. It doesn't create the spike in blood sugar and insulin like other sugars do. At first blush that sounds like a good thing, but that biological mechanism is a protective measure; fructose blows by it, so your body has no way of registering that it's eaten and that it's on its way to being full. To make matters worse, fructose goes directly to your liver, the only organ that can metabolize it. Your liver converts some fructose to glucose (which can then be used as glycogen or converted to fat) and the rest to triglycerides.

Your body breaks all the sugar you eat into glucose or fructose, no matter what the source of the sugar is. But glucose and fructose are metabolized very differently: glucose = fuel; fructose = fat. That's what I mean by Sugar Impact, and that's why I'm going to help you learn to key into how much of which is in the foods you choose.

Now, is fructose always the enemy? No. Remember, it's the primary sugar in fruit, and it's found in other natural, whole foods we eat like some vegetables. But in those cases, it's intertwined with fiber and nutrients. Fiber changes fructose's behavior for the better—it slows digestion in general, so fructose is slower in making its way to the liver, and it makes the fructose harder to access, so we burn some energy getting at it. When fiber and nutrients are absent, which they are in most sources of fructose in our diet—think candy, snack packs, energy drinks—fructose is like a guided missile with nothing to slow it down as it zeroes in on your liver. It's a fat "bombs away."

Most of us already know sugar in processed foods is bad for us, and we try to steer clear of that stuff as much as possible. So what's going on? Well, the truth is, most people don't know how much sugar they're eating. Once you take my Sneaky Sugar Inventory, I bet you're going to be pretty surprised to find out how much sugar is slipping into your diet, even if you consider yourself vigilant about it! It's in a lot of foods we'd never suspect, and some we even consider healthy. So if you're like many people I know, who watch what they eat and have already cut out sweets and the obvious culprits, it's okay to feel confused and frustrated about your expanding waistline and your health issues.

If you feel like you're doing everything right but you're still dealing with the frustration of...

Bloating or gas
Cravings
Inability to lose weight
Increased appetite
Low or unstable energy
Poor mood (unfocused, irritable, depressed)
Stubborn belly fat

. . . you're probably getting way more sugar in your diet than you want or need. We're going to lower your Sugar Impact and take aim at those sneaky sugars and those symptoms!

Sneaky Sugar

You may be eating more sugar than you realize. Here are some sneaky sources that might surprise you!

- Full Original BBQ Chopped Salad (California Pizza Kitchen)—87 grams carbs/23 grams sugar
- Quaker Apples and Cinnamon Oatmeal, 1 packet—33 grams carbs/12 grams sugar
- Venti Starbucks Salted Caramel Mocha with nonfat milk—82 grams carbs/70 grams sugar
- Large Jamba Juice Strawberries Wild Smoothie—130 grams carbs/115 grams sugar
- Ocean Spray Cranberry Juice Cocktail (8 ounces)—28 grams carbs/28 grams sugar
- Vitamin Water "Squeezed" Lemonade (20-ounce bottle)—34 grams carbs/31 grams sugar
- McDonald's Fruit 'N Yogurt Parfait (5.2 ounces)—30 grams carbs/23 grams sugar
- Starbucks Bountiful Blueberry Muffin (127 grams)—55 grams carbs/29 grams sugar

---

IT'S NOT YOUR FAULT

Powering your sugar-burning metabolism with fast-acting sugar and carbs hijacks your ability to keep your appetite in check. It's not your fault—you're no longer in control.

The good news is that you can take control right back—and fast. With the right food—and the right information—your hormones begin to function as they're supposed to and referee the amount of everything you eat. You get your weight, your health, and your life back.

FREE YOURSELF FROM THE SUGAR TRAP

The nice, easy taper and transition from high–Sugar Impact foods to a diet filled with low–Sugar Impact foods will flip your sugar-burning, fat-storing metabolism on its head. The Sugar Impact diet is about to make you a fat burner, which is exactly what you want to lose weight fast and keep it off. When good fats and clean, lean protein become the focus of your diet, you'll trade the roller coaster ride of crashes and quick pick-me-ups for a steady stream of high energy all day long.

When you burn fat, you drop weight fast. And when you're low SI, your other systems, like the hormones in charge of your appetite, are all aligned in lockstep working to keep you losing weight and feeling great. Before you know it, your energy is back, your joint pain is gone, your gastrointestinal distress is in check, and bonus: you'll even burn fat when you sleep!

Here are the obstacles this book will help you understand and overcome if they rear up during your Sugar Impact Diet journey.

Obstacle #1: Cravings

Cravings can be intense and overwhelming, and staving them off is going to be a key part of winning the battle against high-impact sugar. I have a link to Sugar Attack Survival Strategies in the resources section of my website—http://sugarimpact.com/resources—specifically designed to get you through any rough spots, but wouldn't it be better not to experience them at all? Well, that's the goal.

First, you have to figure out where they're coming from. They can be rooted in your genes or your lifestyle (the way you eat), or both. Knowing the source of your cravings is the only way to break their grip.

The other major cause of cravings comes from eating a low-fat diet. No, that was not a typo. Remember, low fat means high sugar, and usually from high-impact sugars. They give you a quick shot of energy, but they set in motion a cycle of cravings for the very foods that *create* cravings. And your system takes a serious beating when you feed the beast of cravings. Your hormones and blood sugar are spiking and cratering in response to whatever you've eaten, but if you aren't aware that you're eating that much sugar, it can feel like punching in the dark. Labels don't aim to help you figure it out; sometimes sugar isn't even listed as sugar on the ingredients list. Barley malt sounds pretty innocent, doesn't it?

The important thing is—and don't lose sight of this—the recipes in this book take care of that for you! They're all lower Sugar Impact, which means they're designed to combat cravings by including the ideal balance of fats, carbs, and protein to keep you full and energized all day long.

Obstacle #2: Addiction

Some of you will flat-out say you're addicted to sugar. And there's real evidence that could be exactly what's going on. We know we're wired to eat sweet, so when it's available every-where all the time, it stands to reason that you could find yourself in a bit of an internal scrap fighting the urge to indulge. The chemicals at war inside you are the very same ones that light up in response to other addictions. As Dr. Pamela Peeke, author of *The Hunger Fix*, explained it to me, "Animal studies have shown that refined sugar is more addictive than cocaine, heroin, or morphine. An animal will choose an Oreo over morphine. Why? This cookie has the perfect combination of sugar and fat to hijack the brain's reward center."

If you're hooked on sugar, you no doubt experience withdrawal when you don't have it. That also means you probably binge when you finally get your hands on it. I have sup-port for that! I'm going to help you cope with any withdrawal symptoms that pop up with my Sugar Withdrawal Strategies (go to http://sugarimpact.com/resources) so you don't experience the defeat of giving in, or the guilt that goes with it.

It's not about "willpower." You're supposed to crave sugar when your blood sugar gets low. The key is to not let that happen—and the Sugar Impact Diet is going to get you out of the high-low blood sugar spin cycle. Once you even out your blood sugar, the rest of you will follow suit.

Obstacle #3: Let's Not Forget Stress

Okay, we've all eaten poorly when we're under stress—myself included. Yes, food is infor-mation for your body, but we have a more complicated relationship with food sometimes: it can also be a comfort when we're stressed out or upset.

Why is it, though, that we can only find comfort in chocolate? Or macaroni and cheese? Why doesn't anyone ever want Brussels sprouts to self-soothe? Well, for one, stress sup-presses the happy hormone serotonin, which is also one of the feel-good neurotransmitters released when you eat sugar. Sweets are just a shortcut to bringing it back, stat.

Knowing what you know now about blood sugar spikes and crashes, it will come as no surprise that stress eating is just a short-term fix that actually leaves us worse off than before. Not to mention that it's a crutch that causes weight gain, fatigue, brain fog, self-esteem issues...should I go on?

So whether you're dealing with cravings, the pull of addiction, or stress eating, high–Sugar Impact foods—and the metabolic havoc they wreak—have had their hooks in you for too long. Going low SI will loosen sugar's grip on you and set your system free.

LET THE HEALING BEGIN

Of the many ways the Sugar Impact Diet takes care of you and ensures your success, the one you'll probably appreciate most (next to 150 high-taste, lower-SI recipes!) is that it doesn't take sugar from you cold turkey. You've been there, done that. You know where that gets you. Amped-up cravings and withdrawal symptoms are a prescription for failure, but when you taper and transition, success is all but guaranteed.

You'll move at your own pace from high-SI to medium-SI to low-SI foods. I'll be there every step of the way to help you ease off the high-SI foods that are hurting you. I also have strategies and Supportive Supplements on the resources section of my website http://sugarimpact.com to help you fight any and all symptoms that make a surprise appearance, so you have smooth sailing on your way to becoming an Impact Player.

One of the things you'll experience as you heal is that you'll retrain your taste buds to be more sensitive to sweetness. The more you're able to subtly tune in to nature's bounty, like the sweetness in berries, the less you'll need of it and the more processed sweets will seem like overkill. Bye-bye cravings!

TASTE IS ALL IT'S CRACKED UP TO BE

As a sugar addict, you may not even realize you're missing out on some spectacular flavors. High-SI foods have paved over your taste buds, and savory and spicy foods may be beyond your notice or desire. But you're about to be introduced to a new world through the flavorful, nutritious recipes in this book. As your taste buds come back to life you'll sense the exquisite sweetness of spices like vanilla and cinnamon, and the satisfying richness of dark chocolate. These recipes have been created to make sure you have no barrier to success—they're easy, fast, and delicious.

And a funny thing happens on your way to becoming low SI—you start to crave the new, healthy, fat-burning foods you've introduced into your diet over the sugar and carbs you're living on now. Once you get into the sensational swaps I'll give you, you won't even miss your high-SI favorites. And why would you? They haven't done you any favors.

I'm willing to bet you like the swaps even more—for the way they taste *and* the way they make you feel.

BASIC TRAINING

The big goal of the Sugar Impact Diet—and this plan—is to eliminate high–Sugar Impact foods. You need to become a sugar sleuth and expose the hidden sources of sugar in your diet. Sticking with the meal plans in this book will take care of you most of the time, so you can exhale. But when you're eating out or at a friend's dinner party, you'll need to be extra vigilant. Refer to the Sneaky Sugar Inventory and the Sugar Impact Scales in this section for helpful guidelines and simple swaps to keep in mind as you transform yourself from a sugar burner to a fat burner.

Commit to becoming a sugar sleuth and eliminating high–Sugar Impact foods, then use these basic principles to give you a rock-solid foundation that removes the guesswork on lowering your SI, so you become lean and healthy *for life*.

Make Breakfast a Protein Shake

Most of us hit the ground running in the morning. You wake up having enough to think about without having to worry about breakfast, right?

A protein shake is a great no-brainer for breakfast: in about the time it takes to pour cereal and milk (a high–Sugar Impact "meal" if ever there was one), you can whip up a delicious, antioxidant-rich, anti-inflammatory, nutrient-dense protein shake.

Blend nondairy, non-soy plant-based or defatted beef protein powder with berries, kale or other leafy greens, flaxseeds or chia seeds, and unsweetened coconut or almond milk for a satisfying, filling breakfast that takes minutes to make but keeps you full for hours. Check out my tips on protein powder on page 39 and some delicious shake recipes beginning on page 65. You can love them as they are, or mix them up to suit your taste. There are also some other awesome low–Sugar Impact breakfast options in the Recipes section if shakes aren't your thing.

Eat by the Sugar Impact Plate

Counting, sorting, and measuring suck all the joy out of eating. Besides, who has the time? The source of your calories is far more important than their number, so I want you to *stop counting them*. How happy are you?! Use my SI Plate (see page 21) and you'll completely eliminate the guesswork for creating fat-burning, filling meals.

Your colorful, nutrient-rich plate will be packed with clean, lean protein; healthy fats; nonstarchy leafy and cruciferous vegetables; and high-fiber, low–Sugar Impact foods. Once you get the hang of it, use the Plate strategy at restaurants, dinner parties, and—yes!—even at fast-food restaurants.

Burst and Resist

One of the things people always ask me—and I know this is on your mind, too—is whether you can lose fat without exercise. Just to let you know, saying "Pretty please?" does not change the answer!

I'm not going to let you completely off the hook when it comes to exercise, but I'm also not expecting you to devote tons of time to it. Nobody has hours to spend on elliptical machines or aerobics classes. And why would you, when you can knock out a fat-blasting, metabolism-boosting workout in just minutes a day? Burst train instead. Burst training is fast, intense exercise that you can do almost anywhere, from a park hill to a hotel stairwell. You go all-out for 30 to 60 seconds, with active recovery of 1 to 2 minutes. During recovery, you should be slowly moving, so you can catch your breath and get your heart rate back down. Set your goal for a total workout of 15 to 30 minutes.

To build strength, boost energy, and blast fat in less time than it takes to drive to the gym, combine burst training with strength training. Lift the heaviest weight you can lift in good form for 8 to 12 reps.

Eliminate Food Intolerances

Even if you're doing everything else right, ignoring food intolerances could mean you'll never get past your weight loss resistance, bloating, gas, and the rest of their unpleasant side effects.

Despite your best efforts, certain foods can derail your chance of success if your body doesn't tolerate them. *The Virgin Diet* targets 7 highly reactive foods—gluten, soy, dairy, eggs, peanuts, corn, and sugar and artificial sweeteners—that could sabotage your fat loss success and send your metabolism into a tailspin.

You already know about the damage high–Sugar Impact foods can create, but even so-called healthy foods like dairy and eggs can create food intolerances if your body just can't handle them. In *The Virgin Diet*, I show you how to eliminate these 7 foods (they can sneak into your diet in really surprising ways!) and then challenge 4 of them to see which ones are doing you harm and keep you clinging to extra pounds.

Supplement Smartly

I wish I had better news on this front, but our food just isn't as nutritious as it used to be. Everything from topsoil erosion to transit times drains minerals from what we eat. Make sure you're getting what you need to support your fast fat loss and give you the strength to fight cravings and hunger. At the very least, take a professional-quality multivitamin/mineral, antioxidant, and an essential fatty-acid formula. If you'd like some recommendations, check out the resources section of my website, http://sugarimpact.com.

Vitamin D is another essential nutrient, and your body makes it when you spend time in the sun. But whether you live in sunny California or a cloudy climate, you're just as likely to test low on vitamin D. Vitamin D is actually a hormone that, among its many benefits, supports bone health and fat loss. Take a 25-hydroxy vitamin D test and work with a practitioner to get your range within 50 and 80 ng/ml. Once you're there, maintain optimal D levels by taking a 2,000 to 5,000 IU daily supplement of vitamin D3 and spending time unprotected in the sun.

You might also consider a digestive enzyme if you're dealing with gas, bloating, and other post-meal issues. Stress and age can deplete your body's ability to make digestive enzymes. That means you don't absorb nutrients or break down your food as well as you used to, and it sets you up for gut-related health conditions.

Beyond that, nearly everyone benefits from extra magnesium and a probiotic supplement.

Get Some Deep Sleep

Insufficient sleep wreaks hormonal havoc and sets you up for an all-day, caffeine-fueled crash-and-burn cycle. Many people say they feel a "new normal" when they finally get enough sleep. Aim for at least 7 hours—and more like 8—every night.

Easier said than done sometimes, right? That's why you need to *prepare* for sleep. It's serious business! About an hour before shut-eye, turn off all your electronics, take a hot bath with a trashy novel and some chamomile tea, and consider herbal sleep formulas if you need them.

Control Your Stress Levels

If you told me to completely eliminate stress, I would ask what planet you want me to vacation on. You could live in the most calming, serene scene and still be a stressed-out mess in your own life. By the same token, you could find your bliss in the center of the craziness in Times Square. It all comes down to perspective and how you handle the curves life throws your way.

We all know you can't completely get rid of stress, so do everything possible to reduce it and its impact on you physically and emotionally. Chronic stress elevates cortisol, a hormone that stores fat and breaks down muscle. That's not what you want!

So make reducing stress a priority. If you can afford massages, schedule them as often as possible. Even dog walks and hanging out with friends can help you de-stress. Figure out what works for *you* and make it a necessity, not a luxury.

THE POWER TOOLS OF SUCCESS

Here's my promise to you: if you bring the commitment, I'll take care of the rest. I've built the Sugar Impact Diet as a program in three cycles, during which you'll travel through the 4Ts (Test, Taper, Transition, Transformed!). The very words *taper* and *transition* give away the approach—you're moving to a low-SI diet without the shock and awe(ful) that usually comes with diets that have you go cold turkey.

On the off chance withdrawal symptoms hit or cravings creep in, don't steel yourself and just try to power through. Why would you do that to yourself, and risk having to start over? I've included a ton of effective strategies in this book to help ease those feelings until they pass, including how to get enough sleep, which supplements to take, proper meal timing and portions, and suggestions for emergency food to carry with you. And trust me, you'll be so glad you stayed the course—the other side is bliss.

To take away any anxiety you may have about what food to pull out of your diet, what food to put in, and when, I've created the following guides to make it super-easy for you:

1. A staples list beginning on page 51, or download it and the Shopping Guides at http://sugarimpact.com/resources

2. Sugar Impact Scales—foods are ranked according to their Sugar Impact (high, medium, and low), and you'll simply move from high-SI choices to medium-SI choices to low-SI choices by following the instructions laid out in the cycles. You're also given an extensive list of swaps for moving from high to medium to low SI to simplify it further.

3. The ideal Sugar Impact Plate, portion sizes, and Meal Timing

4. How to set up your kitchen

5. Meal plans that include the 150 delicious, lower-SI recipes in this book and cover a wide range of eating and lifestyle choices such as being a vegan or vegetarian, or paleo

You can't fail! And the sooner you get started, the sooner you'll be on the other side of Cycle 3, checking your look in the mirror and drinking in the compliments.

THE SUGAR IMPACT SCALES

You're going to love the Sugar Impact Scales! They're easy-to-follow cheat sheets that organize foods according to their impact on your blood sugar—high, medium, or low. No need to memorize and no math. Well, I did the math. I took care of you there, huh? Here's the way a food's SI ranking was determined:

1. Fructose (in grams)
2. Nutrient density
3. Fiber
4. Glycemic load (a measurement of how the food affects your blood sugar that includes typical serving sizes)

I like to think of low-SI foods as having a green light—eat them regularly. The medium-SI foods are yellow—proceed with caution and incorporate only the amount you can have and still feel great. (I'll explain both the best way to taper medium-SI foods out of your diet in Cycle 1 and how to figure out the right amount for you long term in Cycle 3.) When it comes to high-SI foods, no surprise there—stop! They're red. Eat and drink them only rarely.

In short:

- Low Sugar Impact—Go!
- Medium Sugar Impact—Proceed with Caution
- High Sugar Impact—Stop!

The Sugar Impact Scales rank foods within 7 categories to show where hidden sugars tend to be an issue. Some of these may surprise you!

- Grains
- Roots
- Packaged Fruits
- Low- and No-Fat Dairy and Diet Foods
- Sugary Drinks
- Sauces, Dressings, and Condiments
- Sweeteners and Added Sugar

The Sugar Impact Scales within each category will show you which high-SI foods to swap for low- to medium-SI options. I go into more detail about the 7 foods and provide Sugar Impact Scales for each food in the next chapter. They're also available online at http://sugarimpact.com/resources.

TRACK YOUR IMPACT

The journey begins with the first T: Test. What you can measure, you can change. You have to know where you're starting to appreciate where you'll end up. The other benefit of testing is that it's a way of making certain that this program is customized to you, what you're eating, and your triggers. You know as well as I do that a cookie-cutter diet doesn't cut it.

So look at this, the Sugar Impact Quiz, as the beginning of the path to foodie freedom. This quiz focuses on some of the most common symptoms of a high-SI diet.

Your score will be your baseline at the start of the Sugar Impact Diet, but you'll revisit it throughout the cycles to check your progress. Even if you're relatively asymptomatic, you'll see improvement no matter where you start.

Sugar Impact Quiz

Rate each category from 1 to 5, with 1 meaning that the area is a nonissue and 5 meaning that it's a big problem.

Low or Unstable Energy	1	2	3	4	5
Sugar and Carb Cravings	1	2	3	4	5
Appetite	1	2	3	4	5
Poor Mood and Focus	1	2	3	4	5
Gas and Bloating	1	2	3	4	5
Difficulty Losing Weight	1	2	3	4	5
Belly Fat	1	2	3	4	5

- If your total score is 20 or above, or you score a 4 or higher on 2 or more symptoms, you may have to extend Cycle 1 by a week to ease your transition to Cycle 2. Also consider using one or more of the Speed Healing Techniques on the resources section of my website, http://sugarimpact.com.
- If you're struggling with health conditions or you scored 15 or more, you may need to spend a second week in Cycle 1 and taper more slowly so you'll be able to go through Cycle 2 with ease. Use the Sneaky Sugar Inventory (page 17) to identify where medium- and high-SI foods are sneaking into your diet on a regular basis and make those foods the first ones you swap out during Cycle 1.
- If you're starting from the ideal place of a score of 2 or less per symptom and 12 or less overall, good for you! You'll still see a benefit from the program and you'll avoid these symptoms becoming an issue for you later on.

That's an interesting exercise, isn't it? There's no way to ignore the impact of sugar when you see its effects right there in front of you. Now you know you have to act, and you know you're in the right place. That's why this quiz is such a valuable reference point in your quest to kick sugar to the curb. Keep it close!

HOW MUCH SUGAR ARE YOU *REALLY* EATING?

As you begin your Sugar Impact Diet journey, you'll also need to figure out where the sugar in your diet is coming from. So go through this Sneaky Sugar Inventory and circle any foods you eat on a regular basis. Once you've identified them, you'll use the Sugar Impact Scales to swap them out for lower-SI choices. Those changes pay big dividends, and in just 2 weeks. So what are you waiting for?!

Sneaky Sugar Inventory

Circle any food or food ingredient eaten in the last week.

Acesulfame-K (artificial sweetener) | Agave | Almond milk ice cream | Amaranth | Amaranth flour | Animal crackers | Apples | Apricots | Asian dressing | Aspartame | Baked beans | Balsamic vinaigrette | Balsamic vinegar | Bananas | Barley | BBQ sauce | Bean chips | Beer | Beets | Beet juice | Biscotti | Black bean flour | Blue cheese dressing | Brandy | Bread-and-butter pickles | Breakfast bars | Brown rice | Brown sauce | Brown sugar | Buckwheat | Buckwheat flour | Caesar dressing | Cakes and pies | Candy | Cane syrup | Canned fruit cocktail | Capri Sun | Caramel sauce | Carnation Instant Breakfast | Carrot juice | Catalina dressing | Cereals | Champagne | Cherries | Chocolate syrup | Cocktail sauce | Coconut milk creamer, sweetened | Coconut milk ice cream, sweetened | Coconut palm sugar | Coconut sugar | Coffee creamers, refrigerated or dry | Commercial "smoothies" | Cookies | Cool Whip and Lite Cool Whip | Corn | Corn cereals | Corn chips | Cornstarch | Corn syrup | Corn tortillas | Couscous | Crackers | Cream cheese spread | Cream of Wheat | Creamsicles | Crystal Light | Crystalline fructose (artificial sweetener) | <85% dark chocolate | Dates | Diet soda | Dried fruit snacks | Energy bars | English muffins | "Enhanced" waters (that have sweeteners) | Ensure | Farro | Fat-free baked chips | 94% fat-free microwave kettle corn | 94% fat-free microwave popcorn | Fat-free muffin mix | Fat-free pudding | Fat-free or sugar-free Jell-O | Fat-free Twizzlers | Fava bean flour | Fermented soy | Fish sauce | Flavored almond milk yogurt | Flavored coconut yogurt | Flavored kefirs | French dressing | French fries | Fresh figs | Frozen yogurt | Fruit-added cream cheese | Fruit juice concentrates | Fruit juice Popsicles | Fruit juices | Fruit leather | Fudgsicles | Fuze | Garbanzo flour | Gatorade | Gelato | Gin | Glazed nuts | Glucose | Gluten-free beer | Gluten-free flour | Graham crackers | Granola bars | Grapes | Green curry sauce | Grits | Half-and-half | High-fructose corn syrup | Hoisin | Honey | Honey mustard | Honey mustard dressing | Honey-roasted peanuts | Honeydew | Hot and sour sauce | Hot cocoa |

(Continued)

Ice cream | Ice cream sandwiches | Instant oatmeal | Instant rice | Italian dressing | Jams | Ketchup | Kiwi | Kombucha tea | Kool-Aid | Lentil chips | Low-fat cheeses | Low-fat cream cheese spread | Low-fat or lite frozen dinners: Lean Cuisine, Lean Pockets, Lean Gourmet, etc. | Low-fat graham crackers | Low-fat or fat-free ice cream bars | Low-fat or fat-free ice cream | Low-fat Oreos | Low-fat plain yogurt | Macaroni and cheese | Maltodextrin | Mango | Mannitol | Maple syrup | Marinara sauce | Marshmallows | Mashed potatoes | Matzoh | Milk chocolate | Millet | Millet flour | Mixed drinks | Molasses | Mousse | Muesli | Muffins | Mung bean noodles | Nectar | Neotame | Nesquik | Neufchâtel cheese | Nonfat cheeses | Nonfat cream cheese | Nonfat plain yogurt | Nut chips | Oyster crackers | Papaya | Parsnips | Part-skim mozzarella | Part-skim ricotta | Pastas | Peanut sauce | Pears | Pickle relish | Pineapple | Pineapple cottage cheese | Pita | Plain coconut yogurt, sweetened | Plums | Polenta | Pomegranate | Popcorn | Pop-Tarts | Port | Potato chips | Potato starch | Powerade | Preserves | Pretzels | Pudding | Puffed millet | Puffed rice | Quick breads | Quinoa flakes | Quinoa flour | Quinoa pastas | Ranch dressing | Raspberry vinaigrette | Red curry sauce | Reduced-fat cookies | Reduced-fat crackers | Reduced-fat macaroni and cheese | Reduced-fat peanut butter | Reduced-fat Pringles | Rice cakes | Rice chips | Rice crackers | Rice flour | Rice pasta | Rice syrup | Rice tortillas | Risotto | Rockstar energy drink | Root veggie chips | Rum | Rutabaga | Saccharin | Scones | Slimfast | Snack packs | SnackWell's low-fat and fat-free cookies and treats | SoBe | Soda | Sorbet | Sorbitol | Soy cheeses | Splenda | Sprouted whole-grain breads | Steak sauce | Strawberry cream cheese | Sucralose | Sun-dried tomatoes | Sweet chili | Sweet pickles | Sweet pickle relish | Sweet potatoes | Sweet potato fries | Sweet tea | Sweetened coconut water | Sweetened cows' milks—vanilla, chocolate | Sweetened dairy-free milks | Sweetened nut butters | Sweetened whipped cream | Tangerines | Tartar sauce | Tequila | Teriyaki sauce | Thousand Island | Tomato juice | Tomato paste | Tomato sauce | Tortillas | Unsweetened rice milk | Unsweetened soy milk | V8 Juice | Vitamin Water | Vodka | Wasa crackers | Water crackers | Watermelon | Wheat breads | Whipped cream cheese | White flour products | White potatoes | Whole-grain cereal | Wine | Worcestershire sauce | Yams | Yogurts with sugar or artificial sweeteners

How Did You Do?

The Sneaky Sugar Inventory is a shocker, isn't it? I felt pretty good about my SI, but even I found myself circling food after food on the list. There it was, right under my nose—sugar I hadn't invited and didn't want in everything from sun-dried tomatoes to balsamic dressing.

If nothing else, this inventory makes it clear that to really see change in your weight, your energy, and the symptoms of inflammation and chronic conditions you battle every day, it's not only the *amount* of added sugar you're eating that should concern you. The *kinds* of sugar you consume and their impact also have to have a place center stage.

The American Heart Association's guideline for added sugars is that they should only be 5% of your daily discretionary calories. In 2009, the journal *Circulation* broke it down further, setting the limit as 5 teaspoons of added sugar a day for women and 9 teaspoons for men. Notice they're talking added sugar, which leaves out refined grains, fruit juice, and other foods that have a high SI. Most Americans get a lot more than that recommended limit—the average American consumes almost 500 calories of added sugar a day. That amounts to 3 pounds of sugar every week, and thousands of pounds over a lifetime.

Measure Up

Before you dive in, do these few simple things:

- Take a before picture—yes, I know, but you'll thank me soon!
- Take your weight and measure your waist and hips—you'll check in with these numbers throughout the program.
- Journal—I want you to journal every day. A 2008 study in the *American Journal of Preventive Medicine* followed nearly 1,700 people and found that it was the number one factor in predicting their weight loss success. It helps you stay focused on connecting the dots between what you eat, what you weigh, and how you feel.

HOW THE PROGRAM WORKS: THE 3 CYCLES

Your shift from a high-SI diet to a low-SI diet will be gradual—and this is key to the success of the program. It's essential that you not move ahead until you're ready, or you'll open the door to withdrawal and cravings that will derail your progress. Take the three cycles in order, no matter how well you did on the SI Quiz and no matter how much bravado you're feeling. Here's how they work.

Cycle 1—TAPER

After you identify which high-SI foods are wreaking havoc on your weight and health with the Sneaky Sugar Inventory, Cycle 1 will help you let go of those saboteurs slowly. It's designed to ease the grip of high-SI foods with medium-SI swaps, so you won't even feel it. Nothing is cut without being replaced.

Cycle 1 will take you 1 or 2 weeks, depending on how you fared on the Sugar Impact

Quiz. You should take the time you need to make this program work for you—you're laying the foundation for success in Cycle 2, so you can't move on until you're ready. As you swap high-SI foods for medium-SI foods, you're setting the stage for your move from sugar burner to fat burner. Make no mistake, you'll also see big progress here—your metabolism will ramp up, the pounds will start coming off, and you'll get the spring back in your step as your energy gets a boost. You won't want to jeopardize that by jumping ship early!

Cycle 2—TRANSITION

This is where the rubber meets the road. During Cycle 2, you'll swap medium-SI foods for low-SI foods, and your metabolism will make the move from burning sugar to burning fat! That translates into fast weight loss. The average person loses 10 pounds during these 2 weeks! Plus, at the same time your food will begin to taste better than ever—welcome back, taste buds! They're being retrained to have a higher sensitivity to sugar, and that's what will ultimately help you break free of sugar's hold over you.

Cycle 3—TRANSFORMED!

You'll arrive at Cycle 3 a new you. There'll be less of you to love, you'll have more energy and fewer aches, and you'll be more in tune with your body than ever. In Cycle 3, you'll reintroduce some high-SI foods, but I'll understand if you don't want to!

This cycle lets you customize the program to suit your body and your long-term goals. You'll take the Sugar Impact Quiz again to determine how much sugar you can allow back into your diet on a daily basis without undoing all your progress. You'll create a maintenance program that works specifically for you and builds on your success going forward.

CHANGE YOUR IMPACT!

In the next chapter, I'm going to walk you through the Sugar Impact Plate, recommended portion sizes, and the Sugar Impact Clock to take the guesswork out of how much to eat and when. You're certainly not going to go hungry! Your Sugar Impact Diet meals will create a slow, steady rise in blood sugar, so not to worry—I've got your back on their impact. I'm also going to introduce you to the 7 food groups sneaking sugar into your diet, and give you easy swaps to bring your SI down. I've made this as easy as possible so you'll stick with it and focus on the main thing—losing fat fast!

2

THE SUGAR IMPACT PLATE

No matter what you set out to do, you need the right tools to succeed. So to guarantee your swift transformation to a fat-burning machine, you'll need my power tools. They'll help you conquer your sugar addiction, get rid of extra pounds, and restore you to someone you recognize in the mirror.

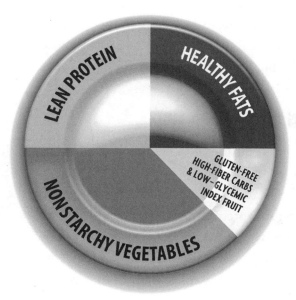

The Sugar Impact Plate

One of the most powerful tools I can offer you is the Sugar Impact Plate. It's designed to leave you happy and satisfied after you eat, to make sure you're not hungry between meals, to feed you with consistent energy and focus, and to help you burn fat for fuel.

The Sugar Impact Plate delivers balanced meals of clean, lean protein, healthy fats, colorful nonstarchy veggies, and a few slow carbs. When you eat by the Plate you won't face the fangs of cravings between meals and you'll feel content with eating less. What you do eat are healing, energizing, nutrient-dense whole foods that burn fat fast.

UNDERSTANDING THE SUGAR IMPACT PLATE

Take a good look at the sections of the Sugar Impact Plate: lean protein, healthy fats, nonstarchy vegetables, and gluten-free high-fiber carbs and fruit. They all work like a symphony to keep your blood sugar nice and even and to propel fast fat loss.

Each macronutrient—protein, fat, and carbs—creates a hormonal response connected to the quality, timing, and amount you eat. Carbs are a source of energy. They trigger the release of insulin to absorb glucose from your blood and move it into your cells where it's used as energy, or stored as glycogen or fat. Proteins are the building blocks of lean muscle tissue, and they keep you full longer by slowing down the time it takes food to leave your stomach. Fat releases chemicals in the small intestine that tell your brain you've had enough to eat. So let's take a look at each of these macronutrients and how they work to pack your Plate with fat-burning fuel.

PROTEIN—PROTEIN BUILDS YOU UP

Protein is great for filling you up and keeping you satisfied, but it's also a quick fix for sugar cravings. When a craving hits, you may just be low in protein, and your system is crying out for it. Protein hardly has any impact on blood sugar, so it doesn't create a big insulin spike. If you go for protein instead of a sugar fix, you'll beat back your craving for sweets by giving your body the building blocks it really needs.

Protein is made up of amino acids, which your body needs to make muscles, hormones, and neurotransmitters. They keep your hair shiny and your skin healthy. They also contribute to healthy bones. Your body can make some amino acids, but others—called the essential amino acids—only come from food, which is why protein is such a key part of the Sugar Impact Diet.

GETTING ENOUGH PROTEIN

I'll get into specific portions of protein for women, men, athletes, and vegans and vegetarians in Cycle 1, but in general, every meal should include 1 serving of clean, lean protein (4 to 6 ounces of fish, chicken, turkey, or grass-fed beef for women, 6 to 8 ounces for men). The average woman should get 75 to 80 grams of protein a day, and most men should get 100 to 120 grams a day. Those figures are based on a 160-pound woman and a 200-pound man. But your protein requirement is dynamic. It's influenced by your weight and body composition, and it will increase if you're under stress, healing, or doing some heavy resistance training. The Sugar Impact Diet is customizable for your needs, so tune in and listen to your body!

I recommend clean animal sources of protein—specifically organic, free-range, cage-free, grass-fed, and no-added-hormone animal protein—whenever possible. If you eat fish, avoid farm-raised fish and fish at risk for high levels of mercury, like ahi tuna and swordfish.

Those guidelines help you avoid animals that are fed genetically modified organisms (GMOs—crops with DNA that has been altered to make them pesticide resistant). Your protein source will also have higher omega-3 fatty acids, higher levels of B12 and other B vitamins, and trace minerals like magnesium and calcium. So always choose meat from an animal that was fed its native diet—its bliss is your bliss, too. And you'll feel even better for supporting farmers who treat their animals humanely.

I've also included vegetarian/vegan protein powder as a choice, but I don't recommend that you get all your protein from plant-based sources. If you're a vegetarian or vegan, be extra diligent about having protein powder, legumes (especially lentils), quinoa, nuts, and/or seeds at each meal. Also, be sure to take a B12 supplement (B12 is only naturally available in animal protein) and an algae-based omega-3 DHA supplement. I've included special vegetarian/vegan meal plans starting on page 276 to make it easy for you to follow the program.

FAT—EAT FAT TO BURN FAT

Here's the skinny: fat doesn't make you fat; sugar makes you fat. I know it's hard to believe this after all those years of conditioning, but fat is your friend! Fat helps curb sugar cravings because it doesn't spike your blood sugar or insulin levels. Even protein raises insulin levels a small amount, and fast carbs can send it soaring, but fat, not so much.

It's worth emphasizing that there are good fats and bad fats, and I'm focusing on the good. Healthy fats like those found in fish, avocados, and olive oil reduce your appetite and stabilize your blood sugar by slowing the release of sugar into your bloodstream. Fat also sends out satiety signals during digestion that tell your brain you're full.

So what's the bottom line? It's this: your body will thrive on a diet rich in more good fat. You'll accelerate your weight loss, lower your blood pressure and your triglycerides, raise your good (HDL) cholesterol, and reduce inflammation. Taken together, those things mean fat is a key weapon in the fight against chronic disease.

But beware of the bad fats, like damaged fats and trans fats. They're gunning for your weight and health—they raise your bad (LDL) cholesterol and lower your good cholesterol. They also increase your risk of developing type 2 diabetes and heart disease, and having a stroke. They're altered during manufacturing specifically to make sure they have a long shelf life, which is why you find them in processed foods that could be passed down for generations: cookies, crackers, cakes, doughnuts, chips, microwave popcorn, and so on... basically any prepared food packaged in a box or bag.

HOW MUCH FAT DO YOU NEED?

I'd like to see you have 2 to 4 servings of healthy fats at every meal. You don't have to remember that, though—the Sugar Impact Plate lays it all out for you. It's as simple as having 1 tablespoon olive oil, ¼ avocado, 4 ounces cold-water fish, 5 to 10 nuts, 1 tablespoon nut butter, or 10 olives. If you're having grass-fed beef or fish, count the fat in that as a serving, too, so you're not doubling up.

If you're vegan or vegetarian and are against taking fish oil, you'll want to focus on ALA-rich foods like flaxseeds and chia seeds, as well as walnuts. You can also find a vegan (algae-derived) DHA supplement to meet your omega-3 needs.

AVOID EATING FAT WITH SUGAR

It turns out there is a way to make a good thing bad. It's if you combine fat with sugar. When fat is combined with high-SI foods, insulin surges to pull excess sugar out of the blood. One of insulin's main jobs is to store the extra sugar as fat, and as it does, it also decreases fat-burning enzymes. Suddenly, you've mixed the perfect, metabolically toxic, fat-storing cocktail.

But don't worry! The recipes in this book will keep you safe on this one; they're full of tasty, rich healthy fats with no high-SI sugars in sight.

CARBS—SUGAR, STARCH, AND FIBER

Sugar, starch, and fiber are all forms of carbohydrates (all sugars are carbs, but not all carbs *start* as sugars). Sugar and carbs get converted into glucose and fructose. All our cells can use glucose, but only the liver processes fructose. And we don't have the digestive enzymes to break down fiber, so it moves slowly through our digestive system, intact. That delivers benefits, too, like keeping our blood sugar stable and helping us feel full longer.

Fast Carbs

I look at sugar based on its impact—how high it raises glucose and insulin or how fast it slams into your liver and starts its fat-making party. Impact is the difference between being lean, sharp, and full of energy, or being overweight, hazy, and exhausted. When you focus on impact, you can divide carbs into two categories: fast or slow, depending on how they affect you.

Fast carbs, like refined sugar, give you a quick hit of energy because they're packed with glucose and little or no fiber to slow down digestion. Your insulin skyrockets and rushes to get your blood sugar down. If all goes well, it's stored in your muscles and liver as fuel for the next time you need it. But space there is limited, and any left over gets stored as fat. Eek!

Starches

Starches move at a different speed. They're plant-based, slow carbs. Slow carbs take longer to digest because they're made up of long chains of sugar, and your body has to work harder to get at the glucose. Once it's accessible, the glucose is again used as energy or stored as glycogen or fat, but because the process of getting to glucose takes longer, your blood sugar and insulin stay low and slow.

Then there's resistant starch, which *resists* digestion (hence its name) and remains intact until it arrives in your colon, which breaks it down into short-chain fatty acids that are used for energy by your colon cells. There are several different sources of resistant starch, from plant walls to chemical synthesis.

Resistant starch is a wellness powerhouse and performs a lot like soluble fiber: it curbs appetite, improves insulin sensitivity, boosts gut function (by feeding good intestinal bugs), and lowers blood sugar response to food. It has some (seemingly minor) potential downsides, one of which is that you may get hit with some gas and bloating. My favorite source of resistant starch is legumes. Legumes provide a double benefit: they're actually high in fiber *and* resistant starch, making them a win-win.

Fiber, Faithful Friend

Fiber, my fave. It's the secret weight loss ninja. You already know that foods dense with fiber make us feel full longer and that fiber maintains blood sugar levels, but it also keeps fat moving through our digestive system so we absorb less of it. *And* it feeds the healthy bacteria in your gut, which are essential for a strong immune system.

I'd like you to get in 50 grams of fiber a day. That only sounds high if you're everyone, because most people only take in 5 to 14 grams a day. But that's just because no one really pays attention to fiber. Now that you know what it can do for you, I hope you start feasting on it! It's so easy to increase, but you have to be patient and do it slowly. If you move too fast, you could invite gas, bloating, diarrhea, or constipation.

On the Sugar Impact Diet, you'll start eating closer to nature, with more whole foods and fewer processed foods, which will bump your fiber intake automatically. Simply put, as your SI goes down, your fiber goes up because low–Sugar Impact foods are usually loaded with fiber. Every meal you eat should include 2 or more servings of nonstarchy vegetables (though the more the better; I'd like to see you having 5 to 10 servings per day!) and up to 2 servings of high-fiber starchy carbs like beans or quinoa.

You can also toss a fiber blend, some chia seeds, or freshly ground flaxseed meal into your breakfast shake, so those two changes alone should get you to 50 grams of fiber a day without breaking a sweat. And as you increase your fiber, bump up the amount of water you drink. It's critical to keep everything moving!

Here are your best choices:

NONSTARCHY VEGETABLES

Arugula
Artichokes
Asparagus
Bamboo shoots
Bean sprouts
Beet greens
Bell peppers (red, yellow, green)
Bok choy
Broccoli
Brussels sprouts
Carrots
Cucumber
Cabbage
Cassava
Cauliflower
Celery
Chicory

Chives
Collard greens
Coriander
Dandelion greens
Eggplant
Endive
Escarole
Fennel
Garlic
Green beans
Jalapeño peppers
Jicama
Kohlrabi
Kale
Leeks
Okra
Onions

Lettuce
Mushrooms
Mustard greens
Parsley
Radishes
Radicchio
Shallots
Snow peas
Spinach
Spaghetti squash
Sugar snap peas
Summer squash
Swiss chard
Turnip greens
Water chestnuts
Watercress
Zucchini

SLOW LOW CARBS

Adzuki beans
Berries (blackberries, blueberries, boysenberries, elderberries, gooseberries, loganberries, raspberries, strawberries, açai)
Black beans
Chickpeas (garbanzo beans)
Cowpeas
Cranberries
French beans
Grapefruit
Great northern beans
Groats
Guava
Kabocha squash

Kidney beans
Leeks
Persimmon
Lentils
Lima beans
Mung beans
Navy beans
Nectarines
Oatmeal—steel cut or rolled
Okra
Oranges
Passion fruit
Peaches
Pinto beans

Pumpkin
Quinoa
Split peas
Star fruit
Squash (acorn, butternut, winter)
Tomatoes
Turnip
White beans
Wild rice

Food Intolerances

Even with the Sugar Impact Plate, be on the lookout for food intolerances. They're usually connected to eggs, dairy, soy, and gluten and cause low-grade symptoms like fatigue, bloating, digestive problems, and joint pain. If you have a food intolerance, you may be missing an enzyme you need to digest a food (as is the case with lactose intolerance) or you may just be sensitive to it. Food intolerances are different from food allergies, which can cause an immediate—and sometimes life-threatening—physical reaction (think peanut allergy).

I've included pastured eggs as a source of clean protein on the Sugar Impact Diet and I've included dairy foods in this book in the recipes, but if you suspect that you have any issues eating these foods, cut them out or replace them!

Now that you have one of the killer Sugar Impact tools, you need to know some of its rules!

EAT BY THE SUGAR IMPACT CLOCK

The Sugar Impact Plate is not only a foolproof way to fill you up and turn you on (your metabolism, that is), but it also guarantees you'll get the nutrition you need to power you through your day. That translates into being able to make it from meal to meal without cravings or a grumbling tummy. If you graze or eat a lot of small meals every day, your blood sugar is on a wild, high-SI ride and your insulin is in fat-storing overdrive. The Sugar Impact Plate will help you transition to three balanced meals every 4 to 6 hours, with an optional snack—without feeling deprived.

The Plate replaces high-SI foods that give you short bursts of energy and punishing crashes with delicious, slow-burn foods like lean protein, nonstarchy veggies, fiber-filled slow carbs, and good fats. They're the mix you need to stabilize your blood sugar, have energy people will envy, and lose weight fast. That sure changes the conversation!

Like every other move on the Sugar Impact Diet, I'll help you make the shift gradually. When you lower your SI and stabilize your blood sugar, you'll stay full longer, which makes stretching out the time between meals a breeze.

Here's the Sugar Impact Clock in a nutshell:

- Breakfast—within 1 hour of waking up. No skipping! When you skip, you spike your blood sugar. Besides, skippers tend to be heavier and less healthy than breakfast eaters.
- Breakfast, Lunch, and Dinner—4 to 6 hours apart, with a snack only if you need it.
- Stop eating 3 hours before bed (no, you cannot just go to bed later!). If you're able to go at least 12 hours between dinner and breakfast, you'll allow your insulin to return to fasting levels, and your body will use stored fat for fuel.

ABOUT THAT SNACK

I'm just going to put this right out there—I'm anti-snacking. There's just no denying that it short-circuits your metabolism and sabotages the path to fat loss. It adds empty calories to your day, and you often eat more than you should, so you end up mindlessly padding your middle.

Snacking keeps insulin elevated, which means fat is getting stored, not burned. Why would your body burn anything other than the sugar it has hanging around? Take a break from noshing and make your body dig into your fat stores to burn what you have packed away. The irony is that snacks, especially sweet and salty ones, don't fend off cravings—they create them! You're snacking throughout the day, never really satisfied but for some reason you're still reaching for more. Sound familiar?

Eat by the Plate to curb hunger between meals, and limit yourself to one snack a day between lunch and dinner if you really need it.

Snack Smartly

The Sugar Impact Diet allows you to have an optional snack, and here's the approved list. These snacks will help you fight the good fight—they're fast, easy, and tasty, and they won't whack your blood sugar or leave you craving more. Crunch away!

- Celery with almond butter
- Homemade kale chips
- Raw veggies with black bean dip
- Hummus with veggies

- Hard-boiled eggs (if not intolerant)
- Slow-roasted or dehydrated nuts and seeds
- Virgin Diet Bar or other approved bars (see Resources on page 299)
- Aseptic-packed wild salmon
- Nitrate-free, no-sugar-added jerky
- Mini protein shake made in a shaker cup with water and protein powder

If you add high-quality supplements (see Supportive Supplements on the resources section of my website, http://sugarimpact.com) you'll be twice armed to resist sugary snacks all day long.

But! Too much food is always too much food, no matter how healthy it is. If you eat more than you need to keep your metabolism revved, the extra will always come home to roost—as fat. So, less is more, even when it's low Sugar Impact.

Lemon-AID

There's an old wives' tale that lemon juice lowers blood sugar. Tim Ferriss, notorious biohacker and author of *The 4-Hour Body*, experimented with it and discovered that having 3 tablespoons lemon juice when he ate lowered his blood sugar peaks by about 10%. Those wives were onto something! Drink Lemon-AID to ease your hunger pangs and stay hydrated:

Zest and juice of 1 lemon or lime
32 ounces water
1 teaspoon glutamine powder
Stevia, monk fruit, xylitol, or erythritol as needed (use as little as possible)
½ thinly sliced lemon
Fiber blend or chia seeds (optional)

In a pitcher, combine the lemon zest and juice with the water. Add the glutamine powder and sweetener (only if needed). Stir well and gently stir in the lemon slices. Think about adding a fiber blend or chia seeds, too. Fiber helps keep your hunger hormone ghrelin suppressed and it reduces the absorption of fat.

P.S. Did you notice the glutamine? Glutamine is an amino acid that helps your body synthesize protein. It also eases sugar cravings and supports gut healing.

Are you ready to fire up your fat loss? Let me see…Plate—check. Meal timing—check. Approved snacks—check. Yep, you're armed and good to go! Let's dig into the 7 foods to swap!

7 FOODS TO SWAP

It's time to get into the very heart of the Sugar Impact Diet—this is what makes it tick. I'm going to take you through the 7 high-SI food categories so you have a clear understanding of the impact each is having on you and how you can make better choices. I'll give you tons of simple swaps to bring your Sugar Impact down, fast. Here they are, again:

- Grains
- Roots
- Packaged Fruit
- Low- and No-Fat Dairy and Diet Foods
- Sauces, Dressings, and Condiments
- Sugary Drinks
- Sweeteners and Added Sugar

This is the most eye-opening part of the journey, and once you have these groups and their high-SI foods laid out in front of you, it will all be smooth sailing. You're going to meet a new you in just 2 weeks!

YOUR SUGAR IMPACT SWAPS: GRAINS

We love grains, right? Aren't they good for us? Not so fast! Don't buy that myth of whole-grain goodness! Sure, whole grains are better than refined grains, which are just sugar in disguise, but grains weren't part of our ancestors' diet at all, so the truth is that we don't need them to survive.

To lower your Sugar Impact, you'll swap grains, especially refined grains (which lack fiber and nutrients and are a main ingredient in many processed foods), for natural, whole foods like beans, nuts, and seeds. Beans, nuts, and seeds are nutrition superheroes, dense with protein, healthy fat, fiber, antioxidants, vitamins, and minerals.

How good does Spaghetti Squash with Capers, Onion, and Bell Pepper (page 185) sound? I know! Don't feel limited by this list, though—play with your food and come up with your own!

Swap Your...	For...
Baked beans	Pinto beans
Bran cereal	Quinoa flakes
Corn soup	White bean soup
Cornstarch	Arrowroot powder
Creamed corn	Black beans
Instant oatmeal	Long-cooking oatmeal
Mashed potatoes	Mashed cauliflower
Nutella	Almond butter
Pasta	Spaghetti squash or shirataki noodles
Peanut butter	Cashew butter
Potato chips	Homemade kale chips
Tofu	Lentils
Tortilla chips	Bean chips or homemade kale chips
Tortillas	Lettuce wraps or coconut wraps
Trail mix	Slow-roasted nut mix
White rice	Wild rice
Whole wheat pasta	Corn-free quinoa pasta

YOUR SUGAR IMPACT SCALE: GRAINS

Here's your Sugar Impact Scale for grains. In Cycle 1, you'll swap high SI for medium SI, then in Cycle 2 you'll swap the medium SIs for lows. You can also download this (and all the Sugar Impact Scales) from http://sugarimpact.com/resources for easy reference. Remember, these foods were assigned their high, medium, or low ranking based on the impact they'll have on you. Any foods that spike your blood sugar and insulin and send your body the message to store more fat are high, and they've been yanked for foods that put your fat-burning metabolism into overdrive.

LOW SUGAR IMPACT

Almond flour
Almonds
Black beans
Black turtle beans
Brazil nuts
Broad beans
Cannellini beans
Cashews
Chia seeds
Chickpeas
Chili—homemade,
   no sugar added
Coconut flour
Coconut wraps
Dehydrated unsweetened
   coconut
Fava beans

Flaxseeds
French green beans
Great northern beans
Green beans
Groats
Hazelnuts
Hempseeds
Hummus
Kidney beans
Lentil soup
Lentils
Lima beans
Long-cooking oatmeal—rolled
   or steel cut
Macadamia nuts
Mung beans
Navy beans

Peanuts*
Peas
Pecans
Pine nuts
Pinto beans
Pistachios
Poppy seeds
Pumpkin seeds
Quinoa
Roasted chestnuts
Sesame seeds
Shirataki noodles
Sunflower seeds
Unsweetened nut butters
Walnuts
Wax beans
Wild rice

* Ideally, choose tree nuts rather than peanuts for their superior fatty-acid profile and lower allergen potential.

Mistaken Identity

Peanuts are not nuts—they're legumes! What's the difference? Legumes have seeds that grow inside pods. Nuts are grown on trees, but peanuts are part of the pea family and grow underground.

MEDIUM SUGAR IMPACT

Amaranth, rice, millet, or buckwheat
   flour
Arrowroot*
Bean chips
Black bean flour
Brown rice
Buckwheat
Chili—store bought, sugar added

Ezekiel sprouted cereal
Fava bean flour
Fermented soy
Garbanzo flour
Lentil chips
Millet
Nut chips
Quinoa flakes

Quinoa flour
Quinoa pasta
Rice chips
Rice crackers
Rice pasta
Rice tortillas
Sprouted whole-grain breads

* If a small amount is used in a recipe—i.e., 1 tablespoon for 4 servings—this is safe for Cycle 2.

HIGH SUGAR IMPACT

Animal crackers	Glazed nuts	Pop-Tarts
Baked beans	Gluten-free flour blend	Potato starch
Barley	Graham crackers	Puffed millet
Biscotti	Grits	Puffed rice
Cakes and Pies	Honey-roasted peanuts	Quick breads
Cookies	Instant oatmeal	Rice cakes
Corn	Instant rice	Risotto
Corn chips	Macaroni and cheese	Scones
Corn tortillas	Matzoh	Soy cheese
Cornbread	Muesli	Sugar cereals
Cornstarch	Muffins	Sweetened nut butters
Couscous	Mung bean noodles	Tortillas
Crackers	Oyster crackers	Wasa crackers
Cream of Wheat	Pasta	Water crackers
Edamame*	Pita	Wheat bread
English muffins	Polenta	White flour
Farro	Popcorn	

This is low sugar, but high in lectins that can cause leptin resistance; choose only organic, fermented soy.

Easy, right? Results will be, too! Now it's time to move on and give high-SI roots the boot.

GIVE HIGH-SI ROOTS THE BOOT

Reducing your SI in root vegetables is easy—just eat from the rainbow, the more color the better. There's no limit to how many low-SI veggies you can have. Nobody ever got fat eating asparagus. Pile them on!

When you ditch high-SI roots, it's going to be in favor of squashes and nonstarchy vegetables—veggies that don't contain much starch. The low-sugar, high-fiber combo means you can eat more—and get fewer carbs—than you would from fruits, whole grains, or starchy vegetables. What does that mean? Less impact! Your blood sugar, insulin, and weight are safe in the hands of nonstarchy vegetables. And they'll give you a big boost toward your goal of 50 grams of fiber a day.

Take a look at some of these delicious swaps for roots. Are you already salivating over having Quinoa Pasta alla Checca (page 144) in place of soggy noodles with sugary marinara from a jar?

Swap Your...	For...
Beet juice	Beets
Beets	Cucumbers
Carrot juice	Green juice
Cooked carrots	Raw carrots
French fries	Baked butternut squash fries
Mashed potatoes	Mashed cauliflower
Parsnips	Cauliflower
Potatoes	Turnips
Sun-dried tomatoes	Chopped fresh tomatoes
Veggie chips	Homemade kale chips
Yams	Pumpkin

YOUR SUGAR IMPACT SCALE: ROOTS

Lean on this Sugar Impact Scale for roots and let it do the heavy lifting for you. It's pulling high-SI carbs off your plate in favor of tasty trades that keep you moving toward your fast fat-loss goals. Don't look back!

LOW SUGAR IMPACT

Acorn squash	Escarole	Pumpkin
Artichoke	Ginger	Radicchio
Asparagus	Homemade kale chips	Radish
Bok choy	Jicama	Snow peas
Broccoli	Kabocha squash	Spaghetti squash
Brussels sprouts	Kale	Spinach
Butternut squash	Leeks	Sprouts
Cabbage	Lettuces	Sugar snap peas
Carrots	Maca	Turnips
Cauliflower	Mushrooms	Water chestnuts
Celery	Mustard greens	Watercress
Chard	Okra	Zucchini
Cucumber	Onions	
Eggplant	Peppers	

MEDIUM SUGAR IMPACT

Beets	Sweet potatoes
Parsnips	Yams
Rutabaga	

HIGH SUGAR IMPACT

Beet juice	Potato chips
Carrot juice	Root veggie chips
French fries	Sweet potato fries
Mashed potatoes	White potatoes

FORBIDDEN FRUIT

Fruit always raises eyebrows, and I get why. I mean, come on—apples are in our national pie! Even if you already know fruit is full of sugar, it doesn't make it any easier to believe one of nature's greatest gifts—colorful, juicy, wholesome fruit—could be doing you any harm. But if you're a sugar addict and a slave to cravings, fruit could very well be keeping you down (and your weight up).

Make the swing from high to low SI in fruit by swapping jams, juice, sorbets, and dried fruit for the real deal. Think of it this way: whole keeps you in control.

Swap Your . . .	For . . .
Apple chips	Homemade kale chips
Apples	Jicama
Canned fruit cocktail	Greek-style yogurt*
Dried cranberries	Fresh cranberries
Dried fruit	Freeze-dried berries
Fruit juice	Lemon-AID
Fruit juice concentrate	Monk fruit, stevia
Fruit-sweetened low-fat or nonfat yogurt	Plain Greek-style yogurt with fresh berries
Grapes	Blueberries
Jamba Juice smoothie	Sugar Impact Shake
Jams	Almond butter
Juice bar	Popsicle made with coconut milk, berries, and vanilla protein powder
Mangoes	Guavas
Pineapple	Grapefruit

Raisins
Sorbet
Sun-dried tomatoes
Tomato bisque

Grapes
Coconut milk ice cream
Fresh tomatoes
Gazpacho

If you're not dairy sensitive.

YOUR SUGAR IMPACT SCALE: FRUIT

The Sugar Impact Scale for fruits will help you quickly see where fruit and fruit-derived goods sneak hidden sugars into your diet and sabotage your good intentions. It's especially handy for Cycles 1 and 3, when you're allowed to have fruit in your shakes.

LOW SUGAR IMPACT

Açai berries (no sugar added)
Avocado*
Blueberries
Cantaloupe
Cranberries
Gazpacho*
Grapefruit

Guava
Lemons*
Limes*
Nectarines
Olives*
Oranges
Peaches

Persimmon
Raspberries
Star fruit
Strawberries
Tomatoes*

0 to 1 gram fructose—safe for Cycle 2.

MEDIUM SUGAR IMPACT

Apples
Apricots
Bananas
Cherries
Dates
Fresh figs
Grapes
Honeydew

Kiwi
Mango
Papaya
Pears
Pineapple
Plums
Pomegranate
Sun-dried tomatoes

Tangerines
Tomato juice
Tomato paste
Tomato sauce
V8 juice
Watermelon

HIGH SUGAR IMPACT

All dried fruit
Canned fruit cocktail
Fruit juice concentrates
Fruit juice Popsicles
Fruit juices

Fruit leather
Jams
Nectar
Preserves and conserves
Sorbet

The transition to low-SI fruits is just one way the Sugar Impact Diet will redefine your relationship with food. While you're preparing for that new you in the mirror, your palate is changing, too. Soon there will be such a thing as too sweet, and that sugary breakfast bun will have no hold over you.

DITCH THE LOW- AND NO-FAT DAIRY AND DIET FOODS

Low- and no-fat dairy and diet foods are huge funnels of sugar into your diet, so you're going to love the fat-loss jump start you'll get when you make changes in this category. The idea that fat is the enemy has its hooks in us deep, and it won't let go without a fight. But a low-fat diet is a high-sugar diet, so it's time to put on the gloves.

I've got plenty of delicious low-SI swaps to help you cut the cravings for low-fat dairy and lose fat fast. Check out this list of nutritious choices to replace those low-fat crutches, and give these tasty treats a try!

Swap Your...	For...
Butter substitute	Coconut cream
Cool Whip	Full-fat coconut milk—whipped
Fat-free pudding	Mousse made with avocado, coconut cream, and coconut milk
Frozen "light" dinner	Lentil soup
Frozen yogurt	Sugar Impact Shake
Fruit on the bottom yogurt	Plain full-fat Greek-style yogurt*
Fudgsicle	Homemade protein Popsicle
Ice cream	Monk fruit–sweetened coconut ice cream
Light cream cheese	Avocado
Low-fat crackers	Bean chips
Low-fat pita chips	Olives
Low-fat potato chips	Homemade kale chips
Margarine	Grass-fed butter
Microwave light popcorn	Roasted chickpeas
Pretzels	Roasted Brussels sprouts
Protein bar	Wild salmon jerky
Skim milk	Full-fat grass-fed milk
Snack packs	Baggie of slow-roasted nuts
Sweetened creamer	Coconut milk creamer—unsweetened
Sweetened soy milk	Unsweetened coconut milk

If you're not intolerant.

Choosing Protein Powder

Protein shakes are an easy way to make sure you're eating by the Sugar Impact Plate, even at breakfast. Here are some general guidelines to follow so shopping for protein powder is pain free.

- Ideally, choose a high-quality protein base: defatted beef- or plant-based powder made from pea, rice, chia, or cranberry protein, or a blend of these.

- Avoid soy, egg, whey or milk protein powders, artificial colors, and sweeteners such as aspartame and sucralose. If there is an added sweetener, it should be no more than 5 grams per serving and it should not be from fructose or high-fructose corn syrup.

- When making your protein shakes, use 1 to 2 scoops of protein powder, according to the package directions.

- To ensure you meet your daily fiber quota (aim for 50 grams), add a fiber blend, which is a mixture of soluble and insoluble fibers. They can be found in most health food stores and online.

- For some of my favorite brands and best recommendations, check out page 306 in the Resources section at the back of the book.

YOUR SUGAR IMPACT SCALE: LOW- AND NO-FAT DAIRY AND DIET FOODS

When you first ditch low-fat diet foods and start eating more healthy fat, you're going to be looking over your shoulder. It feels so decadent you'll be sure you're doing something you shouldn't be. I can't wait to see that smile on your face! Dig into these swaps to see what I'm talking about!

LOW SUGAR IMPACT

Flax milk—unsweetened
Full-fat cheeses (avoid blue cheese due to gluten)
Full-fat cream cheese
Full-fat plain cottage cheese
Monk fruit—sweetened coconut ice cream
Mozzarella
No-sugar-added coconut creamer
No-sugar-added coconut, cashew, or almond milk

No-sugar-added cultured coconut milk
Nut cheese
Organic creamer
Organic plain full-fat Greek-style yogurt
Plain cultured coconut yogurt—no sugar added
Plain dairy or coconut kefir
Protein powder (see above for guidelines)
Ricotta cheese

MEDIUM SUGAR IMPACT

Cream cheese spread
Full-fat grass-fed milk
Full-fat organic milk
Half-and-half
Low-fat cheese
Low-fat cream cheese spread
Neufchâtel cheese
Organic low-fat or nonfat plain Greek-style yogurt

Part-skim mozzarella
Part-skim ricotta
Plain coconut yogurt—sweetened
Soy cheese
Sweetened coconut milk creamer
Unsweetened rice milk
Whipped cream cheese

HIGH SUGAR IMPACT

94% fat-free microwave kettle corn
94% fat-free microwave popcorn
Almond milk ice cream
Blue cheese
Breakfast bars
Carnation Instant Breakfast
Coconut milk ice cream
Creamsicles
Dried fruit snacks
Ensure
Fat-free baked chips
Fat-free muffins
Fat-free pudding
Fat-free sugar-free Jell-O
Fat-free Twizzlers
Flavored almond milk yogurt
Flavored coconut yogurt
Flavored kefirs
Frozen yogurt
Fruit-added cream cheese

Fudgsicles
Gelato
Granola bars
Hot cocoa
Ice cream
Ice cream sandwiches
Lite Cool Whip
Low- or reduced-fat crackers
Low-fat and fat-free cookies
Low-fat graham crackers
Low-fat or fat-free ice cream
Low-fat or fat-free ice cream bars
Low-fat or "light" frozen dinners
Low-fat Oreos
Mousse
Nesquik
Nonfat cheeses
Nonfat cream cheese
Pineapple cottage cheese
Pretzels

Protein bars
Pudding
Reduced-fat macaroni and cheese
Reduced-fat peanut butter
Reduced-fat Pringles
Skim or low-fat milk
Snack packs
SnackWell's low-fat and fat-free
  cookies and treats
Sorbet
Strawberry cream cheese
Sweetened coffee creamers
Sweetened cows' milks—vanilla,
  chocolate
Sweetened dairy-free milks
Sweetened whipped cream
Unsweetened soy milk*
Yogurts with sugar or artificial
  sweeteners

Low sugar but high in lectins that can cause leptin resistance—choose only organic, fermented soy.

Low fat has loosened its grip. Finally! Now you can enjoy the pleasure of nature's brain-fueling, fat-burning, heart-protecting fats—knowing you've also cut off a major point of entry for hidden sugar into your diet.

SO LONG, SWEET DRINKS

After you put all that careful thought and sugar sleuthing into what you eat, it seems a little unfair to discover that something as innocent as your drink could unravel all your good intentions.

Stop drinking your calories, then just sit back and wait for the payoff: fast fat loss, higher energy, and glowing skin. Don't let sugar-sweetened drinks stand between you and any of those things—they're so not worth it! Ditch the high-SI drinks for *anything* on the low-SI list. Bonus points if it's water!

Swap Your...	For...
Beer	Gluten-free beer
Carrot juice	Green juice
Energy drinks	Organic coffee or green tea
Gatorade	Vertical Water
Hot chocolate	Warm coconut milk and chocolate protein powder
Jamba Juice smoothie	Sugar Impact Shake
Latte	Espresso with coconut creamer
Regular/diet soda	Sparkling water
Sweet tea	Brewed tea with lemon
Sweet wine	Pinot noir
Vitamin Water	Hint Water

> Vertical Water is 100% pure maple water tapped fresh from American maple trees. There's nothing added (or taken away)!

YOUR SUGAR IMPACT SCALE: DRINKS

Sweet beverages aren't so sweet to your waistline or your health, but when you kick them to the curb, you'll fast-track fat loss *and* your move from sugar burner to fat burner. I'll drink to that!

LOW SUGAR IMPACT

All teas

Fermented coconut water

Green drinks (greens only, no fruit, carrot, or beet added)*

Green tea—no sugar added

Hint Water

Organic coffee and decaf coffee

Sparkling mineral water

Teeccino

Unsweetened fruit essence teas

Water

Do not drink on their own—add fiber.

MEDIUM SUGAR IMPACT

Dry red wine

Dry white wine

Gin

Gluten-free beer

Kombucha tea—no sugar added

Tequila

Tomato juice

V8 (not with fruit juice)

Vodka

HIGH SUGAR IMPACT

"Enhanced" waters—sweetened

Beer

Brandy

Capri Sun

Carnation Instant Breakfast

Carrot juice

Champagne

Commercial "smoothies"

Crystal Light

Diet soda

Fruit juices

Fuze

Gatorade

Kool-Aid

Mixed drinks

Nesquik

Port

Powerade

Rockstar energy drink

Rum

Slimfast

SoBe

Soda

Sweet tea

Sweetened coconut water

Unsweetened coconut water

Vitamin Water

Wines—sweet, dessert

SAYONARA SUGARY SAUCES, DRESSINGS, AND CONDIMENTS

Remember the Sneaky Sugar Inventory? Back when you thought you weren't eating any sugar? Then, there it was, in black and white. Sneaky sugar was in every sauce, dressing, and dollop. The good news about going low SI in dressings, sauces, and condiments is that you're not likely to even notice the switch. You definitely won't feel robbed of taste or flavor—we're talking about near-even trades delivering a huge Sugar Impact win.

You'll take a big swipe at the high impact of sneaky sugars in sauces, dressings, and condiments just by whipping up your own. It's easier than you think! When you swap out sugar-heavy sauces for rich, natural seasonings, you'll be one step closer to the taste bud turnaround you've been waiting for!

Swap Your...	For...
Balsamic vinegar	Red wine vinegar
BBQ sauce	Dry rub
Cocktail sauce	Horseradish
French dressing	Champagne vinegar and extra-virgin olive oil
Honey mustard	Dijon mustard
Hot-and-sour sauce	Hot sauce
Italian dressing	Extra-virgin olive oil, lemon juice, and oregano vinaigrette
Jellies and jams	Fresh fruit or nut butters
Ketchup	Salsa
Soy-based stir-fry sauce	Homemade coconut aminos–based stir-fry sauce
Steak sauce	Jus
Sweet dressing	Savory dressings like Dijon vinaigrette
Sweet sauces	Savory sauces like pesto
Teriyaki sauce	Coconut aminos with orange zest and stevia

YOUR SUGAR IMPACT SCALE: SAUCES, DRESSINGS, AND CONDIMENTS

The high-SI sugar in sauces, dressings, and condiments can catch you off guard. But it's not the sugar you seek out when you're hit with a craving, is it? So not to worry, you'll let go here without feeling a thing. These low-SI options are full of flavors that will make sure of it.

LOW SUGAR IMPACT

Avocado oil	Mustard	Sour dill pickles
Bragg Liquid Aminos*	Nutritional yeast	Tabasco
Checca sauce	Olive oil	Tapenade
Coconut aminos	Olives	Vinegar
Hot sauce	Pesto	Walnut oil
Macadamia nut oil	Salsa	Wheat-free tamari*
Malaysian red palm fruit oil	Sesame oil	

If not intolerant to soy.

MEDIUM SUGAR IMPACT

Bread-and-butter pickles
Caesar dressing
Fish sauce
Green curry sauce
Italian dressing
Marinara sauce—no sugar added

Pickle relish
Red curry sauce
Sweet pickle relish
Sweet pickles
Tomato sauce

HIGH SUGAR IMPACT

Asian dressing
Balsamic vinaigrette
Balsamic vinegar
BBQ sauce
Blue cheese dressing
Brown sauce
Catalina dressing
Cocktail sauce

French dressing
Hoisin sauce
Honey mustard
Honey mustard dressing
Hot-and-sour sauce
Ketchup
Marinara sauce—sugar added
Peanut sauce

Ranch dressing
Raspberry vinaigrette
Steak sauce
Sweet chili sauce
Tartar sauce
Teriyaki sauce
Thousand Island
Worcestershire sauce

The moves in this category target hidden sugars that slip in on the side and hit you with a high SI you never see coming. So kiss "healthy" dressings good-bye. They've been silently sabotaging your weight and health for years. But now you know that when you block these main portals for sneaky sugars, you'll clear the path for a revved metabolism and fast fat burning. Let these low-SI toppings bring your taste buds to life!

SEE YA, SWEETENERS AND ADDED SUGAR

Remember, this is a low-sugar diet, not a no-sugar diet. So you may be wondering why we're talking about sweeteners—natural or otherwise—at all. What harm could a little honey or calorie-free sweetener do?

High-SI sweeteners are the final frontier. They stoke the fire of your sugar cravings for the very reason you believe they're keeping your sweet tooth at bay—they're causing you to crave more and more sweet. They seem like the perfect solution—they're no- or low-calorie (some are even natural!) and they're not sugar!

Artificial sweeteners are the wolf in sheep's clothing. They are not what they pretend to be! They trigger responses, like cravings, that set up the expectation of calories, and they can drive you to eat more of whatever you've succumbed to. And they're so much sweeter than sugar, they make you crave foods that are super-sweet.

I also get tons of questions about natural sweeteners: Can I have honey? Fruit juice concentrate? How about agave—it's natural, right? Just because it's natural does not make it nirvana. True, natural sweeteners are better than artificial, but it's a game of inches.

As always, you get a cheat sheet! The goal is to lose weight and feel better fast, so I just want to be sure you're crystal clear on which swaps will do that for you. Especially the fast part!

Swap Your...	For...
55% dark chocolate	85% dark chocolate
Agave	Erythritol
Maple syrup	Chicory syrup
Milk chocolate	85% dark chocolate
Nutrasweet	Monk fruit
Processed brown sugar	Raw brown sugar
Processed honey	Raw organic local honey
Processed molasses	Blackstrap molasses
Splenda	Stevia and xylitol
Sugar	Stevia

YOUR SUGAR IMPACT SCALE: SWEETENERS AND ADDED SUGAR

Sweeteners and added sugars keep you chasing sweet, and not the real deal served up by Mother Nature. The shift to low-SI sweeteners will really help you crush your cravings and keep your sweet tooth in check. I can't wait for that moment you sprinkle cinnamon on some Old-Fashioned Oatmeal with Cinnamon, Blueberries, and Raspberries (page 73) and think, "Perfection."

LOW SUGAR IMPACT	
100% dark chocolate	Monk fruit
85% dark chocolate*	Raw cacao (powder and nibs)
Chicory	Stevia
Erythritol	Xylitol
Inulin	

*Stay off in Cycle 2 unless made with low-SI sweetener.

MEDIUM SUGAR IMPACT

70% or higher dark chocolate
Blackstrap molasses
Cane syrup—non-GMO
Coconut palm sugar
Coconut sugar
Glucose (aka dextrose)—non-GMO

Local organic raw honey
Mannitol
Raw brown sugar—nonprocessed
Rice syrup
Sorbitol

HIGH SUGAR IMPACT

<70% dark chocolate
Acesulfame-K
Agave
Aspartame
Candy
Caramel sauce
Chocolate syrup
Corn syrup

Crystalline fructose
Cyclamates
Fruit juice concentrate
High-fructose corn syrup
Honey (processed)
Licorice
Maltodextrin
Maple syrup

Marshmallows
Milk chocolate
Molasses
Neotame
Processed brown sugar
Saccharin
Splenda
Sucralose

Sweeteners and added sugar keep your need for sweet pegged, so lowering your SI here short-circuits a craving and addiction cycle you probably didn't even know you were fueling. Hooray! It means you've conquered the last of the 7 high-SI foods and guarantees dramatic, lifelong results from the Sugar Impact Diet.

It's time to set up your Sugar Impact Kitchen!

3

SETTING UP YOUR SUGAR IMPACT KITCHEN

Let's get your kitchen into tip-top shape so you're ready to whip up all of the spectacular low- and medium-SI recipes to come.

Your kitchen brings your commitment and foundation to life. You'll stock it with all the right foods and tools; it's the place your success starts to take shape. A clear kitchen is about a clear mind—making sure you're faced with only good choices and the weight loss and health-supporting foods you need. Fast fat loss, higher energy, better health, and joie de vivre are the real dishes made in your kitchen.

So first things first. To make room for the good, you have to clear out the bad. It's like any good spring cleaning: you want your bright, shiny, fat-loss foods to take center stage and the stealth saboteurs to hit the highway. Trash those triggers! It's not that I don't trust you but...I don't trust you. That's only because it's impossible to believe you'll win a game of willpower against cravings and addiction. I don't even trust myself! I would never want either of us in a position to be tempted by something that could unravel all our hard work. Get the enemy out of the house.

TIME TO TOSS

Tossing is so liberating. It's like a seesaw in your kitchen. The swing from unhealthy and toxic food to fat burning and healthy food feels like you're being lifted up before you've tasted a thing. Your mouth will be watering to get started as you're stocking the shelves.

Start with the boxes and bags—pitch anything with a long list of unrecognizable ingredients. What you're really doing is denying yourself access to anything that will tempt you and wreck your progress. Don't even have the battle with yourself. If it's not in the house, you'd have to work pretty hard to get it, and my hope is you'll think twice before you do. Besides, you'll be stocked up with lots of terrific swaps with great taste but half or less of the SI. You'll satisfy your craving and not punish your waistline or health in the bargain. Here's a short list to get you started based on what most people have in their kitchen.

Toss It!

- Juice
- Dried fruit
- Bisquick
- Bread
- Sodas—regular or diet
- Splenda or Nutrasweet
- Corn-fed meat
- Trail mix (you know, the kind with peanuts and chocolate)
- Fruit-sweetened yogurt
- Crackers
- Chips
- Pasta
- Baked beans
- Vegetable oils
- Ranch, blue cheese, French dressings
- Milk, soy milk, nondairy creamers
- Mayonnaise
- Cereals
- Snack bars (those candy bars in disguise)
- Frozen "light" dinners
- Agave, honey, maple syrup

As you sweep the shelves, here are some other things that should get tossed: any foods containing artificial sweeteners and colorings, gluten, nonfat dairy, high-fructose corn syrup, and/or partially hydrogenated oils. Also, clear out frozen treats, baked goods, deep-fried foods, candy, soy-based products, and anything that came from a fast-food restaurant.

When in doubt, throw it out. It's going to feel great, I promise! Almost like you're pitching the pounds themselves. Don't let that devil on your shoulder get a foothold! No matter how hard you try to spin it, "fat-free" does not magically make anything a health food. Artificial sweeteners don't give "sweet" a halo. Stay strong!

SHORT AND SWEET LABELS

Have you noticed that you don't see many foods on the high-SI lists that can hit the grocery store without a label? Eating as close to nature as possible means you'll be eating as far from processed as it gets, and the more processed a food, the higher its SI usually is. So steering clear of foods with eye charts for labels is a simple rule of thumb to keep your SI low.

Buy organic whenever you can, but you don't always *have* to buy organic. The nutritional benefit of eating non-organic fruits and veggies outweighs any pesticide risk, and is always better than eating none at all.

There's a cheat sheet that can help you make good choices whether you're on a budget or you just want to be more informed—it's the Environmental Working Group's list of both the "Dirty Dozen Plus" (fruits and veggies dosed with the most pesticides) and the Clean Fifteen (just the opposite). Find it here: www.ewg.org/foodnews/summary .php. But watch out: even organic fruit can carry dirt and germs, or "pesticide drift" from nearby farms, so always wash any produce before you eat it.

Of course, you also need to be on the lookout for GMOs (genetically modified organisms). A GMO is a plant or animal that's been genetically altered to increase its yield or prolong its shelf life. That's done by inserting bacteria, viruses, or other plant and animal genes into the DNA of the organism. There are *serious health risks* associated with genetically modified food, according to the American Academy of Environmental Medicine. Need to know more? Check out www.responsibletechnology.org. You'll find a complete list of foods packing GMOs and a downloadable non-GMO shopping list. You can also look for foods with the certification of the nonprofit organization Non-GMO Project, which gives its approval to brands it determines are GMO free.

STOCKING YOUR SUGAR IMPACT KITCHEN

You may be surprised to learn that stocking your fridge and shelves to the gills with lean protein, healthy fats, slow, low carbs, vegetables, and some fruit doesn't mean you'll be living in a grocery store. Well, unless it's Whole Foods. Whole Foods deserves a moment of wild applause, especially for its 365 brand. If you're lucky enough to have a Whole Foods nearby, you may already know that 365 is GMO free and natural, but priced to compete.

If there's not a Whole Foods within a day's drive of you, that doesn't mean you have to throw in the towel. People who value eating clean and close to nature want to talk about it, whether it's to expand their horizons or yours. So outside of the grocery stores, get online to find your peeps. Join Facebook groups or follow blogs that give you the support you need. Or find a food collective or CSA (community-supported agriculture) in your area so you can support farms directly. And farmers' markets are always—without fail—an amazing source of great, fresh food and fabulous people. You'd be surprised by what you can learn about your food, all while making friends to enjoy it with. You can also always call on the farmers themselves. They'll appreciate the visit, and connecting personally to your food will make you feel that much better about it.

Also, whenever and wherever possible, buy local and in season. We used to do this naturally—it's all we had to choose from!—but now you have to really pay attention to whether that avocado should be in that bin or not. It's worth it, though—food tastes so much better and is more nutritious if it hasn't traveled the globe to get to you. Think about the juicy berries of springtime and the tart, crunchy apples of fall, or the tomatoes popping off your vines in the summer. Well-traveled food is usually packing preservatives for the trip, is wrapped in plastic, and has a higher energy cost than local food. Besides, as soon as fruits and vegetables are harvested, they get more sugary and their nutrients decay. It's why you should also buy your produce whole or as close to it as possible, not cut up—taste and nourishment! I can't think of any better reasons to eat food! To learn more about sourcing seasonal foods, you can visit www.cuesa.org/eat-seasonally/charts/vegetables.

And what about the animals you eat? The benefits of supporting local farms can be huge, for you and for the animals. Farmers who supply their neighborhood supermarkets and butchers depend on those relationships (and your happiness). They tend to the health and meat quality of their animals in ways that factory farmers never will. Patronize those hardworking people who feed us so well!

SHOP 'TIL YOU DROP

Let the fun begin! Shopping can be a blast, especially when you feel so great about every little thing you drop in your cart. When you look at a food and just know that it's the medicine you've been searching for, you can't help but get excited. You're going to want to start digging in before you even check out! Try to hold out and just enjoy the good feeling you get shopping for low-SI food. Imagine your pantry, fridge, and freezer bursting with food that will keep your metabolism revved and burning fat. Foods that do this will be your only choices!

Before you go, make a list to take with you. Do not skip this step! It's mission critical that you give thought to what you're going to buy before you get there and that you stick to your list. I'm only looking out for your best interests—you know the tractor beam–like pull of the end caps in those supermarkets! Once you make eye contact with those bags of popcorn, it can be hard to look away. Check out the Staples Shopping List below, or download a copy to take to the store with you from http://sugarimpact.com/resources.

STAPLES SHOPPING LIST

These are the things I like to keep on hand to be able to make Sugar Impact Diet meals in minutes. You may have some others you'd like to add as well. Use this list as your grocery shopping guide and to keep you on the straight and narrow. Note that I've included dairy and egg options in this list. If you're sensitive or intolerant to those foods, simply don't buy them. Do what works best for you!

SHAKES

_____ Vanilla protein powder

_____ Chocolate protein powder

_____ Fiber blend

_____ _____

_____ _____

_____ _____

OILS & VINEGARS

_____ Extra-virgin olive oil

_____ Olive oil

_____ Coconut oil

_____ Red palm fruit oil

_____ Macadamia nut oil

_____ Asian sesame oil

_____ Red wine vinegar

_____ Rice vinegar—no sugar added

_____ _____

_____ _____

_____ _____

SPICES AND DRIED HERBS

_____ Sea salt

_____ Black peppercorns (to grind fresh)

_____ Ground cumin

_____ Chili powder

_____ Ground cinnamon

_____ Ground nutmeg

_____ Curry powder

_____ Oregano

_____ Basil

_____ Cayenne pepper

_____ Red pepper flakes

_____ Ground chipotle pepper

_____ Onion powder

_____ Garlic powder

_____ Turmeric

_____ Paprika

_____ Rosemary

_____ Mexican seasoning blend

_____ _____

_____ _____

_____ _____

GRAINS/NUTS/SEEDS

_____ Wild rice

_____ Chia seeds

_____ Flaxseeds

_____ Dry quinoa

_____ Almond flour

_____ Coconut flour

_____ Shirataki noodles

_____ Dry sprouted lentils

_____ Almonds, walnuts, cashews, etc.

_____ Long-cooking or steel-cut oats

_____ Groats

_____ Coconut wraps

_____ _____

_____ _____

_____ _____

CYCLES 1 & 3

_____ Quinoa flakes

_____ Quinoa pasta—corn free

_____ Brown rice

_____ Brown rice wraps

_____ Rice pasta

_____ Amaranth, buckwheat, millet

_____ Rice crackers/chips (not cakes)

_____ Bean chips

_____ Arrowroot (small amounts allowable Cycle 2)

JARRED & CANNED

_____ Organic tahini paste (optional, for snack)

_____ Jarred roasted red peppers (optional, for snack)

_____ Cashew or almond butter

_____ Dijon mustard

_____ Coconut aminos

_____ 15-ounce cans organic no-salt-added cannellini beans (or dried)

_____ 15-ounce cans organic no-salt-added black beans (or dried)

_____ 15-ounce cans organic no-salt-added pinto beans (or dried)

_____ 15-ounce cans organic no-salt-added chickpeas (or dried)

_____ 14.5-ounce cans organic diced tomatoes

_____ Organic low-sodium chicken broth

_____ Organic low-sodium vegetable broth

_____ Tabasco or other hot sauce

_____ Kalamata olives

_____ 7-ounce jars marinated artichoke hearts

_____ Bragg Liquid Aminos (if not soy sensitive)

_____ Wheat-free tamari (if not soy sensitive)

_____ Salsa

_____ _____

_____ _____

_____ _____

CYCLES 1 & 3

_____ Tomato sauce, marinara—no sugar added

_____ Tomato juice

MISC

_____ Espresso powder

_____ Organic coffee

_____ Green tea

_____ Sparkling water

_____ Erythritol

_____ Xylitol

_____ Pure stevia

_____ Monk fruit

_____ Chicory

_____ Inulin

_____ 100% dark chocolate

_____ Raw cacao nibs

_____ Vanilla extract, no sugar added

_____ _____

_____ _____

_____ _____

CYCLES 1 & 3

_____ 85% dark chocolate

FRUITS & VEGGIES

_____ Avocado

_____ Lemons

_____ Limes

_____ Lettuces (spinach, arugula, romaine, baby, kale)

_____ Cabbages

_____ Onions

_____ Garlic

_____ Peppers

_____ Broccoli

_____ Asparagus

_____ Spaghetti squash

_____ Cauliflower

_____ Zucchini

_____ Winter squashes

_____ Brussels sprouts

_____ Mushrooms

_____ Celery

_____ Tomatoes

_____ Ginger

_____ Fresh cilantro

_____ _____

_____ _____

_____ _____

CYCLES 1 & 3

_____ Berries—organic frozen for shakes

_____ Grapefruit

_____ Yams, sweet potatoes

_____ Beets

MILKS/DAIRY

_____ Unsweetened coconut, cashew, almond milk

_____ Goat cheese

_____ Coconut kefir

_____ Plain full-fat Greek-style yogurt

_____ Raw cheeses

_____ Kerrygold butter

_____ Grass-fed ghee

_____ _____

_____ _____

_____ _____

PROTEINS

_____ Grass-fed beef

_____ Pastured pork

_____ Pastured eggs

_____ Wild seafood—salmon, halibut, shrimp, scallops, sole, sardines

_____ Free-range chicken—I like Pitman Farms and Rosie brands

_____ Bison

_____ Wild game

_____ Uncured nitrate-free bacon

_____ Turkey breast slices

_____ _____

_____ _____

_____ _____

KITCHEN TOOLS

You may already be master of your domain. But whether you're already accomplished at whirring and whipping and blending or you're a complete newbie, terrified at the thought of slicing or dicing anything, you're about to make big things happen in your kitchen. It all comes down to having the right tools. Check this list against your inventory and add to your drawers and countertops where you see the need. They'll make those beautiful, tasty, low-SI masterpieces seem effortless and fun.

- Blendtec or Vitamix blender
- Box-style grater and Microplane grater
- Can opener
- Cast-iron skillet
- Chef's knife, paring knife, and serrated knives
- Coffee grinder for herbs and spices
- Colander
- Dry and liquid measuring cups, measuring spoons
- Food processor
- Handheld electric mixer
- Heat-resistant spatulas
- Ice cream maker
- Instant-read meat thermometer
- Kitchen scale
- Kitchen shears
- Kitchen timer
- Ladle
- Magic Bullet or NutriBullet for traveling
- Mason jars
- Mixing bowls
- Parchment paper
- Pots and pans: cast-iron, enamel, and/or hard-anodized nonstick skillets; stainless steel pots, saucepans, Dutch oven
- Salad spinner
- Shallow roasting pan or rimmed baking sheet
- Slow cooker/Crock-Pot
- Steamer basket or insert
- Storage containers
- Tongs
- Vegetable peeler and/or spiralizer
- Whisk
- Wooden cutting boards (2)
- Wooden spoons

TIME-SAVING TIPS

We have lives, right?! None of us can afford to spend hour after hour cutting and chopping for every meal. Nothing else would ever get done! So let's promise each other we're only going to spend as much time in the kitchen we absolutely have to, unless we're having fun. Which I hope will be true when you're making Sugar Impact Diet recipes!

It's pretty hard not to be happy with simple, easy meals specifically designed to lower your SI, and help you burn fat fast and feel fabulous. Smart meal prep—including planning ahead and using a few shortcuts—will make you even happier. Let me make certain you use your time well:

1. First, invest a little effort when it's not mealtime; it pays big dividends when you're squeezed. That can be as simple as making sure your pantry, fridge, and freezer are

well stocked with the building blocks of a healthy, energizing, fat-burning meal. Think of them as a safety net. When you always have good ingredients at your fingertips, you can have a Sugar Impact Shake (page 65), a colorful, crisp salad, a soup, or a wrap in front of you *fast*.

2. The best way to be successful at #1 is to make at least one big grocery pilgrimage a week. No more countless runs back to the store. You'll save the time—and gas money—normally chewed up when you shop by pop in, one item at a time.

3. You can also reclaim some time and relieve some stress if you use the weekend to prep meals for the week ahead. Think about taking just a couple of hours on Sunday to make and freeze meals. Then imagine your relief when you find yourself up against dinnertime without a plan—phew! That running start from the weekend is a lifesaver!

4. When you're actually doing the cooking part, double or triple the recipe and freeze the overflow. Or stick the extra in the fridge for tomorrow's lunch. Repurposing can be such a huge help! When you're scheduled wall to wall, there's no relief quite like realizing you have frozen meals or leftovers as emergency bailouts.

But I'm not the only one with ideas—members of my Facebook community are always willing to chime in and share their creative time-saving go-tos...so visit www.facebook .com/jjvirginfanclub to get some extra tips!

BUDGET BACKERS

I get questions all the time about how to do the Sugar Impact Diet on a budget. That's not a small concern, I know! Sometimes a quick look at the shopping list or recipes gives people the impression they'll be shut out of everything this diet has to offer, and I'm here to tell you that is just *not* the case.

It's hard to feed a family well while you're juggling bills and working 'til you drop. It can seem impossible to get a healthy meal on the table every night. Grass-fed beef and wild salmon may not seem to fit in the daily food budget. But I designed the Sugar Impact Diet to be practical and affordable.

In the end, when you tally your bills, I believe you'll save money doing the Sugar Impact Diet. Why? Because you won't be loading your cart with overpriced processed foods or buying trendy, expensive coffee drinks with a side of stale Danish. You're also gaining a lean, healthy physique—and better long-term health—which is priceless.

To help you get even more value out of the weeks you'll spend on the Sugar Impact Diet, here are a whopping twenty strategies to make the most of your food dollar. Pick just a few or use them all and keep your money where it belongs—in your wallet!

1. *Buy in season.* Asparagus peaks in spring, while blueberries are ripest in summer. Besides being fresher and more likely to be locally grown, produce is more affordable in season.

2. *Buy frozen and stock up.* Ever regrettably tossed a head of broccoli that sat in your fridge for a week? Frozen foods eliminate that problem and save you money. You can literally buy months of veggies and other foods to store in your freezer, so you always have organic frozen spinach to toss into soups or stews, or to use as a side dish.

3. *Less meat, more plant-based foods.* I encourage you to only choose the best quality meats, like grass-fed beef and wild-caught salmon. But they aren't cheap, especially if you're trying to feed a family of four or more. Rather than buy lower quality, conventionally produced meats (sorry, but farm-raised salmon is just gross), load your plate with less meat and more green veggies, good fats like avocado, and low-impact, high-fiber carbs.

4. *Start your day with the Sugar Impact Shake.* Occasionally someone will write that they can't afford the protein powder in my online store. A little math solves that problem: even when you add in the coconut milk and other goodies, you'll be spending about 3 to 4 dollars total per Sugar Impact Shake. That's less than you'd spend on a nutrient-empty, fat-storing muffin and a latte.

5. *Don't snack.* I have clients total the money they spend at bodegas, vending machines, and other snack meccas. They're often shocked at the amount. Don't snack unless you absolutely must (and even then, choose wisely). You'll keep your blood sugar stable and save money, too.

6. *Join a farmers' collective or co-op.* More cities now have food co-ops where you volunteer your time for reduced-cost produce and other locally grown and raised foods. Farmers' collectives provide similar opportunities with grass-fed beef and other pasture-raised foods. You probably have a farmers' market during warmer months (which in some places is nearly year round), though some cities now have indoor year-round farmers' markets.

7. *Shop warehouse stores for bulk buys.* This can be a great way to go, but take a list and stick to it, because warehouse stores love to tempt you with "bargains."

8. *Load your plate with high-fiber foods.* Fiber slows stomach emptying, balances blood sugar, curbs cravings, and makes you full faster. What's not to love? Shoot for 2 to 3 high-fiber foods at every meal. Avocados, lentils, and other legumes, nuts, seeds, and leafy greens are all excellent choices.

9. *Prepare ahead of time.* If you know you'll be stuck late at work, prep dinner ingredients in the morning and take away the temptation of delivery or takeout.

10. *Make your own.* Now that you know hidden sugar in your favorite dressing could be stalling your fast fat loss and holding your health hostage, make your own. You'll save money and know exactly what you're getting when dressings, sauces, spice blends, and other condiments come from your kitchen.

11. *Try my stoup recipe.* Stoup is my hybrid of soup and stew. It makes a great fast, economical, hearty meal. You can even toss leftovers into the slow cooker, and voilà! You have dinner waiting when you get home from work. Portion and refrigerate leftovers for office lunches.

12. *Brew your own.* Coffee and tea, that is! Ever tallied how much you spend on those fancy coffee-shop drinks? That doesn't even take into account the sugary pastry or low-fat muffin (aka the adult cupcake) you might have grabbed before you found the Sugar Impact Diet. Become your own barista and brew a cup of organic coffee or green tea for far less than what you'd spend at a coffee shop.

13. *Skip convenience foods.* Supermarkets take advantage of your need to save time, and they sock you in the wallet with presliced veggies, trimmed-and-cleaned chicken breasts, and precooked—well, just about everything. Once I realized prepped broccoli florets cost *twice* as much as organic broccoli heads and that I could buy a whole chicken for the same cost as two tiny breasts, I decided saving a little time wasn't worth spending a lot more money.

14. *Shop day-old foods.* Many grocery stores and butchers discount must-sell-quickly meats and other perishable foods. If you don't see them reduced in the refrigerated aisles, just ask: most stores are happy to get rid of them before their sell-by date. And you'll get good meat cheap. Time for an impromptu cookout!

15. *Buy generics.* Generic foods have evolved since we were kids. Whole Foods 365 products are fabulous and sometimes even less expensive and healthier than the

equivalent conventional store products. Stores often market their own brand, but because they don't have a middleman, you can buy an identical product for less money. You can win in other ways, too. When I compared brand-name and store-brand almond butters, guess what *wasn't* in the store brand? Sugar.

16. *Make spa water or healthy lemonade.* If I had a dollar for every time I heard "I don't like water," I would be on a permanent vacation in Waikiki. For even the most water-phobic, lemonade made with fresh lemons, filtered water, and stevia hits the spot without soda's price or sugar overload. You can also upgrade water by steeping fresh lemon, lime, or orange slices in filtered water. You'll get the spa experience for the cost of a piece of fruit!

17. *Set a budget and make a list.* You've done this and so have I: you realize you're out of something for a meal you're preparing, hop in the car, and, next thing you know, you're swiping your credit card for a triple-digit grocery bill. Wait, how did all that stuff get in your basket? Because you didn't bring a list and stick to it. Plan ahead: determine what you're going to spend, write down everything you need, and *don't deviate.*

18. *Learn the Dirty Dozen and the Clean Fifteen.* In a perfect world, every food would be organic. But in reality, sometimes it's hard to justify spending three times as much for organic produce. So get to know the Dirty Dozen: the 12 most-contaminated foods. Always try to buy those organic. The "Clean 15" are the *least*-contaminated foods. If you're going to buy non-organic, they're your best bets.

19. *Don't overbuy.* Stock up on essentials but don't become swept away by great deals. Know how much you'll use and restrain yourself from overstocking, especially with perishable foods.

20. *Look at the big picture.* When and where you can, invest a little more money in high-quality food. The savings in health care down the road will pay you back in spades—with more quality years in your life! I'd call that a high return on your investment!

I hope you couldn't possibly feel more prepared or inspired. You know just how to set up your kitchen and which nutritious, weight loss–promoting foods to stock it with, and you have the tools to take them to town. The remarkable recipes in this cookbook will come to life in your hands and deliver you from the extra pounds and frustration that have plagued you. You're about to experience weight loss the way it should be—no deprivation, only delicious, energy-fueling, healthy food. You've got nothing to lose, except up to 10 pounds in just 2 weeks!

PART II

SUGAR IMPACT
DIET RECIPES

The straightest path to fast weight loss and reclaiming your energy and health is…eating! And I'm going to make sure you enjoy every forkful. Your plate will be packed with the perfect balance of clean, lean protein, healthy fats, nonstarchy veggies, and slow, low carbs. They'll send your body all the right messages about blood sugar and insulin, fullness and hunger, and mood and energy. But even too much healthy food can be, well, too much, so I'll make sure you're eating the right portions, too. I think you're going to be amazed by how you'll lose weight, look younger, and feel better fast, without feeling hungry or deprived!

I've laid out my program in three easy-to-follow cycles that will attack your weight loss resistance where it lives: in high-SI, hidden sugar—the kind that wrecks your metabolism and hijacks your waistline.

If you're eating high-SI foods, it's no surprise you're having a tough time shaking that stubborn extra weight and that your energy is in the dumps. You're also probably dealing with health issues you're not connecting to what you're eating. When you eliminate high-SI foods, you'll not only lose weight, but you'll have more energy, sleep better, and get back your youthful, glowing skin!

Even if you started the Sugar Impact Diet to lose weight, once you see how good you look and feel, you'll never want to go back to high-SI foods. Never ever.

So if you have any anxiety at all about how the heck you're going to get sugar—your best go-to buddy in times of need—out of your life, rest assured that this cookbook holds your hand every step of the way. My recipes are all medium and low SI, so you can cook and eat worry free (no counting calories!)—all while wondering how such delicious food could be lower sugar!

All my recipes are appropriate for Cycle 2 unless they're specifically designated for Cycles 1 and/or 3.

You'll notice that the go-to sweetener in these recipes is monk fruit. Sometimes, monk fruit can be hard to find (especially pure monk fruit); if you have trouble locating it, try a blend of erythritol (or xylitol) and stevia in the same amount called for in the recipe. One note of caution: I don't recommend using stevia on its own...baking is no time for surprises!

4

SHAKES AND BREAKFASTS

Beware, breakfast skippers! You're working against your fast fat-loss goals and probably don't even know it. You're slowing your metabolism and setting yourself up for a gorge fest in the middle of the day. What you're not doing is helping yourself lose weight.

Research shows that people who eat a protein-packed breakfast lose weight more easily and keep it off longer than those who eat a high-sugar breakfast or skip it all together. So one of the biggest shifts you can make in Sugar Impact is to swap out your "no breakfast" or your high-carb, grab-and-go breakfast for a high-protein, low-SI shake.

Eat within an hour of waking up, and make sure your breakfast (whether it actually is one of those filling, fat-burning shakes or some other tasty low–SI choice) has clean, lean protein, healthy fats, and high–fiber, slow-releasing carbohydrates. A substantial, balanced breakfast will launch you into your day full of energy, with stable blood sugar and nary a craving in sight.

Sugar Impact Shake

If mornings feel like a race against the clock, I'm here to help. There's nothing basic about the fast fat-burning fuel in this easy-to-make shake. Flavorful and protein packed, it will be your gold standard for a quick, on-the-go breakfast.

Makes 1 serving

- 1 to 2 scoops protein blend (any flavor), per package instructions
- 1 to 2 scoops fiber blend
- ½ small avocado
- 1 tablespoon freshly ground chia seeds or flaxseeds
- 8 to 10 ounces unsweetened coconut milk or almond milk
- 5 or 6 ice cubes

In a blender, combine the protein blend, fiber blend, avocado, chia seeds, coconut milk, and ice cubes. Mix on high until smooth. Thin with cold water, if desired.

Nutrient Content per Serving

Calories:	330	**Fat:**	16 grams	**Protein:**	24 grams
Fiber:	15 grams	**Saturated Fat:**	6 grams	**Carbs:**	25 grams
Sodium:	220 mg	**Sugars:**	1 gram		

Super Greens Shake

Your friends will be green with envy wondering your secret. Packed with the perfect combination of protein, fiber, and nutrients, this powerhouse will be just the boost of energy you need to start your day.

Makes 1 serving

- 1 to 2 scoops vanilla-flavored protein blend, per package instructions
- 1 scoop fiber blend
- ¼ small avocado
- 2 cups baby spinach
- 1 to 2 tablespoons maca powder
- ½ teaspoon monk fruit extract
- ⅛ teaspoon ground cinnamon
- 10 ounces unsweetened coconut milk
- 5 or 6 ice cubes

In a blender, combine the protein blend, fiber blend, avocado, spinach, maca powder, monk fruit extract, cinnamon, coconut milk, and ice cubes. Mix on high until smooth. Thin with cold water, if desired.

Nutrient Content per Serving

Calories:	280	**Fat:**	11 grams	**Protein:**	22 grams
Fiber:	14 grams	**Saturated Fat:**	7 grams	**Carbs:**	25 grams
Sodium:	310 mg	**Sugars:**	1 gram		

Pumpkin Spice Shake

Pumpkin spice, in all its slightly sweet, nutty versatility, is no longer relegated to fall, and we're the big winners! All the flavors of pumpkin pie are yours to savor in this nutritious, fiber-rich shake—any time of year.

Makes 1 serving

- 1 to 2 scoops vanilla protein blend, per package instructions
- 1 to 2 scoops fiber blend
- 1 tablespoon freshly ground chia seeds
- 8 to 10 ounces unsweetened coconut milk
- ¼ teaspoon pumpkin pie spice
- 5 to 6 ice cubes

In a blender, combine the protein blend, fiber blend, chia seeds, coconut milk, pumpkin pie spice, and ice cubes. Mix on high until smooth. Thin with cold water, if desired.

Nutrient Content per Serving

Calories:	250	**Fat:**	9 grams	**Protein:**	22 grams
Fiber:	14 grams	**Saturated Fat:**	5 grams	**Carbs:**	21 grams
Sodium:	220 mg	**Sugars:**	1 gram		

Espresso-Almond Shake

Okay, this is just inspired. It combines the pick-me-up of espresso with the nuttiness of almond in a cold, creamy, easy-to-make shake. If only your coffee could be this good!

Makes 1 serving

    1 to 2 scoops vanilla protein blend, per package instructions
    1 scoop fiber blend
    ¼ cup strong-brewed coffee, or a shot of espresso
    1 tablespoon raw almond butter
    2 teaspoons freshly ground flaxseeds
    ¼ teaspoon almond extract
    8 to 10 ounces unsweetened almond milk
    5 or 6 ice cubes

In a blender, combine the protein blend, fiber blend, coffee, almond butter, flaxseeds, almond extract, almond milk, and ice cubes. Mix on high until smooth. Thin with cold water, if desired.

Nutrient Content per Serving

Calories:	320	**Fat:**	16 grams	**Protein:**	25 grams
Fiber:	14 grams	**Saturated Fat:**	6 grams	**Carbs:**	21 grams
Sodium:	220 mg	**Sugars:**	2 grams		

Coconut-Vanilla Shake

You may feel like you should be drinking this creamy, nutrition-packed shake out of a coconut shell, with your toes in the sand. With the added protein and fiber, it will easily keep you satisfied throughout the morning.

Makes 1 serving

    1 to 2 scoops vanilla protein blend, per package instructions
    1 scoop fiber blend
    1 tablespoon raw cashew butter
    2 teaspoons freshly ground flaxseeds
    ¼ teaspoon coconut extract
    8 to 10 ounces unsweetened coconut milk
    5 or 6 ice cubes

In a blender, combine the protein blend, fiber blend, cashew butter, flaxseeds, coconut extract, coconut milk, and ice cubes. Mix on high until smooth. Thin with cold water, if desired.

Nutrient Content per Serving

Calories:	390	Fat:	22 grams	Protein:	26 grams
Fiber:	13 grams	Saturated Fat:	8 grams	Carbs:	32 grams
Sodium:	220 mg	Sugars:	1 gram		

Chocolate, Flax, and Avocado Shake

You only need to try avocado in a shake once to be hooked. This delicious, creamy combination is a nutrient powerhouse, bolstered by the omega-3s from the flaxseed.

Makes 1 serving

- 1 to 2 scoops chocolate protein blend, per package instructions
- 1 scoop fiber blend
- ¼ small avocado
- 2 teaspoons freshly ground flaxseeds
- 2 teaspoons raw almond butter
- 8 to 10 ounces unsweetened coconut milk
- 5 or 6 ice cubes

In a blender, combine the protein blend, fiber blend, avocado, flaxseeds, almond butter, coconut milk, and ice cubes. Mix on high until smooth. Thin with cold water, if desired.

Nutrient Content per Serving

Calories:	350	Fat:	18 grams	Protein:	25 grams
Fiber:	15 grams	Saturated Fat:	6 grams	Carbs:	23 grams
Sodium:	210 mg	Sugars:	2 grams		

Cappuccino Protein Shake

Bellissimo! Coffee and breakfast, all in one. Perfect for a hectic morning, let this delicious and satisfying shake give you an extra bounce in your step. The combination of protein and fiber help keep Sugar Impact low. For a stronger coffee flavor, use ⅓ to ½ cup coffee or stir in 1 to 2 teaspoons freeze-dried espresso powder.

Makes 1 serving

    1 to 2 scoops vanilla protein blend, per package instructions
    1 to 2 scoops fiber blend
    ¼ cup strong-brewed coffee
    1 tablespoon Cinnamon Almond Butter (page 104)
    8 to 10 ounces unsweetened almond milk
    5 or 6 ice cubes

In a blender, combine the protein blend, fiber blend, coffee, almond butter, almond milk, and ice cubes. Mix on high until smooth. Thin with cold water, if desired.

Nutrient Content per Serving

Calories:	290	**Fat:**	14 grams	**Protein:**	24 grams
Fiber:	12 grams	**Saturated Fat:**	6 grams	**Carbs:**	19 grams
Sodium:	220 mg	**Sugars:**	2 grams		

Blueberry-Peach Shake (Cycles 1/3)

Combine the superstar antioxidant attributes of blueberries with the sweet juicy goodness of peaches, and voilà! You'll be so distracted by how good it is, the fact that it's also a low-SI, super-healthy breakfast will slip by unnoticed.

Makes 1 serving

    1 to 2 scoops vanilla protein blend, per package instructions
    1 scoop fiber blend
    ½ cup fresh or frozen blueberries
    ½ fresh medium peach, peeled, pitted, and sliced
    ⅛ teaspoon almond extract
    8 to 10 ounces unsweetened coconut milk
    5 or 6 ice cubes

In a blender, combine the protein blend, fiber blend, blueberries, peach, almond extract, coconut milk, and ice cubes. Mix on high until smooth. Thin with cold water, if desired.

Nutrient Content per Serving

Calories:	270	Fat:	6 grams	Protein:	21 grams
Fiber:	13 grams	Saturated Fat:	5 grams	Carbs:	33 grams
Sodium:	220 mg	Sugars:	14 grams		

Tex-Mex Scrambled Eggs with Avocado and Salsa

Add some gusto to your breakfast. The fresh avocado adds a wonderful texture to the scrambled eggs, in addition to more than 20 vitamins and minerals. For a spicier salsa, stir in 1 teaspoon minced jalapeño pepper.

Makes 2 servings

1 small plum tomato, seeded and chopped (about ½ cup)
2 teaspoons finely chopped red onion
2 teaspoons chopped fresh cilantro
1 teaspoon lime juice
⅛ teaspoon plus ¼ teaspoon sea salt
4 large eggs
1 tablespoon water
½ teaspoon olive oil
½ small avocado, sliced

Combine the tomato, onion, cilantro, lime juice, and ⅛ teaspoon of the salt in a small bowl.

Whisk together the eggs, water, and remaining ¼ teaspoon salt in a bowl. Heat the olive oil in a medium nonstick skillet over medium heat. Add the egg mixture and cook, stirring gently, until the eggs are set, about 2 minutes. Divide the eggs between two plates and top each with half the tomato mixture and half the sliced avocado.

Nutrient Content per Serving

Calories:	190	Fat:	13 grams	Protein:	13 grams
Fiber:	1 gram	Saturated Fat:	3.5 grams	Carbs:	4 grams
Sodium:	590 mg	Sugars:	1 gram		

Pumpkin Bread French Toast with Berry Compote (Cycles 1/3)

I'm going to let you go on believing that I've given you permission to have pumpkin pie for breakfast. The berry compote adds just the right amount of zest. To avoid breaking the bread, be sure to handle it gently when dipping it in the egg.

Makes 4 servings

COMPOTE

1 cup fresh strawberries, hulled and sliced
½ cup fresh blueberries
½ cup fresh raspberries
2 tablespoons orange juice
¼ teaspoon monk fruit extract
1 teaspoon grated orange zest

FRENCH TOAST

3 large eggs, lightly beaten
3 tablespoons whole milk
1 teaspoon vanilla extract
8 (½-inch-thick) slices Coconut-Pumpkin Bread (page 74)
2 teaspoons coconut oil

For the compote, combine the strawberries, blueberries, raspberries, orange juice, and monk fruit extract in a small saucepan. Cook over medium heat, stirring occasionally, until the fruit is just softened, 3 to 4 minutes. Remove from the heat and stir in the orange zest.

For the French toast, whisk together the eggs, milk, and vanilla in a shallow bowl or pie pan. Dip each slice of bread into the egg mixture and allow it to soak up some of the mixture.

Melt 1 teaspoon of the coconut oil in a large nonstick skillet over medium heat. Add 4 bread slices and cook until browned, 3 to 4 minutes per side. Repeat with the remaining coconut oil and bread slices. Serve topped with the compote.

Nutrient Content per Serving

Calories:	370	**Fat:**	29 grams	**Protein:**	12 grams
Fiber:	6 grams	**Saturated Fat:**	17 grams	**Carbs:**	19 grams
Sodium:	360 mg	**Sugars:**	7 grams		

Old-Fashioned Oatmeal with Cinnamon, Blueberries, and Raspberries (Cycles 1/3)

Close your eyes and imagine the sensation of berries popping and squirting over a mouthful of warm oatmeal. Smiling yet? You'll hope there's no bottom to this belly-rubbing, *mmm*-inducing bowl. Be sure to use gluten-free old-fashioned rolled oats.

Makes 2 servings

2½ cups water

¼ teaspoon sea salt

1 cup gluten-free old-fashioned rolled oats

¾ teaspoon ground cinnamon

1½ teaspoons monk fruit extract

½ teaspoon vanilla extract

1 scoop vanilla protein blend

¼ cup fresh blueberries

¼ cup fresh raspberries

1 teaspoon grated orange zest

4 tablespoons slow-roasted almonds (see page 97), coarsely chopped

Bring the water and salt to a boil in a small saucepan over high heat. Stir in the oats, cinnamon, 1 teaspoon of the monk fruit extract, and the vanilla extract; reduce the heat to medium-low and simmer for 15 minutes. Remove from the heat, stir in the protein blend, cover, and let stand for 3 minutes.

Meanwhile, combine the blueberries, raspberries, orange zest, and remaining ½ teaspoon monk fruit extract in a bowl.

Divide the oatmeal between two bowls and top each with ½ cup of the berry mixture and 2 tablespoons almonds.

Nutrient Content per Serving

Calories:	330	**Fat:**	11 grams	**Protein:**	21 grams
Fiber:	9 grams	**Saturated Fat:**	1 gram	**Carbs:**	40 grams
Sodium:	450 mg	**Sugars:**	4 grams		

Goat Cheese and Vegetable Omelet

Goat cheese lends a tangy flavor and a creamy texture for an inspired twist on a high-protein, veggie-filled favorite. If you're dairy sensitive, substitute 2 tablespoons of your favorite nut cheese for the goat cheese.

Makes 1 serving

> 2 large eggs
> ¼ teaspoon plus ⅛ teaspoon sea salt
> ⅛ teaspoon freshly ground black pepper
> 2 teaspoons olive oil
> ⅓ cup finely chopped zucchini
> ¼ cup finely chopped red bell pepper
> ¼ cup finely chopped shallots
> ¼ teaspoon dried basil
> 1 ounce goat cheese, crumbled

Lightly beat together the eggs, ¼ teaspoon of the salt, and the black pepper in a small bowl until well mixed. Set aside.

Heat the olive oil in an 8-inch nonstick skillet over medium-high heat. Add the zucchini, bell pepper, shallots, basil, and remaining ⅛ teaspoon salt. Cook, stirring occasionally, until the vegetables are crisp-tender, 3 to 4 minutes. Reduce the heat to medium. Stir in the eggs and cook until the eggs begin to set in the center, about 3 minutes. Use a spatula to lift up the set edges and allow the uncooked mixture to run underneath. Flip the omelet over; top one half with the goat cheese. Carefully loosen the omelet and fold the empty half over the cheese. Transfer to a plate and let stand for 1 minute before serving.

Nutrient Content per Serving

Calories:	350	**Fat:**	26 grams	**Protein:**	20 grams
Fiber:	3 grams	**Saturated Fat:**	9 grams	**Carbs:**	12 grams
Sodium:	1098 mg	**Sugars:**	6 grams		

Coconut-Pumpkin Bread

Is there anything better than the nostalgic aroma of pumpkin bread as it comes out of the oven? This version, with a touch of coconut, makes any day a holiday. Be sure to purchase canned pumpkin puree, not pumpkin pie mix, to avoid unwanted sugars.

Makes 8 servings

½ cup coconut oil, melted, plus more for the baking pan

4 large eggs

½ cup canned pumpkin puree

½ cup lite culinary coconut milk (see sidebar, page 132)

1 tablespoon vanilla extract

1 cup finely ground almond flour

½ cup coconut flour

2 tablespoons monk fruit extract

2 teaspoons grain-free baking powder

½ teaspoon baking soda

2 teaspoons pumpkin pie spice

1 teaspoon ground cinnamon

¼ teaspoon sea salt

Preheat the oven to 350°F. Grease an 8 x 5-inch glass loaf pan with coconut oil.

Whisk together the melted coconut oil, eggs, pumpkin puree, coconut milk, and vanilla in a bowl. In a separate bowl, combine the almond flour, coconut flour, monk fruit extract, baking powder, baking soda, pumpkin pie spice, cinnamon, and salt and stir well. Add the wet ingredients to the dry and mix until moistened and well combined. Transfer to the prepared loaf pan and smooth the top with a spatula.

Bake until a toothpick inserted into the center of the loaf comes out clean and the outside has lightly browned, 48 to 50 minutes. Remove from the oven and let the bread cool in the pan for 15 minutes. Transfer to a wire rack to cool completely before slicing, about 1 hour. Store wrapped in plastic wrap in a cool place for up to 4 days.

Nutrient Content per Serving

Calories:	290	**Fat:**	26 grams	**Protein:**	8 grams
Fiber:	5 grams	**Saturated Fat:**	15 grams	**Carbs:**	10 grams
Sodium:	350 mg	**Sugars:**	2 grams		

Individual Baked Breakfast Frittatas

Frittatas, which are Italian-style omelets, are staples on most brunch menus. They're also perfect for entertaining or other special occasions because they're fast, easy, and (almost always) universally loved. Enjoy!

Makes 4 servings

Olive oil for the pan
6 slices nitrate-free uncured bacon
1 small red onion, chopped
1 small red bell pepper, finely chopped
1 teaspoon dried basil
8 ounces asparagus, trimmed and cut into ½-inch pieces
12 large eggs
½ teaspoon sea salt
¼ teaspoon freshly ground black pepper

Preheat the oven to 350°F. Lightly dampen a paper towel with a small amount of olive oil and wipe the inside of each cup in a 12-cup muffin pan. Heat a large skillet over medium heat. Add the bacon and cook until crisp, turning once, 6 to 7 minutes. Transfer to a plate lined with a paper towel to drain. When cool enough to handle, chop the bacon and set aside.

Pour off all but 1 tablespoon of the bacon fat from the skillet and return to the stove over medium-high heat. Add the onion, bell pepper, and basil; cook, stirring occasionally, until the vegetables are starting to soften, 2 to 3 minutes. Add the asparagus and cook until bright green, 4 minutes. Remove from the heat and stir in the chopped bacon. Divide the mixture evenly among the prepared muffin cups.

Whisk together the eggs, salt, and black pepper in a bowl. Divide the mixture evenly among the muffin cups.

Bake until the eggs have puffed up and set, 17 to 18 minutes. Remove the frittatas from the muffin pan and serve warm or at room temperature.

Nutrient Content per Serving

Calories:	330	**Fat:**	22 grams	**Protein:**	24 grams
Fiber:	2 grams	**Saturated Fat:**	7 grams	**Carbs:**	9 grams
Sodium:	700 mg	**Sugars:**	3 grams		

5

WRAPS, SALADS, AND SANDWICHES

You may love the handheld ease of eating a wrap, but a lot of the conventional tortillas are high in added sugar and gluten. You can always take them out of the equation and pop out a great salad, but there are ways to enjoy them without wrecking your blood sugar balance.

The fast fat-burning combination of ingredients in this section—whether they're wrapped or not—help you do just that. They also pack a heart-healthy, brain-healthy, anti-inflammatory punch that's hard to top. They're all high in fiber, vitamins, phyto-chemicals, antioxidants, and, of course, protein—so be careful not to transform an otherwise nutrient-rich meal into a sugar-soaked dessert by adding gooey dressing, dried fruit, glazed nuts, or crunchy wontons!

Use the Sugar Impact Plate as your guide for building the best wraps and salads:

1. Start with great greens—the deeper the green color, the better.
2. Add some colorful, nonstarchy veggies—make your plate a rainbow.
3. Include some clean, lean protein.
4. Add a little high-fiber starchy carb.
5. Add some healthy fat.

You can't go wrong!

Turkey, Spinach, and Strawberry Wrap (Cycles 1/3)

The lean, light meat of turkey paired with the sweet juiciness of strawberries makes this a really refreshing spring or summer wrap. Have some fun with the fruit and change it up—try it with raspberries or blueberries in place of the strawberry slices. *Mmmm.*

Makes 2 servings

4 slices nitrate-free uncured bacon
2 brown rice tortillas
2 tablespoons Sugar Impact Mayonnaise (page 197)
1 cup baby spinach
½ cup strawberries, hulled and sliced
6 ounces deli-sliced nitrate-free turkey

Heat a small nonstick skillet over medium heat. Add the bacon and cook until crisp, turning once, 6 to 7 minutes. Transfer to a plate lined with a paper towel to drain.

Spread one side of each tortilla with 1 tablespoon of the mayonnaise. Top each with half of the bacon, spinach, strawberries, and turkey. Roll and serve.

Nutrient Content per Serving

Calories:	380	**Fat:**	17 grams	**Protein:**	2 grams
Fiber:	3 grams	**Saturated Fat:**	3 grams	**Carbs:**	34 grams
Sodium:	808 mg	**Sugars:**	3 grams		

Chicken Cheesesteak Wrap

If the prized food of South Philly is calling your name, this wrap is about to make you very happy. To make it with beef, substitute 8 to 10 ounces thinly sliced flank steak for the chicken. Just don't make it "Whiz wit!"

Makes 2 servings

4 teaspoons olive oil

2 (4- to 5-ounce) boneless skinless chicken breast halves, thinly sliced crosswise

¼ teaspoon sea salt

1 small onion, thinly sliced

2 garlic cloves, minced

½ medium red bell pepper, thinly sliced

¼ teaspoon dried basil

1½ ounces provolone cheese, shredded (about ⅓ cup)

2 coconut wraps (see box, below)

Heat 2 teaspoons of the olive oil in a large nonstick skillet over medium-high heat. Season the chicken with ⅛ teaspoon of the salt; add to the skillet and cook, stirring occasionally, until lightly browned and cooked through, 4 minutes. Transfer the chicken to a plate and set aside.

Add the remaining 2 teaspoons oil to the skillet and heat over medium-high heat. Stir in the onion, garlic, bell pepper, basil, and remaining ⅛ teaspoon salt; cook until the vegetables are beginning to soften, 2 minutes. Reduce the heat to medium and cook until the vegetables are crisp-tender, 3 minutes longer. Stir in the chicken and cook until hot, 1 minute. Remove from the heat and stir in the cheese until melted and well combined. Divide the mixture between the two wraps and serve.

Nutrient Content per Serving

Calories:	390	**Fat:**	23 grams	**Protein:**	31 grams
Fiber:	4 grams	**Saturated Fat:**	10 grams	**Carbs:**	13 grams
Sodium:	590 mg	**Sugars:**	5 grams		

Coconut Wraps

Coconut wraps and other paleo-approved tortilla alternatives are made with coconut meat, coconut water, and coconut oil. If you can't find them at your local health food store, they're easy to order online.

Chicken, Shirataki Noodle, and Snap Pea Salad

Why do noodles still make us feel like kids? At least you can enjoy these without the fear of pasta's carb assault, and instead focus on the fabulous textures and flavors all sharing your plate. Make sure to always give green onions a good rinse before using them in any dish.

Makes 2 servings

1 (8-ounce) bag shirataki noodles, drained and rinsed

8 ounces sugar snap peas (about 1½ cups)

8 ounces asparagus, trimmed and cut into ½-inch pieces (about 2 cups)

2 carrots, thinly sliced on an angle

¼ cup chopped green onions

Olive oil for the pan

2 (6-ounce) boneless skinless chicken breast halves

3 teaspoons Malaysian red palm fruit oil

1 garlic clove, minced

1 teaspoon minced fresh ginger

¼ teaspoon sea salt

2 tablespoons lime juice

2 tablespoons chopped fresh cilantro

2 teaspoons low-sodium wheat-free tamari or coconut aminos

Bring a pot of water to a boil. Cook the noodles according to the package directions. During the last minute of cooking, add the snap peas, asparagus, and carrots. Return the water to a boil and cook for 1 minute longer; drain and rinse under cold water. Transfer to a bowl and add the green onions; set aside.

Lightly dampen a paper towel with a small amount of olive oil and wipe a grill pan with it; heat over medium-high heat. Combine the chicken, 2 teaspoons of the palm fruit oil, the garlic, ginger, and ⅛ teaspoon of the salt in a bowl. Add the chicken to the pan and cook until a thermometer inserted into the thickest part of the chicken registers 165°F, 4 to 5 minutes per side. Transfer to a cutting board and let rest for 2 minutes. Cut the chicken crosswise into thin strips.

Add the remaining 1 teaspoon palm fruit oil, ⅛ teaspoon salt, lime juice, cilantro, and tamari to the noodle mixture and toss well. Divide the noodles between two plates and top each with half of the chicken.

Nutrient Content per Serving

Calories:	300	**Fat:**	11 grams	**Protein:**	34 grams
Fiber:	6 grams	**Saturated Fat:**	4.5 grams	**Carbs:**	18 grams
Sodium:	690 mg	**Sugars:**	6 grams		

Flank Steak and Vegetable Wrap with Chimichurri Sauce

Discover your inner gaucho with the Argentinean flare of this hearty wrap. For an easy shortcut, use nitrate-free deli-sliced roast beef instead of flank steak.

Makes 2 servings

12 ounces flank steak, trimmed

2 teaspoons Smoky BBQ Spice Rub (page 195)

2 teaspoons olive oil, plus more for the pan

½ medium onion, sliced

½ medium zucchini, halved lengthwise and sliced

½ medium yellow squash, halved lengthwise and sliced

⅛ teaspoon sea salt

2 coconut wraps (see box, page 79)

2 tablespoons Chimichurri Sauce (page 190)

Sprinkle the steak all over with the spice rub to coat. Let stand at room temperature for 10 minutes.

Lightly dampen a paper towel with a small amount of olive oil and wipe a grill pan with it; heat over medium-high heat. Add the steak and cook, turning once, until it reaches the desired doneness, 10 to 11 minutes for medium-rare. Transfer the steak to a cutting board and let stand for 5 minutes before thinly slicing.

Meanwhile, heat the 2 teaspoons of olive oil in a large nonstick skillet over medium-high heat. Add the onion and cook, stirring occasionally, until slightly softened, 2 to 3 minutes. Stir in the zucchini and squash and cook until tender and lightly browned, 5 to 6 minutes. Remove from the heat and season with the salt.

Place a wrap on each of two plates. Top each with half of the steak, half of the vegetable mixture, and 1 tablespoon of the chimichurri sauce.

Nutrient Content per Serving

Calories:	420	**Fat:**	25 grams	**Protein:**	37 grams
Fiber:	4 grams	**Saturated Fat:**	10 grams	**Carbs:**	10 grams
Sodium:	600 mg	**Sugars:**	5 grams		

Roasted Beet and Arugula Salad with Shallots and Lemon (Cycles 1/3)

The exquisite simplicity of this salad belies its potent nutritional punch—beets are a great source of fiber and antioxidants, which protect your cells from free radical damage. For even roasting, look for beets around 3 inches in diameter.

Makes 4 servings

1 pound beets (about 4 medium)
8 cups baby arugula
½ avocado, cut into ½-inch pieces
½ medium cucumber, peeled, halved lengthwise, and sliced
2 tablespoons lemon juice
¼ cup finely chopped shallots
2 tablespoons extra-virgin olive oil
¼ teaspoon sea salt
⅛ teaspoon freshly ground black pepper

Preheat the oven to 425°F. Position a rack in the center.

Place the beets on a rimmed baking sheet. Roast until the beets can be easily pierced with a knife, 55 to 60 minutes. Remove from the oven and let cool for 10 minutes. Peel the beets and cut each into 8 wedges; transfer to a bowl and add the arugula, avocado, and cucumber.

Combine the lemon juice, shallots, oil, salt, and pepper in a bowl. Pour over the beet mixture and toss well to coat. Divide among four plates and serve.

Nutrient Content per Serving

Calories:	150	**Fat:**	9 grams	**Protein:**	4 grams
Fiber:	3 grams	**Saturated Fat:**	1 gram	**Carbs:**	16 grams
Sodium:	430 mg	**Sugars:**	9 grams		

Shrimp Caesar Salad

Grilled shrimp change up this timeless salad and give you an antioxidant and anti-inflammatory boost to boot. Choose wild, cold-water shrimp if you can. Romano cheese is made from sheep's milk and has a slightly sharp and nutty flavor. If you're intolerant to dairy, leave it out or substitute an equivalent amount of nut or vegan cheese.

Makes 4 servings

⅓ cup Sugar Impact Mayonnaise (page 197)

2 tablespoons grated Pecorino Romano cheese

1 oil-packed anchovy, drained and mashed to a paste

2 teaspoons lemon juice

½ teaspoon low-sodium wheat-free tamari or coconut aminos

¼ teaspoon Tabasco sauce

¼ teaspoon freshly ground black pepper

8 cups torn romaine lettuce

2 teaspoons olive oil, plus more for the pan

1½ pounds jumbo shrimp (16 to 20 per pound), peeled and deveined

¼ teaspoon sea salt

Combine the mayonnaise, cheese, anchovy, lemon juice, tamari, Tabasco sauce, and pepper in a bowl. Place the lettuce in a separate large bowl. Add the mayonnaise mixture to the lettuce and toss well.

Lightly dampen a paper towel with a small amount of olive oil and wipe a grill pan with it; heat over medium-high heat. Combine the 2 teaspoons of the olive oil, shrimp, and salt in a bowl. Place the shrimp on the grill pan and cook until opaque and cooked through, 2 to 3 minutes per side.

Divide the lettuce mixture among four plates. Top each with one-quarter of the shrimp.

Nutrient Content per Serving

Calories:	190	**Fat:**	16 grams	**Protein:**	7 grams
Fiber:	2 grams	**Saturated Fat:**	2.5 grams	**Carbs:**	6 grams
Sodium:	440 mg	**Sugars:**	2 grams		

Southwest Grilled Steak Salad on Crisped Rice Tortillas (Cycles 1/3)

I'm serving up a festival of southwestern flavor, so get in the spirit! Throw the flank steaks on the grill and enjoy some music by the backyard fireplace as the sun goes down. Allowing the meat to stand at room temperature before cooking allows it to cook more evenly and faster than throwing it right on the grill straight out of the fridge.

Makes 4 servings

1 teaspoon ground cumin

1 teaspoon garlic powder

1 teaspoon ground coriander

1 teaspoon chili powder

½ teaspoon sea salt

¼ teaspoon ground chipotle pepper

1½ pounds flank steak, trimmed

8 cups chopped romaine lettuce

1 medium cucumber, peeled and chopped

1 orange bell pepper, chopped

1 cup grape tomatoes, halved

½ medium avocado, cut into ¼-inch pieces

1 teaspoon grated lime zest

1 tablespoon lime juice

1 tablespoon olive oil, plus more for the pan

⅛ teaspoon freshly ground black pepper

4 brown rice tortillas

Prepare the grill for direct-heat cooking over medium-high heat, 350 to 400°F.

Combine the cumin, garlic powder, coriander, chili powder, ¼ teaspoon of the salt, and the chipotle pepper in a small bowl. Rub the mixture all over the steak to coat; let stand at room temperature for 20 minutes.

Meanwhile, combine the lettuce, cucumber, bell pepper, tomatoes, avocado, lime zest, lime juice, the 1 tablespoon of the olive oil, remaining ¼ teaspoon salt, and the black pepper in a large bowl and toss well.

Lightly oil the grill grates and place the steak on the grill. Cover and cook with the lid closed, turning once, for 8 to 10 minutes for medium-rare or until the desired doneness. Remove the steak from the grill and let stand for 5 minutes before slicing. Place the tortillas on the grill and cook, turning occasionally, until lightly browned and crisp, 2 to 3 minutes.

Place one tortilla on each of four plates. Top evenly with the romaine mixture and sliced steak.

Nutrient Content per Serving

Calories:	480	**Fat:**	19 grams	**Protein:**	41 grams
Fiber:	8 grams	**Saturated Fat:**	4.5 grams	**Carbs:**	36 grams
Sodium:	540 mg	**Sugars:**	5 grams		

Asian Confetti Quinoa Salad with Almonds

Quinoa is actually a seed, not a grain, and it's worth working into your diet as often as possible—it's high in protein, rich in fiber, and packed with minerals. This simple and versatile salad is a tasty way to help you do that. Look for tricolor quinoa in your market, and make sure to thoroughly rinse quinoa before cooking to avoid a bitter taste.

Makes 2 servings

½ cup red quinoa, rinsed
½ cup tricolor or other quinoa, rinsed
2 cups water
1 small red bell pepper, chopped
1 small green bell pepper, chopped
½ cup slow-roasted almonds (see page 97)
½ cup chopped green onions
1 tablespoon low-sodium wheat-free tamari or coconut aminos
1 tablespoon rice vinegar
2 tablespoons chopped fresh cilantro
1 teaspoon toasted sesame oil
¼ teaspoon sea salt

Combine the quinoas and the water in a small saucepan and cook according to the package directions. Transfer to a bowl and let cool for 5 minutes.

Fluff the quinoa with a fork and stir in the bell peppers, almonds, green onions, tamari, vinegar, cilantro, sesame oil, and salt.

Nutrient Content per Serving

Calories:	500	**Fat:**	19 grams	**Protein:**	19 grams
Fiber:	8 grams	**Saturated Fat:**	1 gram	**Carbs:**	69 grams
Sodium:	780 mg	**Sugars:**	6 grams		

Pan-Seared Seafood Salad with Tomatoes and Fennel

This salad is just screaming to be a part of a beach party. It can be made several hours ahead and tossed just before serving, to make sure it doesn't cut into your playtime near the surf. Serve over baby spinach or arugula, if desired.

Makes 4 servings

  2 teaspoons olive oil

  12 ounces sea scallops

  12 ounces large shrimp, peeled and deveined

  ¼ teaspoon freshly ground black pepper

  ½ medium fennel bulb, thinly sliced (about ¾ cup)

  2 celery stalks, thinly sliced

  1 cup grape tomatoes, halved

  1 carrot, thinly sliced

  ½ small red onion, thinly sliced (about ¼ cup)

  4 teaspoons lemon juice

  2 tablespoons extra-virgin olive oil

  3 tablespoons chopped fresh basil

  ⅛ teaspoon sea salt

Heat 1 teaspoon of the olive oil in a large nonstick skillet over medium-high heat. Keeping them separated, season the scallops and shrimp with ⅛ teaspoon of the pepper. Add the scallops to the skillet and cook until browned and cooked through, 3 to 4 minutes per side; transfer to a large bowl and set aside. In the same skillet, heat the remaining 1 teaspoon olive oil. Add the shrimp and cook until lightly browned and cooked through, 2 to 3 minutes per side; transfer to the bowl with the scallops.

Add the fennel, celery, tomatoes, carrot, onion, lemon juice, extra-virgin olive oil, basil, salt, and remaining ⅛ teaspoon pepper to the bowl and toss well.

Nutrient Content per Serving

Calories:	230	**Fat:**	10 grams	**Protein:**	23 grams
Fiber:	2 grams	**Saturated Fat:**	1.5 grams	**Carbs:**	10 grams
Sodium:	618 mg	**Sugars:**	2 grams		

Goat Cheese Burger Wrap

Okay, this is delicious genius, if I do say so myself. Goat cheese–filled burgers! You can already imagine that cheesy sensation when you sink your teeth into one, can't you?! Substitute nut cheese for the goat cheese if you're dairy sensitive. And for extra flavor, grill the tomato slices for 1 minute per side before adding them to your wrap.

Makes 4 servings

1½ pounds lean ground beef

1 teaspoon chopped fresh thyme

1 teaspoon garlic powder

1 tablespoon Dijon mustard

½ teaspoon sea salt

¼ teaspoon freshly ground black pepper

2 ounces goat cheese

4 coconut wraps (see box, page 79)

4 Boston lettuce leaves

4 slices tomato

4 tablespoons Sugar Impact Mayonnaise (page 197)

Combine the beef, thyme, garlic powder, mustard, salt, and pepper in a large bowl and gently mix. Using your hands, form the mixture into four equal balls, and with your index finger make an indentation into the center of each. Fill each with one-quarter of the goat cheese, then pinch the meat to seal. Form each ball into a ¾-inch-thick patty.

Heat a grill pan over medium-high heat and add the patties. Cook, turning once, 5 to 6 minutes total for medium-rare or longer for your desired doneness.

Place one wrap on each of four plates. Top each wrap with a lettuce leaf, a tomato slice, and a burger. Spread the top of each burger with 1 tablespoon of the mayonnaise. Fold the wrap up and over the burger and serve.

Nutrient Content per Serving

Calories:	440	**Fat:**	30 grams	**Protein:**	32 grams
Fiber:	3 grams	**Saturated Fat:**	13 grams	**Carbs:**	10 grams
Sodium:	640 mg	**Sugars:**	4 grams		

Lamb Souvlaki with Cultured Coconut Milk Tzatziki

I'm going to go out on a lamb (boo!) and say this popular Greek fast food is about to become a new family favorite. The seasoned lamb is perfectly complemented by the fresh and tangy homemade tzatziki (but hey, the Greeks knew that already!). If you're okay with dairy, you can sub in an equal amount of plain full-fat Greek-style yogurt for the cultured coconut milk. If you're using wooden skewers, soak them in warm water for 30 minutes to prevent burning.

Makes 4 servings

    1½ pounds lean leg of lamb, trimmed and cut into 32 even cubes

    4 teaspoons olive oil, plus more for the pan

    3 garlic cloves, minced

    2 tablespoons plus 1 teaspoon lemon juice

    1 teaspoon dried oregano

    ⅛ teaspoon freshly ground black pepper

    ½ cup unsweetened cultured coconut milk (such as So Delicious brand)

    ½ medium cucumber, peeled, seeded, grated, and excess liquid squeezed out

    ½ teaspoon grated lemon zest

    ½ teaspoon sea salt

    8 cups mixed baby greens

    3 tablespoons Dijon Vinaigrette (page 193)

Combine the lamb, 2 teaspoons of the oil, 2 garlic cloves, 2 tablespoons of the lemon juice, the oregano, and the pepper in a medium bowl; refrigerate for 30 minutes.

Meanwhile, make the tzatziki sauce by combining the remaining 2 teaspoons oil, remaining garlic clove, remaining 1 teaspoon lemon juice, the coconut milk, cucumber, lemon zest, and ⅛ teaspoon of the salt in a small bowl. Refrigerate until ready to serve.

Preheat the broiler. Lightly dampen a paper towel with olive oil and wipe a broiler pan with it.

Thread the lamb onto four 12-inch skewers. Sprinkle with the remaining ¼ teaspoon plus ⅛ teaspoon salt. Set the skewers on the broiler pan. Broil the lamb 5 inches from the heat, turning occasionally, until cooked through, 8 minutes.

Meanwhile, combine the baby greens and the vinaigrette in a large bowl. Divide the salad among four plates and top with the lamb. Spoon the tzatziki over the lamb and serve.

Nutrient Content per Serving

Calories:	520	**Fat:**	39 grams	**Protein:**	34 grams
Fiber:	3 grams	**Saturated Fat:**	13 grams	**Carbs:**	9 grams
Sodium:	570 mg	**Sugars:**	4 grams		

Mediterranean Salmon Wrap with Caper Dressing

This is just about as exotic as a wrap can get, so treat yourself to the richness of salmon and capers, and don't even think about the big nutritional boost you're getting in the bargain. As an alternative, stir 1 teaspoon drained capers, 1 teaspoon chopped shallots, and 1 teaspoon grated lemon zest into 2 tablespoons Sugar Impact Mayonnaise (page 197) for a quick tartar sauce.

Makes 2 servings

1 teaspoon olive oil

2 (6-ounce) skinless wild king or sockeye salmon fillets

¼ teaspoon sea salt

⅛ teaspoon freshly ground black pepper

2 tablespoons pitted Kalamata olives, chopped

½ small jarred roasted red pepper, rinsed, drained, and chopped

4 teaspoons Caper Vinaigrette (page 192)

1 teaspoon grated lemon zest

2 coconut wraps (see box, page 79)

12 fresh basil leaves

Heat a grill pan over medium-high heat. Rub the oil over the salmon fillets and season with the salt and pepper. Add the salmon to the pan and cook, turning once, until the fish flakes easily with a fork, 9 to 10 minutes. Transfer to a bowl and break the salmon into chunks with a fork. Fold in the olives, red pepper, dressing, and lemon zest.

Place one wrap on each of two plates. Top each with half the basil leaves, then spoon half the salmon mixture over the top. Fold the sides of the wrap up and over the salmon mixture and serve.

Nutrient Content per Serving

Calories:	400	**Fat:**	21 grams	**Protein:**	36 grams
Fiber:	2 grams	**Saturated Fat:**	7 grams	**Carbs:**	13 grams
Sodium:	920 mg	**Sugars:**	3 grams		

BLT Wedge Salad with Avocado and Dijon Vinaigrette

This salad version of the classic sandwich meets the criteria for nostalgic satisfaction but adds avocado for a contemporary (and nutritional) touch. Be sure to buy organic iceberg, and if you want a more nutrient dense take on this salad, sub in romaine or butter lettuce (also known as Boston lettuce).

Makes 4 servings

8 slices nitrate-free uncured bacon

1 medium head iceberg lettuce

2 plum tomatoes, seeded and chopped

4 tablespoons Dijon Vinaigrette (page 193)

½ medium avocado, cut into 12 slices

Heat a large skillet over medium heat. Cook the bacon until crisp, turning once, 6 to 7 minutes. Transfer to a plate lined with a paper towel to drain. When cool enough to handle, chop the bacon and set aside.

Cut the lettuce head into four wedges and place them in a large bowl. Add the tomatoes and 3 tablespoons of the vinaigrette and toss well.

Place a lettuce wedge and one-quarter of the tomatoes on each of four plates. Place 3 avocado slices on each plate, then sprinkle the lettuce with the chopped bacon. Drizzle the remaining 1 tablespoon vinaigrette over the avocado on each plate.

Nutrient Content per Serving

Calories:	220	**Fat:**	19 grams	**Protein:**	8 grams
Fiber:	2 grams	**Saturated Fat:**	3.5 grams	**Carbs:**	7 grams
Sodium:	410 mg	**Sugars:**	3 grams		

Ham, Cheddar, Onion, and Jalapeño Quesadillas (Cycles 1/3)

Ham and cheese have a long, happy history together in everything from sandwiches to omelets, but the jalapeños in these quesadillas really add a nice touch of heat to a familiar pairing. If you're not a fan of cheddar, substitute an equal amount of Jack, Swiss, or goat cheese.

Makes 2 servings

   2 teaspoons Malaysian red palm fruit oil
   1 medium red onion, thinly sliced
   3 garlic cloves, minced
   ½ jalapeño pepper, seeded and finely chopped
   2 brown rice tortillas
   2 ounces natural cheddar cheese, shredded
   4 ounces nitrate-free deli-sliced ham, cut into ¼-inch-wide strips
   12 fresh cilantro leaves

Heat the oil in a large nonstick skillet over medium-high heat. Add the onion, garlic, and jalapeño and cook, stirring occasionally, until slightly softened, 3 to 4 minutes. Transfer the mixture to a bowl.

Place the tortillas on a work surface. Sprinkle one-quarter of the cheese over the lower half of each tortilla. Top the cheese evenly with the onion mixture, ham, and 6 cilantro leaves each, then sprinkle each with half of the remaining cheese. Fold the empty half of each tortilla over the filling to form a half-moon.

Heat the same skillet in which you cooked the onion mixture over medium and add the quesadillas. Cook until the tortillas are lightly browned, the filling is hot, and the cheese has melted, 3 to 4 minutes per side. Transfer to a cutting board and let stand for 1 minute. Cut each quesadilla into three wedges and serve hot.

Nutrient Content per Serving

Calories:	400	**Fat:**	20 grams	**Protein:**	23 grams
Fiber:	3 grabs	**Saturated Fat:**	9 grams	**Carbs:**	32 grams
Sodium:	820 mg	**Sugars:**	3 grams		

Classic Greek Salad with Pan-Grilled Chicken and Feta Cheese

Feta cheese usually gets its tangy flavor from sheep's milk, but it's sometimes made with goat's milk, which tends to have a slightly creamier texture. If you're dairy intolerant, substitute your favorite nut cheese for the feta.

Makes 4 servings

1 tablespoon olive oil, plus more for the pan
4 (6-ounce) boneless skinless chicken breast halves, pounded to an even thickness
½ teaspoon sea salt
¼ teaspoon freshly ground black pepper
1 pint grape tomatoes, halved
1 seedless cucumber, peeled, halved lengthwise, and cut into ¾-inch pieces
1 green bell pepper, sliced
1 small red onion, thinly sliced
⅓ cup feta cheese, crumbled
¼ cup fresh parsley leaves
¼ cup pitted Kalamata olives, sliced
1 tablespoon red wine vinegar
¾ teaspoon dried oregano
1 tablespoon extra-virgin olive oil

Combine the 1 tablespoon of olive oil with the chicken in a large bowl. Season the chicken with ¼ teaspoon of the salt and ⅛ teaspoon of the black pepper. Lightly dampen a paper towel with a small amount of olive oil and wipe a grill pan with it; heat over medium-high heat. Add the chicken and cook until a thermometer inserted into the thickest part of the chicken registers 165°F, 5 to 6 minutes per side. Transfer to a cutting board and let rest for 5 minutes.

Meanwhile, combine the tomatoes, cucumber, bell pepper, onion, feta, parsley, and olives in a large bowl. Add the vinegar, oregano, extra-virgin olive oil, ¼ teaspoon salt, and ⅛ teaspoon black pepper and toss well. Cut the chicken into ¾-inch pieces and add to the bowl; toss well, then divide among four plates and serve.

Nutrient Content per Serving

Calories:	250	**Fat:**	16 grams	**Protein:**	17 grams
Fiber:	3 grams	**Saturated Fat:**	4 grams	**Carbs:**	12 grams
Sodium:	790 mg	**Sugars:**	5 grams		

6

___

SNACKS

If I had my way, there would be no such thing as snacking, but I'm realistic enough to know that healthy snacks can be a necessary crutch on the journey to extending time between meals and making the transition from sugar burner to fat burner.

So go ahead and snack (well, only if you're truly hungry!). Use the following recipes to graduate from the Sugar Impact Diet as a smart, low–SI snacker.

White and Red Bean Salsa with White Onion, Tomato, and Cilantro

Salsa is a hit no matter what the occasion. The beauty of this light, fresh sauce is that it can be made up to 4 hours ahead. Serve it with celery stalks, endive, Bibb lettuce cups, or purchased lentil chips (Cycles 1/3).

Makes 8 servings

1 (15-ounce) can organic no-salt-added cannellini beans, drained and rinsed

1 (15-ounce) can organic no-salt-added red kidney beans, drained and rinsed

2 plum tomatoes, seeded and chopped

½ medium avocado, cut into ¼-inch pieces

1 jalapeño pepper, seeded and finely chopped

⅓ cup finely chopped white onion

2 tablespoons chopped fresh cilantro

1 tablespoon lime juice

¾ teaspoon sea salt

Combine the cannellini beans, kidney beans, tomatoes, avocado, jalapeño, onion, cilantro, lime juice, and salt in a bowl. Gently mix and let stand for 15 minutes to allow the flavors to meld before serving.

Nutrient Content per Serving

Calories:	80	**Fat:**	2.5 grams	**Protein:**	4 grams
Fiber:	4 grams	**Saturated Fat:**	0 grams	**Carbs:**	12 grams
Sodium:	290 mg	**Sugars:**	2 grams		

Fresh-Baked Gluten-Free Sesame "Pretzels"

Craving a crunch? You can feel good about your family munching on these—they have none of the corn syrup, enriched flour, or inflammation-inducing oils you'll find in most packaged pretzels. For a more aromatic pretzel, add ½ teaspoon ground cinnamon to the almond meal.

Makes 8 servings (16 pretzels)

1¼ cups almond meal or almond flour

½ teaspoon sea salt

1 tablespoon coconut butter

2 large eggs

2 tablespoons plus 2 teaspoons coconut flour

1 large egg white, beaten with 1 teaspoon water

2 teaspoons sesame seeds

Preheat the oven to 350°F. Line a large baking sheet with parchment paper.

Combine the almond meal and salt in a medium bowl. Add the coconut butter and rub it into the mixture with your fingertips. Stir in the eggs and mix well. Add the coconut flour and knead the dough until well combined. Let rest for 10 minutes.

Divide the dough into 16 pieces. Working with one piece at a time, roll the dough out into a 7- to 8-inch-long rope. Twist the dough rope into your desired pretzel shape and place on the prepared baking sheet. Repeat with the remaining dough.

Brush the pretzels with the egg white mixture and sprinkle evenly with sesame seeds. Bake until the pretzels are lightly browned, 23 to 25 minutes. Let cool before serving.

Nutrient Content per Serving

Calories:	150	**Fat:**	12 grams	**Protein:**	6 grams
Fiber:	3 grams	**Saturated Fat:**	2.5 grams	**Carbs:**	6 grams
Sodium:	180 mg	**Sugars:**	1 gram		

Lemon-Chili Roasted Almonds

You don't just want to eat more almonds because they're high in healthy fats and a good source of fiber. You want them to taste amazing, too! So sass them up now and then to keep them interesting. This take on roasted almonds adds just the right combination of zest and spice to do the trick. Make a double or triple batch and keep them in an airtight container in the refrigerator to maintain freshness. They can keep in the fridge for up to 2 months and in the freezer for up to 6 months.

Makes 12 servings (about 3 tablespoons per serving)

1 egg white
1 tablespoon lemon juice
2 cups raw almonds
1 teaspoon chili powder
½ teaspoon ground coriander
¾ teaspoon sea salt
⅛ teaspoon cayenne pepper
1 tablespoon grated lemon zest

Preheat the oven to 225°F.

Whisk the egg white with the lemon juice in a medium bowl until frothy. Add the almonds and toss to coat. Transfer the almonds to a colander and let drain for 5 minutes.

Meanwhile, combine the chili powder, coriander, salt, and cayenne pepper in a separate medium bowl. Add the nuts to the bowl and toss well. Transfer to a large rimmed baking sheet.

Bake the almonds, stirring after 15 minutes, until lightly roasted, 45 to 50 minutes. Remove from the oven, transfer to a bowl, and toss with the lemon zest. Let cool completely before serving.

Nutrient Content per Serving

Calories:	120	**Fat:**	10 grams	**Protein:**	5 grams
Fiber:	3 grams	**Saturated Fat:**	0.5 grams	**Carbs:**	5 grams
Sodium:	150 mg	**Sugars:**	1 gram		

Lime and Jalapeño Hummus

Hummus is hard to beat when you're in the mood to dip, but you have to be wary of what you'll find in expensive packaged brands. Take control and make this spiced-up version instead! It's fast, easy, fresh—and oh, so much tastier.

Makes 8 servings (3 tablespoons per serving)

1 (15-ounce) can organic no-salt-added chickpeas, drained
1 jalapeño pepper, seeded
1 small garlic clove
3 tablespoons chopped fresh cilantro
4 teaspoons tahini paste
2 teaspoons raw almond butter
Grated zest of 1 lime
2 tablespoons lime juice
2 tablespoons water, plus more as needed
2 tablespoons olive oil
¼ teaspoon sea salt

Combine the chickpeas, jalapeño, garlic, cilantro, tahini, almond butter, zest, lime juice, and water in the bowl of a food processor and process to a puree. Transfer to a medium bowl and stir in the oil and salt. For a slightly thinner consistency, stir in an additional 1 to 2 tablespoons water. Store in an airtight container in the refrigerator for up to 4 days.

Nutrient Content per Serving

Calories:	90	**Fat:**	6 grams	**Protein:**	3 grams
Fiber:	2 grams	**Saturated Fat:**	0.5 grams	**Carbs:**	7 grams
Sodium:	80 mg	**Sugars:**	0 grams		

Smoky Baba Ghanoush

Baba ghanoush is a Middle Eastern favorite that always delivers on the promise of its flavorful ingredients. It also has the added benefit of being rich in protein, vitamins, and minerals. Select eggplants that are firm and heavy for their size. Serve with celery and carrot sticks for a little crunch!

Makes 8 servings (about ¼ cup per serving)

2 (1-pound) eggplants, pricked all over with the tip of a sharp knife
2 tablespoons tahini paste
2 tablespoons extra-virgin olive oil
1 tablespoon lemon juice
2 teaspoons smoked paprika
1 garlic clove
½ teaspoon sea salt
¼ teaspoon freshly ground black pepper

Preheat the oven to 375°F.

Place the eggplants on a large baking sheet. Roast until the eggplant is very soft, 45 to 50 minutes. Turn on the broiler, place the eggplant 4 to 5 inches from the heat source, and cook, turning occasionally, until the skin is slightly charred, 7 to 8 minutes. Remove from the oven and let cool for 30 minutes, or until cool enough to handle. Cut the eggplants in half and scoop out the flesh with a spoon discarding the skins. Place the eggplant in a mesh sieve or colander and let any excess liquid drain for 20 minutes.

Transfer the eggplant to a food processor and add the tahini, oil, lemon juice, paprika, garlic, salt, and pepper. Process until the mixture is well combined but not a completely smooth paste. Transfer to a serving bowl. Store in a covered container in the refrigerator for up to 1 week.

Note: If the whole eggplant won't fit under your broiler, then increase the oven temperature to 450°F and bake for an additional 12 to 15 minutes to brown the skin to give it a slightly smoky flavor.

Nutrient Content per Serving

Calories:	90	**Fat:**	6 grams	**Protein:**	2 grams
Fiber:	4 grams	**Saturated Fat:**	1 gram	**Carbs:**	9 grams
Sodium:	150 mg	**Sugars:**	2 grams		

Slow-Roasted Nuts

Slow roasting is sort of like the culinary equivalent of "handled with care"; it lowers anti-nutrients, improves digestibility, and makes the nuts tastier all at the same time. Nuts are the perfect nutrient-dense, fat-burning fuel, so carry a handful with you to beat back cravings and get an on-the-go energy boost. Make sure your oven can be set at 140°F; otherwise, use a dehydrator.

Makes 8 servings (about 3 tablespoons per serving)

1½ cups raw nuts (cashews, walnuts, almonds, pecans, macadamias)
½ teaspoon sea salt

Place the nuts in a large bowl and add enough water to cover by 3 inches, then stir in the salt. Let the nuts soak overnight at room temperature.

Preheat the oven to 140°F.

Drain the nuts and spread them on a rimmed baking sheet or dehydrator trays. Bake the nuts for 8 hours or dehydrate for 8 hours. Remove from the oven or dehydrator and let cool completely (the nuts will crisp up as they cool). Store in a resealable plastic bag in the refrigerator for up to 3 months.

(Almonds)
Nutrient Content per Serving

Calories:	210	**Fat:**	19 grams	**Protein:**	8 grams
Fiber:	4 grams	**Saturated Fat:**	1.5 grams	**Carbs:**	7 grams
Sodium:	200 mg	**Sugars:**	2 grams		

(Cashews)

Calories:	160	**Fat:**	12 grams	**Protein:**	5 grams
Fiber:	1 gram	**Saturated Fat:**	2 grams	**Carbs:**	8 grams
Sodium:	200 mg	**Sugars:**	2 grams		

(Pecans)

Calories:	190	**Fat:**	20 grams	**Protein:**	2 grams
Fiber:	3 grams	**Saturated Fat:**	1.5 grams	**Carbs:**	4 grams
Sodium:	190 mg	**Sugars:**	1 gram		

Roasted Spiced Chickpeas

Chickpeas have been a dietary staple for thousands of years, and for good reason. These buttery, protein-rich legumes offer digestive support and blood sugar control and are so satisfying they're eaten daily in some parts of the world. To help the spices stick, make sure you toss them with the chickpeas as soon as they come out of the oven. After they have cooled completely, store them in an airtight container for days of enjoyment.

Makes 4 servings (about ¼ cup per serving)

> 1 (15-ounce) can organic no-salt-added chickpeas, drained and rinsed
> 1 tablespoon Malaysian red palm fruit oil
> ½ teaspoon ground cumin
> ¼ teaspoon garlic powder
> ⅛ teaspoon ground cinnamon
> ¼ teaspoon sea salt
> ⅛ teaspoon cayenne pepper

Preheat the oven to 400°F.

Line a rimmed baking sheet with paper towels and spread the chickpeas over the top. Place more paper towels over the chickpeas and gently rub the chickpeas to thoroughly dry them. Discard any loose skins and transfer the chickpeas to a bowl and toss with the palm fruit oil.

Discard the paper towels and line the baking sheet with aluminum foil. Pour the chickpeas onto the baking sheet and roast, shaking the pan every 10 minutes, until the chickpeas are browned and crunchy, 33 to 35 minutes. Transfer to a bowl and gently stir in the cumin, garlic powder, cinnamon, salt, and cayenne pepper. Let cool completely before serving.

Nutrient Content per Serving

Calories:	100	**Fat:**	4 grams	**Protein:**	4 grams
Fiber:	3 grams	**Saturated Fat:**	2 grams	**Carbs:**	12 grams
Sodium:	160 mg	**Sugars:**	1 gram		

Grilled Nectarine Salsa (Cycles 1/3)

Refreshingly juicy nectarines make this sweet and tangy salsa a wonderful alternative to its run-of-the-mill cousin. Enjoy it as a snack or as the perfect complement to pork chops, tuna, salmon, or chicken. Save time and make it ahead—you can refrigerate it for up to a day.

Makes 8 servings (about 2 cups)

> 1 tablespoon olive oil, plus more for the pan
> 3 large ripe but firm nectarines, pitted and quartered
> ½ medium red onion, halved lengthwise through the root end
> ½ red bell pepper, finely chopped
> 1 teaspoon grated lemon zest
> 1 tablespoon lemon juice
> 1 small serrano pepper, finely chopped
> 2 tablespoons chopped fresh mint
> ½ teaspoon sea salt
> 3 ounces bean chips

Lightly dampen a paper towel with a small amount of olive oil and wipe a grill pan with it; heat over medium-high heat.

Gently toss the nectarines and onion with the tablespoon of oil, then place on the grill pan. Grill the nectarines and onion until well marked and beginning to soften, 4 minutes per side. Transfer to a cutting board and let cool for 5 minutes.

Coarsely chop the nectarines and onion and transfer to a medium bowl. Stir in the bell pepper, lemon zest, lemon juice, serrano pepper, mint, and salt. Let stand for at least 15 minutes before serving with the bean chips.

Nutrient Content per Serving

Calories:	100	**Fat:**	4.5 grams	**Protein:**	2 grams
Fiber:	3 grams	**Saturated Fat:**	0 grams	**Carbs:**	14 grams
Sodium:	180 mg	**Sugars:**	5 grams		

Garlic Hummus with Lentil Chips (Cycles 1/3)

I believe garlic makes everything better, so you can do the math on my feelings about garlic + hummus! As ubiquitous as hummus is, it can be easy to dismiss until you make your own. That's when you discover the deep, rich, authentic experience hummus is meant to deliver. For a little more zest, increase the Tabasco sauce to 1½ teaspoons.

Makes 8 servings (3 tablespoons per serving)

   3 tablespoons extra-virgin olive oil
   4 garlic cloves, thinly sliced
   1 (15-ounce) can organic no-salt-added chickpeas, drained
   4 teaspoons tahini paste
   Grated zest of 1 lemon
   2 tablespoons lemon juice
   ½ teaspoon Tabasco sauce
   2 tablespoons water, plus more as needed
   ¼ teaspoon sea salt
   4 ounces lentil chips

Heat the oil in a small skillet over medium heat. Add the garlic and cook, stirring, until lightly browned, 1½ to 2 minutes. Transfer the garlic and any oil in the pan to a bowl and let cool for 2 minutes.

Combine the chickpeas, tahini, lemon zest, lemon juice, Tabasco sauce, water, and the garlic and oil in a food processor and process to a puree. Transfer to a bowl and stir in the salt. For a slightly thinner consistency, stir in an additional 1 to 2 tablespoons water. Serve with the lentil chips.

Nutrient Content per Serving

Calories:	160	**Fat:**	8 grams	**Protein:**	4 grams
Fiber:	2 grams	**Saturated Fat:**	1 gram	**Carbs:**	17 grams
Sodium:	190 mg	**Sugars:**	1 gram		

Cucumber Chips with Guacamole

Holy guacamole! I don't know if I can offer enough reverence for the avocado, but the transformation this low–Sugar Impact, nutrient-packed fruit makes when it becomes guacamole is just magical. When selecting your avocados, gently press the bottom with your thumb, and if it yields to light pressure, it's ready for your fiesta.

Makes 8 servings

⅓ cup finely chopped white onion
½ jalapeño pepper, finely chopped
3 tablespoons chopped fresh cilantro
½ teaspoon sea salt
2 medium avocados, pitted and peeled
½ plum tomato, seeded and chopped
1 tablespoon lime juice
2 medium cucumbers, peeled and cut into 24 slices total (about ½ inch thick)

Combine 2 tablespoons of the onion, 1 teaspoon of the jalapeño, 1 tablespoon of the cilantro, and ¼ teaspoon of the salt in a medium bowl. With a wooden spoon, mash the ingredients six times to help release their flavors. Add the avocado and coarsely mash with a fork. Stir in the remaining onion, jalapeño, cilantro, salt, tomato, and lime juice. Place the cucumber slices on a large plate or serving platter and top each slice with about 1 tablespoon of the guacamole.

Nutrient Content per Serving

Calories:	70	**Fat:**	6 grams	**Protein:**	2 grams
Fiber:	2 grams	**Saturated Fat:**	0.5 grams	**Carbs:**	6 grams
Sodium:	150 mg	**Sugars:**	1 gram		

Spicy Black Bean Dip with Celery

Packed with protein and fiber, black beans are low Sugar Impact and can easily stand on their own as a meal. But that's not always the most flavorful way to enjoy them. This dip will instantly get the undivided attention of your taste buds. If you'd prefer a milder flavor, substitute ½ teaspoon smoked paprika for the chipotle.

Makes 4 servings (about 5 tablespoons per serving)

   1 (15-ounce) can organic no-salt-added black beans, drained
   2 tablespoons lime juice
   2 tablespoons olive oil
   ½ teaspoon ground coriander
   ½ teaspoon ground cumin
   ¼ teaspoon ground chipotle pepper
   2 tablespoons water
   3 tablespoons chopped fresh cilantro
   ½ teaspoon sea salt
   20 celery sticks

Combine the beans, lime juice, oil, coriander, cumin, chipotle pepper, and water in a food processor and process to a puree. Transfer to a bowl and stir in the cilantro and salt. Serve with the celery sticks. Store in an airtight container in the refrigerator for up to 5 days.

Nutrient Content per Serving

Calories:	130	**Fat:**	7 grams	**Protein:**	5 grams
Fiber:	6 grams	**Saturated Fat:**	1 gram	**Carbs:**	16 grams
Sodium:	430 mg	**Sugars:**	1 gram		

Chipotle Deviled Eggs

The devil of these eggs is in the details—the spices have been chosen with care to make sure they work together to deliver a heavenly experience. Eggs have been called nature's perfect food because they provide an unbeatable source of protein and essential vitamins. For spicier palates, increase the chipotle to ¼ teaspoon. For bigger crowds, this recipe can be easily doubled or tripled.

Makes 4 servings

   5 large eggs
   3 tablespoons Sugar Impact Mayonnaise (page 197)
   ¾ teaspoon Dijon mustard
   ½ teaspoon grated lime zest
   ⅛ teaspoon ground chipotle pepper
   ⅛ teaspoon paprika
   ⅛ teaspoon sea salt
   2 teaspoons chopped fresh cilantro

Place the eggs in a medium saucepan and add enough cold water to cover them by 2 inches. Bring the water to a boil over high heat; cover the pan, remove from the heat, and let stand for 12 minutes. Meanwhile, fill a bowl with ice and water. Transfer the eggs to the bowl of ice water and let cool for 15 minutes.

Peel the cooled eggs and halve each lengthwise. Place the yolks in a bowl with one whole egg white; set the remaining whites aside. Mash together the yolks and white with a fork until fairly smooth. Stir in the mayonnaise, mustard, lime zest, chipotle pepper, paprika, and salt; mix well. Set the reserved egg whites on a plate, cut-side up, and spoon the filling into each half. Cover with plastic wrap and chill for at least 1 hour before serving. Sprinkle evenly with the cilantro before serving.

Nutrient Content per Serving

Calories:	160	**Fat:**	13 grams	**Protein:**	8 grams
Fiber:	0 grams	**Saturated Fat:**	3 grams	**Carbs:**	3 grams
Sodium:	250 mg	**Sugars:**	0 grams		

Chipotle Kale Chips

Warning! You won't be able to stop at just one. But you'll make more! (Remember that I warned you.) Even the most finicky snacker will ditch the potato chip like, well, a hot potato, once they savor this nutrition-packed, low-calorie treat. For a milder flavor, substitute smoked paprika for the ground chipotle.

Makes 4 servings

   1 bunch kale (about 1 pound), washed and thoroughly dried
   1 tablespoon olive oil
   ¼ teaspoon ground coriander
   ¼ teaspoon ground cumin
   ¼ teaspoon ground chipotle pepper
   ¼ teaspoon sea salt

Preheat the oven to 325°F.

Remove and discard the tough kale stems; tear the leaves into 1½-inch pieces. Toss the kale in a large bowl with the oil, gently rubbing the leaves with your fingers to help spread the oil evenly. Add the coriander, cumin, chipotle pepper, and salt and toss well.

Arrange the kale in a single layer on two large baking sheets. Bake one batch at a time, until crisp, turning the leaves once, 16 to 18 minutes. Repeat with the second batch. Let cool on the pan. Serve immediately or store in a covered container at room temperature for up to 2 days.

Nutrient Content per Serving

Calories:	60	**Fat:**	4 grams	**Protein:**	3 grams
Fiber:	2 grams	**Saturated Fat:**	0.5 grams	**Carbs:**	6 grams
Sodium:	170 mg	**Sugars:**	0 grams		

Cinnamon Almond Butter

I've got mad love for almond butter, and the intense aromatics of cinnamon make this version irresistible. Don't worry if you're right there with me—this butter offers some pretty sweet benefits, from healthy fats to blood sugar control. For a little variety, swap cashews or pecans for the almonds.

Makes 12 servings

1 cup slow-roasted almonds (see page 97)
4 teaspoons coconut butter
1½ teaspoons monk fruit extract
¼ teaspoon ground cinnamon
⅛ teaspoon almond extract (optional)

Combine the almonds, coconut butter, monk fruit extract, cinnamon, and almond extract (if using) in a food processor. Process until a smooth paste forms. Transfer to a covered container and store in the refrigerator for up to 3 months. Let stand at room temperature to soften slightly before serving.

Nutrient Content per Serving

Calories:	70	**Fat:**	6 grams	**Protein:**	2 grams
Fiber:	1 gram	**Saturated Fat:**	1.5 grams	**Carbs:**	2 grams
Sodium:	50 mg	**Sugars:**	1 gram		

7

MAINS

The mains are the celebrity of the dish. They're the centerpiece of your meals, a front row reminder of the low-SI, fast fat-loss road you're on. Let them fuel you and keep you full and happy and coming back for more. You have to eat to lose weight, and these spectacular choices will make sure you do.

BEEF, PORK, AND LAMB

Clean, lean protein is a warrior in the battle of the bulge. It's essential for managing hunger and keeping blood sugar levels stable. Beef, pork, and lamb are protein titans that do that. They also contain other significant nutrients, including iron, zinc, and the B vitamins.

But the source of your meat matters! Factory-farmed animals can be high in saturated fat and pumped full of antibiotics and hormones. Support your own health—and humane, sustainable farming—by voting with your dollars for grass-fed, clean, lean cuts.

Slow-Cooker Tomato-Braised Lamb Shanks (Cycles 1/3)

Patience pays dividends, especially when it comes to cooking. Drench these lamb shanks in the tomato-based sauce and let the slow cooker work its magic. If you have an intolerance to dairy, just leave out the grated cheese. This dish is also great for leftovers—so don't be afraid to freeze any extra for up to 6 months.

Makes 4 servings

> 1 tablespoon olive oil, plus more for the slow cooker
> 4 (12-ounce) lamb shanks, trimmed
> ½ teaspoon sea salt
> ¼ teaspoon freshly ground black pepper
> 4 garlic cloves, minced
> ½ cup chopped shallots
> 1 teaspoon dried basil
> ½ cup dry red wine
> 1 (14.5-ounce) can diced tomatoes
> 3 tablespoons organic tomato paste
> 2 tablespoons grated Parmesan cheese

Lightly dampen a paper towel with a small amount of olive oil and wipe a 5- to 6-quart slow cooker with it. Heat the 1 tablespoon of oil in a large nonstick skillet over medium-high heat. Season the lamb shanks with ¼ teaspoon of the salt and ⅛ teaspoon of the pepper. Add the lamb to the skillet and cook, turning occasionally, until browned, 6 to 8 minutes. Transfer the lamb to the prepared slow cooker.

Return the skillet to the heat and add the garlic, shallots, and basil; cook, stirring occasionally, until the garlic and shallots are beginning to soften, 1 to 2 minutes. Pour in the wine, bring the mixture to a boil, and cook until the wine has almost evaporated, 2 to 3 minutes. Stir in the tomatoes, tomato paste, remaining ¼ teaspoon salt, and remaining ⅛ teaspoon pepper. Cook for 3 minutes; stir in the cheese, then pour the mixture over the lamb shanks.

Cover the slow cooker and cook on low until the lamb is very tender, 7 to 8 hours.

Nutrient Content per Serving

Calories:	360	**Fat:**	18 grams	**Protein:**	32 grams
Fiber:	3 grams	**Saturated Fat:**	7 grams	**Carbs:**	12 grams
Sodium:	650 mg	**Sugars:**	5 grams		

Roasted Pork Tenderloin with Basil Vinaigrette

Clean and lean is the goal, for you and your meat. Pork tenderloin is the very essence of clean, lean protein, but that "lean" also means you have to be careful not to overcook it, as it will dry out very easily.

Makes 4 servings

1 teaspoon ground coriander

½ teaspoon paprika

½ teaspoon sea salt

¼ teaspoon freshly ground black pepper

1 tablespoon olive oil

1½ pounds pork tenderloin, trimmed

8 cups mixed baby greens, baby arugula, baby spinach

5 tablespoons Basil Vinaigrette (page 197)

Preheat the oven to 500°F.

Combine the coriander, paprika, salt, and pepper in a small bowl.

Heat the oil in a large ovenproof skillet over medium-high heat. Rub the pork with the coriander mixture to coat. Add the pork to the skillet and cook until browned, about 4 minutes. Transfer the skillet to the oven and cook for 20 to 22 minutes, until a thermometer inserted into the thickest part of the pork registers 145°F. Remove the pork from the pan and let stand for 5 minutes, then cut crosswise into 12 slices.

While the pork rests, toss the baby greens with 3 tablespoons of the dressing in a large bowl. Divide the greens among four plates and top each with three slices of the pork. Drizzle ½ tablespoon of the dressing over each serving of the pork.

Nutrient Content per Serving

Calories:	290	**Fat:**	19 grams	**Protein:**	25 grams
Fiber:	3 grams	**Saturated Fat:**	3.5 grams	**Carbs:**	6 grams
Sodium:	720 mg	**Sugars:**	3 grams		

Mustard and Garlic–Marinated Pork Chops

The combination of flavors in this infusion packs a punch—let your chops soak up the marinade for up to 4 hours, if you'd like. They may also be cooked on an outdoor grill or broiled.

Makes 4 servings

  4 (8-ounce) bone-in pork chops, about ¾ inch thick

  2 tablespoons olive oil, plus more for the pan

  1 tablespoon Dijon mustard

  2 teaspoons chopped fresh thyme

  3 garlic cloves, minced

  1 tablespoon red wine vinegar

  ½ teaspoon freshly ground black pepper

  ½ teaspoon sea salt

Combine the pork chops, the 2 tablespoons of oil, mustard, thyme, garlic, vinegar, and pepper in a medium bowl; mix well to coat. Cover and refrigerate the pork chops for 1 hour.

Remove the bowl from the refrigerator and allow the pork chops to stand at room temperature for 15 to 20 minutes.

Lightly dampen a paper towel with a small amount of olive oil and wipe a grill pan with it; heat over medium-high heat.

Remove the pork chops from the bowl and wipe off any excess marinade with paper towels. Season the pork with the salt. Place the chops on the grill pan and cook until well marked and cooked through, 6 to 8 minutes per side.

Nutrient Content per Serving

Calories:	250	**Fat:**	14 grams	**Protein:**	29 grams
Fiber:	0 grams	**Saturated Fat:**	3 grams	**Carbs:**	1 gram
Sodium:	280 mg	**Sugars:**	0 grams		

Marinated Pork Skewers with Lemon Vinaigrette

Finding easy ways to get more pork in rotation is a must. Lean cuts of pork are high in protein, low in fat, and loaded with B vitamins, which you need to keep your low-SI metabolism revved. Marinate these in the morning to make dinner a breeze. If you're using wooden skewers, be sure to soak them in warm water for 30 minutes first to prevent burning.

Makes 4 servings

1 tablespoon olive oil, plus more for the pan

1½ pounds lean pork tenderloin, trimmed and cut into 32 cubes

1 small yellow or orange bell pepper, cut into 16 pieces

16 cherry tomatoes

1 tablespoon chopped shallots

1 tablespoon lemon juice

3 tablespoons Cilantro Pesto (page 196)

½ teaspoon sea salt

¼ teaspoon freshly ground black pepper

4 tablespoons Easy Lemon Vinaigrette (page 193)

Preheat the broiler. Lightly dampen a paper towel with olive oil and wipe a broiler pan with it.

Combine the pork, bell pepper, cherry tomatoes, the 1 tablespoon of oil, shallots, lemon juice, and pesto in a bowl; mix to coat well. Let stand at room temperature for 30 minutes. Thread the pork, bell peppers, and cherry tomatoes onto eight skewers, dividing each ingredient evenly among the skewers.

Place the skewers on the prepared pan and season with the salt and pepper. Broil the pork and vegetables 4 inches from the heat, until cooked through, about 8 minutes, turning every 2 minutes. Spoon the vinaigrette over the skewers to serve.

Nutrient Content per Serving

Calories:	430	**Fat:**	28 grams	**Protein:**	38 grams
Fiber:	2 grams	**Saturated Fat:**	6 grams	**Carbs:**	6 grams
Sodium:	550 mg	**Sugars:**	3 grams		

Strip Steaks with Tomatoes, Olives, and Parsley

You'll get credit for working a lot harder than you did on this dinner—I call that a win-win! It's a well-dressed spread that can be ready in less than 30 minutes.

Makes 4 servings

4 (6-ounce) boneless strip steaks, preferably grass fed, trimmed

1 teaspoon dried basil

½ teaspoon dried oregano

¾ teaspoon sea salt

¼ teaspoon freshly ground black pepper

4 medium plum tomatoes (about 1 pound), seeded and chopped

⅓ cup pitted Kalamata olives, halved

3 tablespoons finely chopped shallots

3 tablespoons chopped fresh parsley

1 tablespoon red wine vinegar

1 tablespoon extra-virgin olive oil, plus more for the pan

Season the steak with the basil, oregano, ½ teaspoon of the salt, and the pepper. Combine the tomatoes, olives, shallots, parsley, vinegar, extra-virgin olive oil, and remaining ¼ teaspoon salt in a medium bowl.

Lightly dampen a paper towel with a small amount of olive oil and wipe a grill pan with it; heat over medium-high heat. Add the steaks and cook until the beef is cooked to medium-rare, 5 to 6 minutes per side, or longer for your desired doneness. Serve topped with the tomato mixture.

Nutrient Content per Serving

Calories:	320	**Fat:**	17 grams	**Protein:**	36 grams
Fiber:	1 gram	**Saturated Fat:**	4.5 grams	**Carbs:**	5 grams
Sodium:	740 mg	**Sugars:**	2 grams		

Ginger Beef Tenderloin Kebabs over Cucumber Salad

The flavorful marinade makes this elegant salad sing—and yes, you'll impress your guests. If you're using wooden skewers, be sure to soak them in warm water for at least 30 minutes first to prevent burning.

Makes 4 servings

Olive oil for the pan

SALAD

1 medium cucumber, peeled, halved lengthwise, and sliced

1 medium red bell pepper, cut into thin strips

1 carrot, thinly sliced

1 small red onion, thinly sliced

2 tablespoons unseasoned rice vinegar

½ teaspoon monk fruit extract

¼ teaspoon sea salt

1 tablespoon Malaysian red palm fruit oil

KEBABS

1½ pounds beef tenderloin, preferably grass fed, trimmed and cut into 24 cubes

1 tablespoon Malaysian red palm fruit oil

1½ tablespoons minced fresh ginger

1 tablespoon lemon juice

2 garlic cloves, minced

1 tablespoon low-sodium wheat-free tamari

3 green onions, cut into 24 pieces (total)

½ teaspoon sea salt

¼ teaspoon freshly ground black pepper

Preheat the broiler. Lightly dampen a paper towel with olive oil and wipe a broiler pan with it.

For the salad, combine the cucumber, bell pepper, carrot, red onion, vinegar, monk fruit extract, salt, and oil in a large bowl; refrigerate until ready to serve.

For the kebabs, combine the beef, oil, ginger, lemon juice, garlic, and tamari in a large bowl. Let stand at room temperature for 30 minutes.

Alternately thread the beef and green onions onto four skewers, threading the green onions horizontally. Season with the salt and pepper. Place the kebabs on the prepared pan. Broil the kebabs 5 inches from the heat source until the beef is cooked to medium-rare, 8 to 10 minutes, or longer for your desired doneness, turning every 2 minutes. Divide the cucumber salad among four plates and top each with a kebab.

Nutrient Content per Serving

Calories:	520	**Fat:**	40 grams	**Protein:**	32 grams
Fiber:	3 grams	**Saturated Fat:**	17 grams	**Carbs:**	9 grams
Sodium:	700 mg	**Sugars:**	4 grams		

Easy Mozzarella Burgers on Lettuce with Tomato Sauce (Cycles 1/3)

Capers add a touch of sophistication, and tomato sauce subs for ketchup in this grilled classic. Be sure to purchase a tomato sauce made without sugar to keep your burgers lower SI. Swap nut cheese for mozzarella if you're dairy sensitive.

Makes 4 servings

1½ pounds lean ground beef
2 teaspoons drained capers
1 teaspoon garlic powder
1 teaspoon dried basil
½ teaspoon sea salt
¼ teaspoon freshly ground black pepper
4 slices fresh mozzarella (2 ounces)
4 Boston lettuce leaves
½ cup prepared no-sugar-added tomato-basil sauce

Combine the beef, capers, garlic powder, basil, salt, and pepper in a large bowl and gently mix with your hands. Form the mixture into four ¾-inch-thick patties. Heat a grill pan over medium-high heat and add the patties. Cook, turning once, 4 to 5 minutes for medium-rare or longer for your desired doneness. During the last minute of cooking, top each burger with one slice of the cheese and cover loosely with aluminum foil to melt the mozzarella.

Place one lettuce leaf on each of four plates. Heat the tomato sauce in a small saucepan over medium heat for 1 minute until warm. Place a burger on each lettuce leaf and spoon 2 tablespoons of the tomato sauce over the top.

Nutrient Content per Serving

Calories:	320	**Fat:**	18 grams	**Protein:**	36 grams
Fiber:	1 gram	**Saturated Fat:**	8 grams	**Carbs:**	3 grams
Sodium:	510 mg	**Sugars:**	1 gram		

Coffee-Rubbed Flank Steak

This rub will bring your steak to life just the way your morning cup perks you up. You'll enjoy the earthy taste of this rub so much that you'll want to make a double batch to keep on hand.

Makes 4 servings

1 tablespoon finely ground coffee

2 teaspoons paprika

2 teaspoons ground cumin

½ teaspoon monk fruit extract

¼ teaspoon dried thyme

¾ teaspoon sea salt

¼ teaspoon freshly ground black pepper

1½ pounds flank steak, preferably grass fed, trimmed of visible fat

2 teaspoons olive oil, plus more for the pan

Combine the coffee, paprika, cumin, monk fruit extract, thyme, salt, and pepper in a small bowl. Brush the steak all over with the 2 teaspoons of oil, then rub the coffee mixture over both sides to coat.

Lightly dampen a paper towel with a small amount of olive oil and wipe a grill pan with it; heat over medium-high heat. Place the steak in the pan and cook, 5 to 6 minutes per side for medium-rare or longer for your desired doneness. Transfer the steak to a cutting board and let stand for 5 minutes before cutting across the grain on an angle into thin slices.

Nutrient Content per Serving

Calories:	290	**Fat:**	14 grams	**Protein:**	35 grams
Fiber:	1 gram	**Saturated Fat:**	5 grams	**Carbs:**	2 grams
Sodium:	510 mg	**Sugars:**	0 grams		

Broiled Herb and Pepper–Crusted Lamb Chops

You may not think of lamb chops often, but I hope this recipe will change that. Lamb is a staple in Mediterranean diets, which is often linked to lower risk of cardiovascular disease. As with red meat, protein in lamb is considered nutritionally complete—it has all 8 essential amino acids, and it's also high in vitamins and minerals. For an added flavor boost, add 1 tablespoon grated orange zest (still makes it Cycle 1 approved!) to the parsley mixture.

Makes 4 servings

   1 tablespoon olive oil, plus more for the pan
   1 tablespoon chopped fresh parsley
   2 teaspoons chopped fresh oregano
   1 teaspoon Dijon mustard
   1 teaspoon coarsely ground black pepper
   ½ teaspoon garlic powder
   8 (¾-inch-thick) lean bone-in loin lamb chops (about 1½ pounds)
   ½ teaspoon sea salt

Combine the 1 tablespoon of oil, parsley, oregano, mustard, pepper, and garlic powder in a medium bowl. Add the lamb chops and toss well to coat; let stand at room temperature for 20 minutes.

   Meanwhile, preheat the broiler. Lightly dampen a paper towel with olive oil and wipe a broiler pan with it.

   Season the lamb with the salt and place it on the prepared broiler pan. Broil the lamb 4 inches from the heat, turning once, 5 to 6 minutes for medium-rare or longer for your desired doneness.

Nutrient Content per Serving

Calories:	310	**Fat:**	24 grams	**Protein:**	20 grams
Fiber:	0 grams	**Saturated Fat:**	11 grams	**Carbs:**	1 gram
Sodium:	360 mg	**Sugars:**	0 grams		

Beef and Pork Meat Loaf

The very thought of meat loaf probably transports you back to some comforting childhood scene (unless you think of the singer, which is something else entirely). You may not have known what a delicate hand this protein-rich dish requires—when you combine the ingredients be careful not to overwork the mixture or the meat loaf could become tough.

Makes 6 servings

1 tablespoon olive oil, plus more for the pan

1 medium onion, finely chopped

2 tablespoons chopped fresh oregano

1¾ pounds lean ground beef

½ pound lean ground pork

½ cup gluten-free old-fashioned rolled oats, soaked in water for 10 minutes and drained

1 large egg

2 tablespoons Dijon mustard

⅓ cup chopped fresh parsley

1 tablespoon garlic powder

2 teaspoons ground coriander

1¼ teaspoons sea salt

½ teaspoon freshly ground black pepper

Preheat the oven to 350°F. Lightly dampen a paper towel with olive oil and wipe a large rimmed baking sheet with it.

Heat the 1 tablespoon of oil in a medium nonstick skillet over medium-high heat. Add the onion and oregano and cook, stirring occasionally, until the onion is slightly softened, 4 to 5 minutes. Transfer to a large bowl and add the beef, pork, oats, egg, mustard, parsley, garlic powder, coriander, salt, and pepper; mix well. Transfer the meat mixture to the prepared baking sheet and form it into an 8 x 4 x 2-inch loaf.

Bake the meat loaf until a thermometer inserted into the center registers 165°F, 48 to 50 minutes. Remove from the oven and let cool for at least 10 minutes before slicing.

Nutrient Content per Serving

Calories:	340	**Fat:**	17 grams	**Protein:**	37 grams
Fiber:	2 grams	**Saturated Fat:**	6 grams	**Carbs:**	10 grams
Sodium:	710 mg	**Sugars:**	2 grams		

Beef Pepper Steak–Broccolini Stir-Fry

Everyone loves Chinese food, and this Asian-inspired dish is so quick and easy to make, there's no point in hassling with takeout. The ingredients are straightforward, too, but if you're not familiar with broccolini, it's a cross between broccoli and Chinese broccoli (*gai-lan*).

Makes 4 servings

1¼ pounds flank steak, trimmed and cut crosswise into ¼-inch-thick slices

2 tablespoons low-sodium wheat-free tamari or coconut aminos

5 teaspoons Malaysian red palm fruit oil

1 medium red onion, sliced

1 medium red bell pepper, sliced

1 tablespoon minced fresh ginger

2 garlic cloves, minced

1 bunch broccolini (about 8 ounces), trimmed and cut into 2-inch pieces

¼ cup water

⅓ cup chopped green onions

Combine the flank steak and 1 teaspoon of the tamari in a large bowl; toss well.

Heat 2 teaspoons of the oil in a large nonstick skillet over medium-high heat. Add half of the beef and cook until no longer pink, about 2 minutes. Transfer the steak to a plate. Return the skillet to the stove and repeat with 1 teaspoon of the oil and the remaining steak.

Pour off any liquid from the skillet and heat the remaining 2 teaspoons oil over medium-high heat. Add the onion and cook until starting to soften, 1 to 2 minutes. Stir in the bell pepper, ginger, and garlic; cook for 2 minutes. Add the broccolini and water; cook, stirring occasionally, until the broccolini is crisp-tender, about 3 minutes. Stir in the beef and any juices that have accumulated on the plate and cook until hot, about 1 minute. Remove from the heat and stir in the remaining 5 teaspoons tamari and the green onions.

Nutrient Content per Serving

Calories:	310	**Fat:**	16 grams	**Protein:**	32 grams
Fiber:	2 grams	**Saturated Fat:**	7 grams	**Carbs:**	9 grams
Sodium:	440 mg	**Sugars:**	3 grams		

Onion and Tomato–Smothered Pork Cutlets (Cycles 1/3)

These pork cutlets will serve up a down-home meal without the usual sugar shock of a breaded coating. If thin, sliced pork chops aren't available, place your pork chops between two sheets of plastic wrap and pound with a meat mallet or rolling pin to a thickness of ¼ inch. Heck, if you've had a frustrating day, you may just want to buy them thicker and pound away!

Makes 4 servings

2 tablespoons olive oil, plus more for the pan

8 thinly sliced boneless center-cut pork loin chops (1½ pounds), trimmed

½ teaspoon sea salt

¼ teaspoon freshly ground black pepper

3 medium onions, thinly sliced

1 tablespoon chopped fresh oregano

6 garlic cloves, sliced

1 cup Homemade Chicken Stock (page 194) or low-sodium store-bought chicken broth

⅓ cup tomato paste

Preheat the oven to 350°F. Lightly dampen a paper towel with olive oil and wipe a 13 x 9-inch baking dish with it.

Heat 1 tablespoon of the oil in a large skillet over medium-high heat. Season the pork with ¼ teaspoon of the salt and ⅛ teaspoon of the pepper. Add the pork to the skillet and cook until browned, 2 minutes per side; transfer to the prepared baking dish.

Return the skillet to the stove and heat the remaining 1 tablespoon oil over medium-high heat. Add the onions and oregano and cook, stirring occasionally, until the onions are slightly softened, 2 to 3 minutes. Add the garlic and cook until the onions are tender, 4 to 5 minutes longer. Stir in the stock and tomato paste; bring to a boil and cook for 3 minutes. Remove from the heat and stir in the remaining ¼ teaspoon salt and ⅛ teaspoon pepper. Spoon the onion mixture over the pork.

Bake until the pork is cooked through, 10 minutes.

Nutrient Content per Serving

Calories:	350	**Fat:**	15 grams	**Protein:**	35 grams
Fiber:	4 grams	**Saturated Fat:**	3.5 grams	**Carbs:**	18 grams
Sodium:	450 mg	**Sugars:**	9 grams		

POULTRY

Poultry is an easy-to-cook canvas that makes it a go-to meal for people with busy lives (who did I leave out?). Sauces, marinades, and rubs transform chicken, duck, and turkey into sophisticated meals. But they're also versatile enough to make great leftovers!

Poultry is also one of the more budget-friendly ways to make sure clean, lean protein takes center stage on your Sugar Impact Plate. Plus, it's a good source of vitamins (B6 and

B12) and minerals (selenium) that support strong bones, heart health, and fast fat loss by keeping your metabolism humming.

Remember, you'll get the biggest health bang for your buck from organic, pasture-raised, hormone- and antibiotic-free poultry. Industrial chicken, turkey, and duck are pumped full of antibiotics and added hormones, which all end up in you. Eek!

Chinese Black Bean, Turkey, and Almond Stir-Fry

Look for genuine fermented black beans that have no added ingredients (they're available in Asian food markets). They're slightly salty and have a strong scent, and they add a savory depth to this meal.

Makes 4 servings

1¼ pounds turkey breast cutlets, cut crosswise into ¾-inch pieces

1 teaspoon Asian sesame oil

3 teaspoons macadamia nut oil

2 garlic cloves, minced

1 tablespoon minced fresh ginger

1 medium red onion, chopped

12 ounces baby bok choy, coarsely chopped

⅓ cup slow-roasted almonds (see page 97)

1½ tablespoons fermented black beans, mixed with 3 tablespoons water

1 tablespoon low-sodium wheat-free tamari or coconut aminos

Combine the turkey breast cutlets and sesame oil in a large bowl.

Heat 1 teaspoon of the macadamia nut oil in a large nonstick skillet over medium-high heat. Add half of the turkey and cook until browned, 3 minutes. Transfer to a plate. Repeat with 1 teaspoon of the macadamia nut oil and the remaining turkey.

Wipe the skillet clean, return it to the heat and add the remaining 1 teaspoon macadamia nut oil. Add the garlic and ginger and cook until fragrant, 15 seconds. Add the onion and cook until starting to soften, 1 to 2 minutes. Add the bok choy and almonds; cook, stirring often, until the bok choy is crisp-tender, 1 to 2 minutes. Add the turkey, black beans, and tamari; cook until hot, 1 to 2 minutes. Divide among four plates or bowls.

Nutrient Content per Serving

Calories:	290	Fat:	11 grams	Protein:	39 grams
Fiber:	2 grams	Saturated Fat:	1 gram	Carbs:	10 grams
Sodium:	290 mg	Sugars:	1 gram		

Duck Breast Fajitas

A sophisticated take on the traditional steak version, and a low-SI way to get your fajita fix! Duck breasts without skin and bone also have fewer calories and less overall fat than a boneless, skinless chicken breast, so eat up!

Makes 4 servings

4 teaspoons olive oil, plus more for the pan

1 medium red onion, sliced

1 yellow bell pepper, sliced

1 teaspoon chili powder

1 cup grape tomatoes, halved

2 teaspoons low-sodium wheat-free tamari or coconut aminos

1 tablespoon chopped fresh cilantro

4 (7-ounce) boneless duck breast halves, skin removed

¼ teaspoon sea salt

⅛ teaspoon freshly ground black pepper

4 coconut wraps (see box, page 79)

½ medium avocado, cut into 8 slices

¼ cup unsweetened cultured coconut milk

Heat 1 tablespoon of the oil in a large nonstick skillet over medium-high heat. Add the onion and cook until slightly softened, 2 to 3 minutes. Add the bell pepper and chili powder; cook until the bell pepper is slightly softened, 3 to 4 minutes. Stir in the tomatoes and cook until just starting to wilt, 2 minutes. Add the tamari and cook for 30 seconds longer. Remove from the heat and stir in the cilantro.

Meanwhile, combine the duck breasts and remaining 1 teaspoon oil in a large bowl and season with the salt and pepper. Lightly dampen a paper towel with a small amount of olive oil and wipe a grill pan with it; heat over medium-high heat. Add the duck breasts to the pan and cook, loosely covered with aluminum foil, until a thermometer inserted into the thickest portion of the duck registers 165°F, 6 to 7 minutes per side. Transfer to a cutting board and let stand for 2 minutes. Thinly slice the duck across the grain.

Place one coconut wrap on each of four plates. Top each evenly with the duck, bell pepper mixture, avocado, and coconut milk.

Nutrient Content per Serving

Calories:	270	**Fat:**	16 grams	**Protein:**	19 grams
Fiber:	4 grams	**Saturated Fat:**	7 grams	**Carbs:**	14 grams
Sodium:	340 mg	**Sugars:**	7 grams		

Pepper-Crusted Turkey Paillards over Spinach with Dijon Vinaigrette

Paillard is a French culinary term that refers to a quick-cooking piece of meat, and you'll want just that so you can be eating this salad as soon as possible! It's satisfying, nutrient rich, and full of sophisticated flavors. The spice from the pepper complements the turkey perfectly. If you'd like a subtler flavor, cut back on the pepper by ¼ to ½ teaspoon.

Makes 4 servings

4 (6-ounce) turkey cutlets
1 tablespoon plus 1 teaspoon olive oil
¼ teaspoon sea salt
1¼ teaspoons coarsely ground black pepper
8 cups baby spinach
⅓ cup Dijon Vinaigrette (page 193)

Brush the turkey with 1 teaspoon of the oil. Season with the salt, then press the pepper onto both sides of each cutlet.

Heat the remaining 1 tablespoon oil in a large skillet over medium-high heat. Add the turkey and cook until browned and cooked through, 4 to 5 minutes per side. Remove from the skillet.

Combine the spinach and 4 tablespoons of the vinaigrette in a bowl. Divide the mixture among four plates. Top each with one turkey cutlet, then drizzle each portion with 1 teaspoon of the vinaigrette.

Nutrient Content per Serving

Calories:	310	**Fat:**	18 grams	**Protein**	33 grams
Fiber:	2 grams	**Saturated Fat:**	2 grams	**Carbs:**	6 grams
Sodium:	540 mg	**Sugars:**	0 grams		

Pounded Chicken Breasts with Roasted Peppers and Capers

You may have had a hard day, but don't take it out on your protein. You want to make sure it loves you back. *Gently* pounding the chicken to an even thickness ensures even cooking. Look for bottled roasted peppers packed in brine—water and salt. Be sure to rinse them well and pat dry with paper towels.

Makes 4 servings

CHICKEN

2 teaspoons olive oil, plus more for the pan

1 tablespoon lemon juice

1 teaspoon dried basil

¼ teaspoon sea salt

⅛ teaspoon freshly ground black pepper

4 (6-ounce) boneless skinless chicken breast halves

TOPPING

1 (12-ounce) jar roasted peppers, drained, rinsed, patted dry, and sliced

6 cups baby kale salad mix

½ medium Vidalia or other sweet onion, thinly sliced (about ½ cup)

¼ cup Caper Vinaigrette (page 192)

For the chicken, combine the 2 teaspoons of oil, lemon juice, basil, salt, and black pepper in a large bowl and set aside. Sandwich one chicken breast half between two pieces of plastic wrap and use a meat mallet with a smooth surface or a rolling pin to gently pound the chicken to an even ¼-inch thickness. Repeat with the remaining chicken breast halves. Add the chicken to the bowl and turn once to coat with the mixture. Let stand at room temperature for 10 minutes.

Preheat the broiler. Lightly dampen a paper towel with a small amount of olive oil and wipe a broiler pan with it.

Meanwhile, for the topping, combine the roasted peppers, kale salad, onion, and vinaigrette in a bowl and toss well.

Place the chicken under the broiler, 4 to 5 inches from the heat, and cook until a thermometer inserted into the thickest part registers 165°F, 4 to 5 minutes, turning once. Serve the chicken topped with the roasted pepper mixture.

Nutrient Content per Serving

Calories:	170	**Fat:**	6 grams	**Protein:**	27 grams
Fiber:	0 grams	**Saturated Fat:**	1 gram	**Carbs:**	0 grams
Sodium:	290 mg	**Sugars:**	0 grams		

Turkey and Vegetable Skillet

Your Sugar Impact Plate is going to be very happy to see this coming—clean, lean protein and lots of colorful veggies in one fell swoop. Turkey cutlets are sometimes labeled as turkey chops, so don't let that fool you when you're shopping.

Makes 4 servings

> 2 tablespoons olive oil
> 1¼ pounds turkey cutlets, cut crosswise into ½-inch-thick strips
> 2 teaspoons Dijon mustard
> 2 teaspoons grated lemon zest
> ½ teaspoon sea salt
> ¼ teaspoon freshly ground black pepper
> ½ cup chopped shallots
> 3 garlic cloves, minced
> 1½ teaspoons chopped fresh thyme
> 8 ounces Brussels sprouts, quartered
> 1 red bell pepper, sliced
> 8 ounces sugar snap peas
> ½ cup Homemade Chicken Stock (page 194) or low-sodium store-bought chicken broth

Heat 2 teaspoons of the oil in a large nonstick skillet over medium-high heat. Combine the turkey with the mustard, lemon zest, ¼ teaspoon of the salt, and ⅛ teaspoon of the black pepper. Add half of the turkey and cook, stirring occasionally, until lightly browned, 2 to 3 minutes. Transfer to a plate. Heat 1 teaspoon of the oil and repeat with the remaining turkey.

Heat the remaining 1 tablespoon oil in the skillet over medium-high heat. Add the shallots, garlic, and thyme; cook, stirring occasionally, for 1 minute. Add the Brussels sprouts and cook for 2 minutes. Stir in the bell pepper and cook for 2 minutes longer. Add the sugar snap peas and cook until bright green, 1 minute. Add the chicken stock and bring to a boil. Stir in the turkey and cook until hot, 1 to 2 minutes. Stir in the remaining ¼ teaspoon salt and ⅛ teaspoon black pepper. Divide among four bowls and serve.

Nutrient Content per Serving

Calories:	290	**Fat:**	8 grams	**Protein:**	39 grams
Fiber:	5 grams	**Saturated Fat:**	1 gram	**Carbs:**	15 grams
Sodium:	500 mg	**Sugars:**	6 grams		

BBQ-Rubbed Whole Roasted Chicken

This roasted chicken is great for a Sunday night supper and leftovers are terrific in a salad the next day (if there are any!). Be generous with the rub both inside and outside the bird's cavity so the seasonings are absorbed into the meat during roasting.

Makes 6 servings

1 tablespoon olive oil, plus more for the pan
1 (4-pound) whole chicken
1 tablespoon lemon juice
2 tablespoons Smoky BBQ Spice Rub (page 195)

Preheat the oven to 400°F. Position a rack in the center. Set a wire rack in a shallow roasting pan. Lightly dampen a paper towel with a small amount of olive oil and wipe both the roasting pan and rack with it.

Loosen the skin over the breasts, legs, and thighs of the chicken with your fingers. Rub the chicken all over and under the skin with the 1 tablespoon of oil and lemon juice. Sprinkle the spice rub over the skin and sprinkle some in the cavity. Set the chicken on the rack in the roasting pan, breast-side up. Tuck the wing tips under the body and tie the legs together with kitchen twine, if desired.

Roast the chicken until an instant-read thermometer inserted into the thickest part of the thigh without hitting the bone registers 165°F, about 1 hour 10 minutes. Transfer the chicken to a cutting board. Let stand for 10 minutes before carving.

Nutrient Content per Serving

Calories:	370	**Fat:**	22 grams	**Protein:**	40 grams
Fiber:	0 grams	**Saturated Fat:**	6 grams	**Carbs:**	1 gram
Sodium:	250 mg	**Sugars:**	0 grams		

Jerk-Spiced Chicken Thighs with Roasted Pineapple Chutney (Cycles 1/3)

This dish will transport you to da islands, mon! A tropical treat for your taste buds, this meal is a perfect blend of spicy and sweet. The chutney can be made up to 3 days ahead and kept in the refrigerator. It's also great on pork.

Makes 4 servings

> Olive oil for the pan
> ½ pineapple, peeled, cored, and cut into ½-inch-thick slices
> 1 tablespoon plus 1 teaspoon coconut oil
> ¼ cup finely chopped red bell pepper
> 2 tablespoons chopped green onion
> ½ teaspoon minced fresh ginger
> 1 tablespoon chopped fresh mint
> ⅛ teaspoon sea salt
> 8 bone-in skinless chicken thighs (about 2¼ pounds), trimmed
> 2½ tablespoons Jerk Rub (page 195)

Preheat the oven to 425°F. Lightly dampen a paper towel with a small amount of olive oil and wipe two rimmed baking sheets with it.

Brush the pineapple with 1 teaspoon of the coconut oil and place on one of the baking sheets. Roast until the pineapple is tender and lightly browned, turning once, 15 minutes. Remove from the oven and let cool for 10 minutes. Cut the cooled pineapple into ½-inch pieces and transfer to a bowl; stir in the bell pepper, green onion, ginger, mint, and salt and set aside until ready to serve.

Melt the remaining 1 tablespoon coconut oil and combine it with the chicken in a large bowl. Rub the chicken all over with the jerk rub and place on the remaining baking sheet. Roast the chicken for 25 to 28 minutes, until a thermometer inserted into the thickest portion of the leg without hitting the bone registers 165°F. Serve the chicken with the chutney.

Nutrient Content per Serving

Calories:	380	**Fat:**	17 grams	**Protein:**	36 grams
Fiber:	3 grams	**Saturated Fat:**	7 grams	**Carbs:**	18 grams
Sodium:	640 mg	**Sugars:**	12 grams		

Lime-Marinated Chicken Kebabs with Cilantro Pesto

These light and healthy kebabs are perfect for a backyard BBQ on a summer evening. The lime marinade and Cilantro Pesto (page 196) intermingle to create a fiesta of flavor. Having the cilantro pesto on hand makes this recipe a snap. Don't be afraid to try it with the Chimichurri Sauce (page 190) as well. If you're using wooden skewers, be sure to soak them in warm water for 30 minutes first to prevent burning.

Makes 4 servings

1½ pounds boneless skinless chicken thighs, trimmed and cut into 32 pieces

1 medium red bell pepper, cut into 16 pieces

1 medium yellow bell pepper, cut into 16 pieces

1 tablespoon olive oil, plus more for the pan

1 garlic clove, minced

1 tablespoon grated lime zest

2 tablespoons lime juice

1 teaspoon dried oregano

½ teaspoon sea salt

¼ teaspoon freshly ground black pepper

½ cup Cilantro Pesto (page 196)

Combine the chicken, bell peppers, the 1 tablespoon of oil, garlic, lime zest, lime juice, and oregano in a large bowl. Refrigerate for 30 minutes.

Preheat the broiler. Lightly dampen a paper towel with a small amount of olive oil and wipe a broiler pan with it.

Alternately skewer 4 chicken pieces and 4 bell pepper pieces on each of eight skewers. Season with salt and black pepper and set the skewers on the prepared pan.

Broil the chicken and peppers 5 inches from the heat source until cooked through, 8 to 10 minutes, turning every 2 minutes. Serve the skewers with the cilantro pesto.

Nutrient Content per Serving

Calories:	400	**Fat:**	28 grams	**Protein:**	30 grams
Fiber:	2 grams	**Saturated Fat:**	5 grams	**Carbs:**	6 grams
Sodium:	550 mg	**Sugars:**	3 grams		

Slow Cooker–Braised Chicken Legs with Rosemary, Onions, and Celery

Because it's braised and infused with savory seasonings and vegetables for hours, this succulent slow-cooked chicken will fall right off the bone! Makes great leftovers for tomorrow's lunch.

Makes 4 servings

1 tablespoon olive oil, plus more for the slow cooker

8 bone-in skin-on chicken legs (about 2½ pounds)

½ teaspoon salt

¼ teaspoon freshly ground black pepper

4 garlic cloves, minced

1 medium onion, chopped

3 celery stalks, cut into ¾-inch slices

1 small fennel bulb, cored and sliced

2 teaspoons chopped fresh rosemary

½ cup Homemade Chicken Stock (page 194) or low-sodium store-bought chicken broth

2 teaspoons arrowroot

Lightly dampen a paper towel with a small amount of olive oil and wipe a 5- to 6-quart slow cooker with it.

Heat the 1 tablespoon of oil in a large nonstick skillet over medium-high heat. Season the chicken with ¼ teaspoon of the salt and ⅛ teaspoon of the pepper. Add the chicken to the skillet and cook, turning occasionally, until browned, 4 to 6 minutes. Transfer the chicken to the prepared slow cooker.

Return the skillet to the heat and add the garlic, onion, celery, fennel, and rosemary and cook, stirring occasionally, until the vegetables are starting to soften, 2 to 3 minutes. Pour in the chicken stock and cook for 1 minute. Remove from the heat and stir in the arrowroot and remaining ¼ teaspoon salt and ⅛ teaspoon pepper.

Pour the vegetable mixture into the slow cooker, cover, and cook on low until the chicken is tender, 6 to 7 hours.

Nutrient Content per Serving

Calories:	450	**Fat:**	30 grams	**Protein:**	32 grams
Fiber:	4 grams	**Saturated Fat:**	8 grams	**Carbs:**	13 grams
Sodium:	520 mg	**Sugars:**	3 grams		

Turkey Meatballs with Parmesan and Tomato Sauce (Cycles 1/3)

Meatballs! Fun to say, fun to make! Some say that the rounder they are, the better they taste, so grab the kids and make it a contest to see who can make the best one. The meatballs can be made up to 2 days ahead and reheated in the sauce. If you're dairy intolerant, skip the Parmesan cheese.

Makes 4 servings

2 tablespoons olive oil

1 medium onion, finely chopped

3 garlic cloves, minced

1 teaspoon dried basil

1 (14.5-ounce) can no-salt-added petite diced tomatoes

3 tablespoons tomato paste

½ teaspoon sea salt

¼ teaspoon freshly ground black pepper

1½ pounds lean ground turkey

¼ cup gluten-free old-fashioned rolled oats

1 teaspoon garlic powder

1 teaspoon dried oregano

1 large egg

⅓ cup grated Parmesan cheese

Quinoa pasta or spaghetti squash, for serving (optional)

Shredded parsley, for garnish

Heat 1 tablespoon of the oil in a medium nonstick skillet over medium-high heat. Add the onion, garlic, and basil; cook until the onion and garlic are starting to soften, 1 to 2 minutes. Add the tomatoes and tomato paste; reduce the heat to medium and cook, stirring occasionally, until slightly thickened, 10 to 12 minutes. Season the sauce with ¼ teaspoon of the salt and ⅛ teaspoon of the pepper. Remove from the heat.

Combine the turkey, oats, garlic powder, oregano, egg, cheese, and remaining ¼ teaspoon salt and ⅛ teaspoon pepper in a large bowl; mix well with your hands. Form the turkey mixture into 16 balls and set aside on a plate.

Heat the remaining 1 tablespoon oil in a large nonstick skillet over medium heat. Add the meatballs and cook, turning occasionally, until browned and cooked through, 16 to 18 minutes. Transfer the meatballs to the skillet with the sauce and bring to a simmer over medium heat. Cook for 3 minutes.

Serve the meatballs and sauce in a bowl as-is, or on top of quinoa pasta (Cycle 1/3) or spaghetti squash for a heartier meal. Garnish with shredded parsley.

Nutrient Content per Serving

Calories:	370	**Fat:**	21 grams	**Protein:**	31 grams
Fiber:	3 grams	**Saturated Fat:**	5 grams	**Carbs:**	16 grams
Sodium:	520 mg	**Sugars:**	5 grams		

Slow Cooker Moroccan Chicken Tagine

Tagine is perhaps Morocco's most famous culinary export. After slow cooking this dish for hours, come home to your reward—a symphony of deliciously exotic aromas!

Makes 4 servings

1 tablespoon olive oil, plus more for the slow cooker

8 bone-in skinless chicken thighs (2 pounds), trimmed

½ teaspoon sea salt

¼ teaspoon freshly ground black pepper

1 medium onion, chopped

6 garlic cloves, minced

1 green bell pepper, chopped

1 teaspoon ground coriander

½ teaspoon paprika

¼ teaspoon saffron threads, crushed

¼ teaspoon ground ginger

1 cinnamon stick

¾ cup Homemade Chicken Stock (page 194) or low-sodium store-bought chicken broth

1 cup organic no-salt-added chickpeas, drained and rinsed

¼ cup pitted Kalamata olives, halved

3 tablespoons chopped fresh cilantro

1 tablespoon grated orange zest

1 tablespoon grated lemon zest

Lightly dampen a paper towel with a small amount of olive oil and wipe a 5- to 6-quart slow cooker with it.

Heat the 1 tablespoon of oil in a large skillet over medium-high heat. Season the chicken with ¼ teaspoon of the salt and ⅛ teaspoon of the black pepper. Add 4 chicken thighs to the skillet and cook until browned, 8 minutes, turning once. Transfer the chicken to a plate and repeat with the remaining thighs.

Reduce the heat to medium and add the onion and garlic; cook, stirring, for 1 minute. Add the bell pepper and cook for 1 minute. Stir in the coriander, paprika, saffron, ginger, and cinnamon stick; cook for 30 seconds. Pour in the stock and cook for 1 minute, scraping up any browned bits that have stuck to the bottom of the pan. Add the chickpeas and cook for 1 minute. Transfer the vegetables to the prepared slow cooker. Stir in the olives and remaining ¼ teaspoon salt and ⅛ teaspoon pepper. Set the chicken thighs on top of the chickpea mixture, cover, and cook on low until the chicken is very tender, 6 to 7 hours.

Transfer the chicken to a serving platter and stir the cilantro, orange zest, and lemon zest into the chickpea mixture. Spoon the chickpea mixture over the chicken and serve.

Nutrient Content per Serving

Calories:	350	**Fat:**	13 grams	**Protein:**	38 grams
Fiber:	5 grams	**Saturated Fat:**	3.5 grams	**Carbs:**	17 grams
Sodium:	580 mg	**Sugars:**	4 grams		

Tandoori Chicken

This dish gets its name from the traditional tandoor ovens from India and Pakistan, so that may explain the pull you feel to cook it on the outdoor grill. Let this mix and mingle of exotic spices transport you to a faraway land!

This dish will need to be refrigerated overnight before cooking. If you do prefer to grill the chicken, grill over indirect medium-high heat (400 to 450°F) for 25 to 28 minutes, or until the internal temperature of the chicken reaches 165°F.

Makes 4 servings

    1 cup cultured unsweetened coconut milk
    2 tablespoons lemon juice
    3 garlic cloves, minced
    1 tablespoon minced fresh ginger
    2 teaspoons paprika
    1 teaspoon ground cumin
    ¼ teaspoon saffron threads, crushed
    ¼ teaspoon ground cinnamon
    ¼ teaspoon cayenne pepper
    8 bone-in skinless chicken thighs (2¼ pounds), trimmed
    Olive oil for the pan
    ¾ teaspoon sea salt

Combine the coconut milk, lemon juice, garlic, ginger, paprika, cumin, saffron, cinnamon, and cayenne in a large bowl. Add the chicken and toss well to coat. Cover with plastic wrap and refrigerate overnight.

Preheat the oven to 450°F. Lightly dampen a paper towel with a small amount of olive oil and wipe a large rimmed baking sheet with it.

Remove the chicken from the marinade and season with the salt. Place the chicken on the prepared baking sheet. Roast until a thermometer inserted into the thickest part of the chicken registers 165°F, 25 to 28 minutes.

Nutrient Content per Serving

Calories:	190	**Fat:**	7 grams	**Protein:**	27 grams
Fiber:	1 gram	**Saturated Fat:**	2.5 grams	**Carbs:**	4 grams
Sodium:	560 mg	**Sugars:**	2 grams		

Turkey Cutlets with Marsala and Shiitake Mushrooms (Cycles 1/3)

The shiitake mushrooms add a rich, smoky depth to this dish that will have your taste buds singing *arigatō*! Make sure to use dry Marsala wine and not the sweet version.

Serves 4

- 4 (6-ounce) turkey breast cutlets
- ¼ teaspoon plus ⅛ teaspoon sea salt
- ¼ teaspoon freshly ground black pepper
- 2 tablespoons arrowroot powder
- 2 tablespoons olive oil
- 8 ounces shiitake mushrooms, stems removed and thinly sliced
- 3 garlic cloves, minced
- ¾ cup Homemade Chicken Stock (page 194) or low-sodium store-bought chicken broth
- ½ cup Marsala wine
- 2 tablespoons chopped fresh parsley

Season the turkey with ¼ teaspoon of the salt and ⅛ teaspoon of the pepper. Spread the arrowroot on a large plate and lightly dredge both sides of each turkey cutlet in the arrowroot.

Heat 1 tablespoon of the oil in a large nonstick skillet over medium-high heat. Add the turkey and cook until lightly browned, 3 to 4 minutes per side. Transfer to a plate and set aside.

Wipe the skillet clean, then in the same skillet, heat the remaining 1 tablespoon oil; add the mushrooms and cook, stirring occasionally, until lightly browned and softened, 5 minutes. Stir in the garlic and cook until slightly softened, 1 to 2 minutes. Pour in the stock and wine; bring to a boil and cook until the mixture begins to thicken, about 2 minutes. Reduce the heat to medium and add the turkey. Cook, turning occasionally, until the turkey is hot and cooked through, about 3 minutes. Remove from the heat and stir in the parsley and remaining ⅛ teaspoon salt and ⅛ teaspoon pepper.

Nutrient Content per Serving

Calories:	300	**Fat:**	8 grams	**Protein:**	39 grams
Fiber:	2 grams	**Saturated Fat:**	1 gram	**Carbs:**	12 grams
Sodium:	350 mg	**Sugars:**	4 grams		

Easy Weeknight Curried Chicken Breasts with Cashews and Green Onions

Curry and fresh spices transform an everyday chicken dinner into an exotic experience. To expand your repertoire, try this recipe with boneless center-cut pork chops.

Makes 4 servings

  3 teaspoons coconut oil
  4 (6-ounce) boneless skinless chicken breast halves
  ¼ teaspoon plus ⅛ teaspoon sea salt
  ¼ teaspoon freshly ground black pepper
  1 medium red onion, thinly sliced
  1 medium red bell pepper, thinly sliced
  1 tablespoon minced fresh ginger
  3 garlic cloves, minced
  1 tablespoon curry powder
  1 cup unsweetened lite culinary coconut milk (such as So Delicious brand) (see box, page 132)
  ½ cup sliced green onions
  ⅓ cup slow-roasted cashews (see page 97), coarsely chopped
  ¼ cup sliced fresh basil leaves

Heat 2 teaspoons of the oil in a large nonstick skillet over medium-high heat. Season the chicken with ¼ teaspoon of the salt and ⅛ teaspoon of the black pepper; add to the skillet and cook until browned on both sides, about 6 minutes. Transfer the chicken to a plate and set aside.

Return the skillet to the heat and add the remaining 1 teaspoon oil. Stir in the onion and bell pepper; cook, stirring occasionally, until the vegetables are slightly softened, 2 to 3 minutes. Add the ginger and garlic; cook for 1 minute. Add the curry powder and cook, stirring, for 30 seconds. Reduce the heat to medium and pour in the coconut milk; simmer for 1 minute. Add the chicken and cook, turning occasionally, until a thermometer inserted into the thickest part of the chicken registers 165°F, 11 to 12 minutes. Remove from the heat and stir in the green onions, cashews, basil, and remaining ⅛ teaspoon salt and ⅛ teaspoon black pepper.

Nutrient Content per Serving

Calories:	330	**Fat:**	15 grams	**Protein:**	39 grams
Fiber:	3 grams	**Saturated Fat:**	8 grams	**Carbs:**	10 grams
Sodium:	470 mg	**Sugars:**	4 grams		

Culinary coconut milks are intended for use in recipes that call for canned cooking milks. They're higher in fat than the packaged coconut milk you drink. You can find them in the Thai section or baking aisle in grocery stores.

Warm Chicken Salad with Pecans, Basil, and Caper Vinaigrette

Warm chicken and green beans certainly elevate the standard lunchtime fare of cold chicken over plain old lettuce. But if you're having a day where "easy" trumps "sophisticated," don't rule out this salad—the chicken can also be served at room temperature, so make all the components ahead of time and toss just before serving.

Makes 4 servings

8 ounces green beans, halved crosswise
2 teaspoons olive oil
1½ pounds boneless skinless chicken thighs (about 5 thighs)
½ teaspoon sea salt
¼ teaspoon freshly ground black pepper
4 celery stalks, cut into ½-inch-thick slices
2 carrots, thinly sliced
1 large orange bell pepper, chopped
⅓ cup slow-roasted pecans (see page 97)
3 cups baby spinach
¼ cup sliced fresh basil leaves
¼ cup Caper Vinaigrette (page 192)

Bring a medium saucepan of lightly salted water to a boil over high heat. Add the green beans, return the water to a boil, and cook for 1 minute; drain and set aside.

Heat the oil in a large nonstick skillet over medium-high heat. Season the chicken with the salt and black pepper. Add the chicken to the skillet; cook until a thermometer inserted into the thickest part of the thigh registers 165°F, 7 to 8 minutes per side. Transfer the chicken to a cutting board and let rest for 2 minutes. Cut the chicken into strips and transfer to a bowl. Add the green beans, celery, carrots, bell pepper, pecans, spinach, basil, and vinaigrette; toss well and serve.

Nutrient Content per Serving

Calories:	360	**Fat:**	22 grams	**Protein:**	28 grams
Fiber:	6 grams	**Saturated Fat:**	2 grams	**Carbs:**	15 grams
Sodium:	690 mg	**Sugars:**	6 grams		

FISH AND SHELLFISH

Seafood lovers, rejoice! You win. Your favorites are low in saturated fat, packed with protein, iron, and B vitamins, and are the richest source of omega-3 fatty acids of any food on the planet. And, as you now know, the more healthy fat you eat, the better—it helps prevent heart disease and reduce high blood pressure and inflammation. It also boosts brain power, improves immune function, and eases joint pain.

For the most concentrated nutritional benefit among already great choices, go for cold-water wild fish, starting with those lowest on the food chain (like sardines and anchovies). But if those aren't your bag, don't sweat it. These mouthwatering recipes offer you plenty of choices, and all of them make exquisite meals.

Simply Grilled Shrimp with Lime

According to Leonardo da Vinci, "Simplicity is the ultimate sophistication," and this recipe is certainly both (don't worry, you can still grill the shrimp in your flip-flops). Cook over direct high heat for 2 to 3 minutes per side on a gas or charcoal grill.

Makes 4 servings

1½ pounds large shrimp, peeled and deveined
1 tablespoon olive oil
¼ teaspoon ground coriander
¼ teaspoon sea salt
¼ teaspoon freshly ground black pepper
1 tablespoon grated lime zest
1 tablespoon chopped fresh cilantro
1 lime, quartered

Preheat a grill pan over medium-high heat.

Toss the shrimp with the oil, coriander, salt, and pepper; let stand for 5 minutes.

Add the shrimp to the grill pan and cook until marked and cooked through, 3 to 4 minutes per side. Transfer to a bowl and toss with the lime zest and cilantro. Serve with the lime quarters.

Nutrient Content per Serving

Calories:	180	**Fat:**	6 grams	**Protein:**	32 grams
Fiber:	0 grams	**Saturated Fat:**	0 grams	**Carbs:**	0 grams
Sodium:	510 mg	**Sugars:**	0 grams		

Herbed Salmon Cakes with Tartar Sauce

The Sugar Impact Plate has a spot for clean, lean protein at every meal, and wild, cold-water fish is a great way to fill it. If you want to mix it up from time to time, swap salmon for fresh tuna in this recipe—it's just as to die for.

Makes 4 servings

TARTAR SAUCE

¼ cup Sugar Impact Mayonnaise (page 197)
2 tablespoons finely chopped shallots
2 tablespoons finely chopped cucumber
2 teaspoons chopped drained capers

SALMON CAKES

1½ pounds skinless salmon fillet, cut into 1-inch chunks
1 tablespoon chopped drained capers
1 large egg, lightly beaten
3 tablespoons chopped fresh parsley
1 tablespoon chopped fresh basil
1 teaspoon Dijon mustard
1 tablespoon olive oil

For the tartar sauce, combine the mayonnaise, shallots, cucumber, and capers in a small bowl; set aside.

For the salmon cakes, place the salmon in a food processor and pulse until chopped. Transfer to a bowl and stir in the capers, egg, parsley, basil, and mustard. With moist hands, form the mixture into four ¾-inch-thick patties.

Heat the oil in a large nonstick skillet over medium heat. Add the salmon patties and cook, turning once, until browned and cooked through, 8 to 10 minutes. Serve the salmon cakes topped with the tartar sauce.

Nutrient Content per Serving

Calories:	350	**Fat:**	20 grams	**Protein:**	37 grams
Fiber:	0 grams	**Saturated Fat:**	3.5 grams	**Carbs:**	3 grams
Sodium:	370 mg	**Sugars:**	1 gram		

Blackened Salmon with Basil Aioli

Salmon may be well known for its high protein and omega-3 content, but it's packed with other nutrients, too, including vitamin D. Choose wild-caught Alaskan salmon and make it a crunchy treat—keep the skin on the fillets and cook on the skin side two-thirds of the way through.

Makes 4 servings

¼ cup Sugar Impact Mayonnaise (page 197)
½ small garlic clove, crushed to a paste
2 tablespoons chopped fresh basil
1 teaspoon lemon juice
1 teaspoon sweet paprika
½ teaspoon ground cumin
½ teaspoon ground coriander
½ teaspoon garlic powder
¼ teaspoon dried thyme
¾ teaspoon sea salt
¼ teaspoon ground chipotle pepper
4 (6-ounce) skin-on salmon fillets
1 teaspoon Malaysian red palm fruit oil

Combine the mayonnaise, garlic, basil, and lemon juice in a small bowl. Set aside.

Combine the paprika, cumin, coriander, garlic powder, thyme, salt, and chipotle pepper in a small bowl. Rub the mixture over the salmon fillets.

Heat the oil in a large nonstick skillet over medium-high heat. Add the salmon and cook for 4 to 5 minutes per side, until the fish flakes easily with a fork. Serve topped with the mayonnaise mixture.

Nutrient Content per Serving

Calories:	310	**Fat:**	17 grams	**Protein:**	35 grams
Fiber:	1 gram	**Saturated Fat:**	3.5 grams	**Carbs:**	3 grams
Sodium:	620 mg	**Sugars:**	0 grams		

Thai Coconut Steamed Mussels

Bathing mussels in a rich, slightly sweet coconut bath brings out the best in them (and you, too, I hope!). Prior to cooking, any open mussels should close when lightly tapped. Discard any that don't close or have cracked or broken shells. Rinse the shells before cooking.

Makes 4 servings

  1 tablespoon coconut oil
  1 medium onion, chopped
  4 garlic cloves, minced
  1 serrano pepper, seeded and finely chopped
  1 cup lite culinary coconut milk (see box, page 132)
  4 tablespoons chopped fresh cilantro
  2 tablespoons lime juice
  ¼ teaspoon monk fruit extract
  1 teaspoon low-sodium wheat-free tamari or coconut aminos
  3 pounds mussels, scrubbed and debearded

Heat the oil in a Dutch oven over medium-high heat. Add the onion, garlic, and serrano pepper; cook, stirring often, until slightly softened, 3 to 4 minutes. Stir in the coconut milk, 2 tablespoons of the cilantro, the lime juice, monk fruit extract, and tamari. Bring the mixture to a boil and cook for 1 minute. Add the mussels, cover, return to a boil, and cook until the shells open, 4 to 5 minutes. Remove from the heat and discard any unopened mussels.

Divide the mussels among four bowls. Spoon sauce from the pan over each serving and sprinkle with the remaining 2 tablespoons cilantro.

Nutrient Content per Serving

Calories:	360	**Fat:**	12 grams	**Protein:**	41 grams
Fiber:	1 gram	**Saturated Fat:**	5 grams	**Carbs:**	19 grams
Sodium:	1040 mg	**Sugars:**	4 grams		

Plank-Roasted Salmon

Plank roasting is a great way to add an earthy, smoky quality to your fish. If you don't have a plank, you don't have to skip this recipe—simply cook the salmon on a baking sheet instead.

Makes 4 servings

1 tablespoon plus 2 teaspoons olive oil

4 (6-ounce) skin-on salmon fillets

1 tablespoon lemon juice

2 teaspoons Dijon mustard

¼ teaspoon sea salt

⅛ teaspoon freshly ground black pepper

Preheat the oven to 350°F.

Lightly brush one side of a large alder wood or cherry wood plank with 2 teaspoons of the oil. Set in the center of the oven, oiled-side up, and bake for 20 minutes.

Rub the salmon with the remaining 1 tablespoon oil. Combine the lemon juice and mustard in a small bowl and brush over the salmon. Season with the salt and pepper.

Place the salmon fillets skin-side down on the plank and roast until the fish is firm and flakes easily with a fork, 14 to 15 minutes.

Nutrient Content per Serving

Calories:	250	**Fat:**	12 grams	**Protein:**	34 grams
Fiber:	0 grams	**Saturated Fat:**	2.5 grams	**Carbs:**	1 gram
Sodium:	290 mg	**Sugars:**	0 grams		

Bacon-Wrapped Scallops

Or, as I prefer to think of it, "Bacon Hugs Scallops." If you're paleo or low carb, take note—paleo-style bacon won't work in this recipe, so choose regular nitrate-free bacon instead. And look for regular, not jumbo, "dry" sea scallops rather than wet scallops, which are packed in brine.

Makes 4 servings

1½ pounds sea scallops, preferably wild caught (20 pieces)

¼ teaspoon freshly ground black pepper

10 slices nitrate-free uncured bacon, halved crosswise

1 teaspoon olive oil

Season the scallops with the pepper.

Lay the bacon slices on a work surface. Place a scallop on half of each bacon slice, then roll the bacon around the scallop and set aside on a plate, seam-side down.

Heat the oil in a large nonstick skillet over medium-high heat. Add half of the scallops, placing them seam-side down in the pan, and cook until the bacon is browned and the scallops are cooked through, 4 minutes per side. Repeat with the remaining scallops. Serve hot or at room temperature.

Nutrient Content per Serving

Calories:	310	**Fat:**	19 grams	**Protein:**	18 grams
Fiber:	1 gram	**Saturated Fat:**	5 grams	**Carbs:**	17 grams
Sodium:	998 mg	**Sugars:**	0 grams		

Lettuce-Wrapped Steamed Halibut with Chimichurri Sauce

Wrapping the halibut in lettuce for steaming gives it the fresh flavor of your garden and adds moisture. If you don't have a bamboo steamer, you can place the fish on a wire rack set over the pot and cover with foil.

Makes 4 servings

4 large romaine lettuce leaves
4 (6-ounce) halibut fillets, preferably wild caught
¼ teaspoon sea salt
⅛ teaspoon freshly ground black pepper
¼ cup Chimichurri Sauce (page 190)

Bring a large pot of salted water to a boil. Fill a large bowl with water and ice. Drop the lettuce leaves into the boiling water and cook for 30 seconds. Immediately transfer to the ice water to stop the cooking; drain. Reserve the pot of boiling water.

Arrange the lettuce leaves on a work surface. Season the halibut with the salt and pepper. Place one fillet on each lettuce leaf, then fold the lettuce around the halibut to enclose it completely.

Return the pot of water to a boil. Place the wrapped halibut in a bamboo steamer and set the steamer over the boiling water. Cover and cook until the fish is firm and flakes easily with a fork, about 10 minutes.

Place one halibut fillet on each of four plates and serve with the chimichurri sauce.

Nutrient Content per Serving

Calories:	210	**Fat:**	8 grams	**Protein:**	32 grams
Fiber:	1 gram	**Saturated Fat:**	1.5 grams	**Carbs:**	2 grams
Sodium:	410 mg	**Sugars:**	0 grams		

Peppered Shrimp with Mango (Cycles 1/3)

I'm already in the islands—how about you? And this will make you feel even better—shrimp are high in omega-3s and are a concentrated source of antioxidants. Sweeten them up with mangoes that are fragrant and yield to light pressure (do not mash the mangoes!).

Makes 4 servings

1½ pounds large shrimp, peeled and deveined
¼ teaspoon sea salt
¼ teaspoon coarsely ground black pepper
1½ tablespoons coconut oil
1 red onion, thinly sliced
1 tablespoon minced fresh ginger
1 garlic clove, minced
1 cup sliced mango
1 tablespoon chopped fresh mint
1 tablespoon chopped green onion
1 tablespoon unsweetened coconut flakes

Season the shrimp with the salt and pepper. Heat 1 tablespoon of the oil in a large nonstick skillet over medium-high heat. Add the shrimp, working in two batches if necessary to avoid overcrowding, and cook until browned and cooked through, 2 to 3 minutes per side; transfer to a plate.

Return the skillet to the heat and add the remaining ½ tablespoon oil. Stir in the onion, ginger, and garlic and cook until slightly softened, 3 to 4 minutes. Add the mango and cook for 2 minutes longer. Add the shrimp and cook until hot, 1 minute. Remove from the heat and stir in the mint, green onion, and coconut flakes.

Nutrient Content per Serving

Calories:	220	**Fat:**	8 grams	**Protein:**	24 grams
Fiber:	2 grams	**Saturated Fat:**	5 grams	**Carbs:**	13 grams
Sodium:	490 mg	**Sugars:**	8 grams		

Seared Halibut with Lemon-Basil Gremolata

If you're not familiar with the Italian condiment gremolata, you'll be surprised at how much its few, simple ingredients sass up this halibut. Gremolata is traditionally made with parsley, lemon, and raw garlic, but I've refined it by using fresh basil and cooking the garlic to take the edge off.

Makes 4 servings

> 4 (6-ounce) skinless halibut fillets
> 1 tablespoon Dijon mustard
> ½ teaspoon sea salt
> ¼ teaspoon freshly ground black pepper
> 2 tablespoons olive oil
> 3 garlic cloves, minced
> 1 large plum tomato, seeded and chopped
> 3 tablespoons chopped fresh basil
> 1 tablespoon grated lemon zest

Brush the halibut fillets with the mustard and season with the salt and pepper.

Heat 1 tablespoon of the oil in a large nonstick skillet over medium-high heat. Add the halibut and cook for 5 minutes. Turn the halibut over and cook until the fish flakes easily with a fork, about 5 minutes longer. Transfer to a plate.

In the same skillet, heat the remaining 1 tablespoon oil and stir in the garlic; cook, stirring, until fragrant, 30 seconds. Add the tomato and cook until starting to wilt, 1 to 2 minutes. Remove from the heat and stir in the basil and lemon zest. Spoon the tomato mixture over the halibut and serve.

Nutrient Content per Serving

Calories:	230	**Fat:**	9 grams	**Protein:**	32 grams
Fiber:	0 grams	**Saturated Fat:**	1.5 grams	**Carbs:**	2 grams
Sodium:	500 mg	**Sugars:**	0 grams		

Fillet of Sole Piccata

You probably think of chicken when you think of piccata, but its flavors suit white fish to a T. If you can't find sole, you can substitute flounder for this light, elegant dish.

Makes 4 servings

2 teaspoons olive oil

4 (6-ounce) skinless sole fillets

½ teaspoon sea salt

¼ teaspoon freshly ground black pepper

3 tablespoons lemon juice

2 teaspoons drained capers, chopped

2 tablespoons extra-virgin olive oil

Heat the olive oil in a large nonstick skillet over medium-high heat. Season the sole fillets with ¼ teaspoon of the salt and ⅛ teaspoon of the pepper. Add to the skillet and cook until lightly browned, 3 minutes. Turn the fillets over and cook until the fish flakes easily with a fork, 1 to 2 minutes longer. Transfer the sole to a platter.

Return the skillet to the stove over medium-high heat and add the lemon juice and capers; cook for 20 seconds. Remove from the heat and whisk in the extra-virgin olive oil, remaining ¼ teaspoon salt and ⅛ teaspoon pepper; spoon the sauce over the sole and serve.

Nutrient Content per Serving

Calories:	140	**Fat:**	11 grams	**Protein:**	11 grams
Fiber:	0 grams	**Saturated Fat:**	1.5 grams	**Carbs:**	1 gram
Sodium:	580 mg	**Sugars:**	0 grams		

MEATLESS MAINS

I haven't been shy about recommending you include animal protein in your diet, and having been a vegetarian, I come at that from personal experience. Animal protein fuels a high-functioning metabolism that burns fat fast. But you can still get the essential nutrition you need, lose fat fast, and stay supercharged without eating meat (work with me here—just promise you won't give high-SI processed foods a pass as "vegetarian"!).

A plant-based diet is often really high in fiber, something that's hard for most people to get enough of. Vegetables, beans and legumes, and nuts all make a big contribution on the fiber front, so vegetarians tend to get a lot of digestive support. Plants, nuts, and seeds are also dense with other nutrients like vitamins and antioxidants, which ward off cancer and other chronic conditions. People who choose to eat *less* meat will gain a heart-protective benefit, but all the antioxidants in vegetables also actively work on behalf of the heart, so if they're the centerpiece of your diet, that's great news!

Each of these recipes also includes plenty of protein—so there's one less thing that requires your attention.

Mushroom, Cashew, Spinach, and Lentil Skillet

French lentils, which are also known as lentils du Puy, are small green lentils with a rich flavor. They were once grown only in the volcanic soils of Puy, France, but now they're also grown in North America and Italy. They work great in salads and other dishes and hold their shape much better than regular green or brown lentils.

Makes 4 servings

>   2 tablespoons coconut oil
>   8 ounces white mushrooms, sliced
>   ¾ teaspoon sea salt
>   2 medium onions, chopped
>   2 carrots, chopped
>   3 celery stalks, chopped
>   6 garlic cloves, minced
>   1 teaspoon chopped fresh thyme
>   1 cup French lentils, picked over, rinsed, and drained
>   4 cups water
>   ¼ teaspoon smoked paprika
>   1 cup quinoa, rinsed
>   4 cups baby spinach
>   ¼ cup slow-roasted cashews (see page 97)
>   ¼ teaspoon freshly ground black pepper

Heat 1 tablespoon of the oil in a large nonstick skillet over medium-high heat. Add the mushrooms and ¼ teaspoon of the salt; cook, stirring occasionally, until the mushrooms are browned, 6 to 7 minutes. Transfer the mushrooms to a bowl and set aside.

Return the skillet to the stove and add the remaining 1 tablespoon oil. Stir in the onions, carrots, celery, garlic, and thyme; cook until tender and lightly browned, 6 to 7 minutes. Add the lentils, water, and paprika; bring to a boil, reduce the heat to medium-low, cover, and simmer until tender, 28 to 30 minutes.

Meanwhile, cook the quinoa according to the package directions.

Uncover the lentils and stir in the mushrooms, spinach, cashews, remaining ½ teaspoon salt, and the pepper. Serve over the quinoa.

Nutrient Content per Serving

Calories:	470	**Fat:**	13 grams	**Protein:**	20 grams
Fiber:	15 grams	**Saturated Fat:**	7 grams	**Carbs:**	73 grams
Sodium:	590 mg	**Sugars:**	9 grams		

Portobello Pizzas (Cycles 1/3)

You don't have to be a vegetarian to appreciate the dense, meaty texture of portobellos. They're a hefty, filling, low-calorie, and low-sugar alternative to the tired old greasy pizza crust. As a vegan alternative, mash 1 cup drained cannellini beans with 2 tablespoons olive oil to substitute for the ricotta cheese, and top with nut cheese instead of mozzarella.

Makes 4 servings

1 tablespoon olive oil, plus more for the pan

8 large portobello mushroom caps

¼ teaspoon sea salt

1 cup ricotta cheese

½ cup no-sugar-added prepared tomato sauce

8 fresh basil leaves

4 ounces fresh mozzarella, thinly sliced

Preheat the oven to 425°F. Lightly dampen a paper towel with a small amount of olive oil and wipe a large baking sheet.

With a spoon, scrape out and discard the dark brown gills from the mushrooms. Lightly brush the mushroom caps with the 1 tablespoon of oil and sprinkle with the salt. Set on the prepared baking sheet, gill-side up, and roast for 15 minutes. Turn the mushrooms over and cook until the caps are tender but still hold their shapes, 5 minutes longer. Remove from the oven and turn the caps over. Let cool for 5 minutes. Reduce the oven temperature to 350°F.

Top each mushroom cap with 2 tablespoons of the ricotta, 1 tablespoon of the tomato sauce, 1 basil leaf, and ½ ounce of the mozzarella. Place in the oven and bake until the cheese has melted, 5 minutes.

Nutrient Content per Serving

Calories:	280	**Fat:**	18 grams	**Protein:**	16 grams
Fiber:	3 grams	**Saturated Fat:**	10 grams	**Carbs:**	13 grams
Sodium:	240 mg	**Sugars:**	5 grams		

Quinoa Pasta alla Checca (Cycles 1/3)

Quinoa Pasta alla Checca is gorgeous in its simplicity. It lets the freshness of every ingredient take center stage and guarantees you'll never want to see another high-SI jar of marinara again. Be sure to look for quinoa pasta that's made without corn products, so you avoid issues with intolerance and high Sugar Impact. For a vegan version, omit the mozzarella and pecorino and sub in your favorite nut cheese.

Makes 4 servings

8 ounces gluten-free quinoa fusilli or other pasta shape

3 tablespoons extra-virgin olive oil

½ small garlic clove, minced

5 plum tomatoes, seeded and chopped

5 ounces fresh mozzarella cheese, cut into ½-inch cubes

¼ cup thinly sliced fresh basil leaves

2 tablespoons grated Pecorino Romano cheese

¾ teaspoon sea salt

¼ teaspoon freshly ground black pepper

Bring a large pot of lightly salted water to a boil over high heat. Add the pasta and cook according to the package directions; drain and transfer to a large bowl.

Add the oil, garlic, tomatoes, mozzarella, basil, pecorino, salt, and pepper to the pasta; toss well.

Nutrient Content per Serving

Calories:	420	**Fat:**	21 grams	**Protein:**	13 grams
Fiber:	5 grams	**Saturated Fat:**	7 grams	**Carbs:**	50 grams
Sodium:	550 mg	**Sugars:**	2 grams		

Easy Vegetarian White Chili

Proof that vegetarians and carnivores *can* find common ground! Cannellini beans (technically white kidney beans) are a filling source of fiber and protein, so no one is going to feel like they got robbed of a hearty meal just because this chili is sans meat. For a little creamy richness, top each serving with a tablespoon of unsweetened cultured coconut milk.

Makes 4 servings

1 cup dry quinoa, rinsed

2 tablespoons olive oil

2 medium onions, chopped

4 garlic cloves, minced

1 medium red bell pepper, chopped

1 medium green bell pepper, chopped

1 jalapeño pepper, seeded and finely chopped

1 tablespoon chili powder

2 teaspoons dried oregano

1 teaspoon ground coriander

½ teaspoon smoked paprika

2 (15-ounce) cans organic no-salt-added cannellini beans, drained and rinsed

2 cups Homemade Vegetable Stock (page 191) or low-sodium store-bought vegetable broth

¼ cup chopped fresh cilantro

¾ teaspoon sea salt

Cook the quinoa according to the package directions.

Meanwhile, heat the oil in a Dutch oven over medium-high heat. Add the onion, garlic, red and green bell peppers, and jalapeño; cook, stirring occasionally, until the vegetables are slightly softened, 4 to 5 minutes. Stir in the chili powder, oregano, coriander, and paprika; cook, stirring, for 1 minute. Add the beans and stock and bring the mixture to a boil. Cover, reduce the heat to medium-low, and simmer, stirring occasionally, until the vegetables are tender, 18 to 20 minutes. Remove from the heat and stir in the cilantro and salt. Divide the quinoa among four bowls and top each with one-quarter of the chili.

Nutrient Content per Serving

Calories:	380	**Fat:**	12 grams	**Protein:**	14 grams
Fiber:	12 grams	**Saturated Fat:**	1.5 grams	**Carbs:**	57 grams
Sodium:	510 mg	**Sugars:**	8 grams		

Spicy Black Bean Burgers with Goat Cheese and Wilted Tomato Salsa

Warm spices and tangy goat cheese are throwing a party for your taste buds! So toss out all those sad, flat, processed patties and rediscover the pure joy of this grown-up American burger with cheese. They can be made ahead and refrigerated for up to 8 hours before cooking. For a vegan version, substitute 1 vegan egg for the regular egg and omit the goat cheese. To make a vegan egg substitute, mix 3 tablespoons warm water with 1 tablespoon ground chia seeds and let stand until the mixture has the texture of a raw egg, about 10 minutes.

Makes 4 servings

   1 tablespoon olive oil, plus more for the pan

   ½ cup dry quinoa, rinsed

   1 (15-ounce) can organic no-salt-added black beans, drained and rinsed

   1 large egg

   1 teaspoon garlic powder

   ½ teaspoon ground cumin

   ¼ teaspoon red pepper flakes

   ¾ teaspoon sea salt

   ½ cup sliced shallots

   4 garlic cloves, sliced

   3 large plum tomatoes (about 1 pound), seeded and chopped

   2 teaspoons white wine vinegar

   3 tablespoons thinly sliced fresh basil leaves

   2 ounces goat cheese, crumbled

Preheat the oven to 375°F. Lightly dampen a paper towel with a small amount of olive oil and wipe a large baking sheet with it.

Cook the quinoa according to the package directions.

Place half of the beans in a bowl and mash with a fork. Stir in the remaining beans, cooked quinoa, egg, garlic powder, cumin, red pepper flakes, and ½ teaspoon of the salt. Mix well and let stand for 15 minutes.

Meanwhile, heat the 1 tablespoon of oil in a medium nonstick skillet over medium-high heat. Add the shallots and garlic and cook, stirring occasionally, until starting to brown, 3 to 4 minutes. Add the tomatoes and cook until wilted, about 2 minutes. Stir in the vinegar and cook for 30 seconds. Remove from the heat and stir in the basil and remaining ¼ teaspoon salt; set aside.

With slightly damp hands, form the bean mixture into eight patties, each about 3 inches in diameter. Place the patties on the prepared baking sheet. Bake for 10 minutes, then turn the patties over and bake for 7 minutes longer. Top each patty with some of the goat cheese and bake until the cheese melts slightly and the patties are crisp around the edges, 3 minutes. Serve the patties topped with the tomato mixture.

Nutrient Content per Serving

Calories:	450	**Fat:**	10 grams	**Protein:**	12 grams
Fiber:	8 grams	**Saturated Fat:**	3.5 grams	**Carbs:**	33 grams
Sodium:	600 mg	**Sugars:**	5 grams		

8

SOUPS AND STEWS

There's something about soup that's tied to an emotional experience. It's hard to think about soup without feeling warm, cozy, or über-satisfied. No matter what the weather (though, I admit, nothing beats warm soup on a chilly day!), soup is a unique way to bring together subtle flavors and the satisfying heft of a full meal.

The water base of soups and stews makes them hydrating right out of the gate (win!). I've also taken care to make sure these are packed with protein, to support your bone health and lean muscle mass. The high-fiber veggies and other nutrient-rich ingredients fuel your body's fat-burning and disease-fighting machinery, too.

The flavor of these soups is brought to life with herbs rather than a lot of added salt. Store-bought soups can be high in sodium, so my hope is that once you see how easy and satisfying it is to make your own, you'll never go back.

Turkey-Bean Chili with Crispy Coconut Wrap Strips

Perfect for a cool evening, this healthy and hearty chili will shower your palate with flavor with each savory bite. If turkey isn't for you, this chili works great with ground beef or bison. The addition of dark chocolate lends an additional layer of depth and richness.

Makes 4 servings

1 tablespoon olive oil

1 medium white onion, chopped

3 garlic cloves, minced

1 large green bell pepper, chopped

1 pound natural lean ground turkey

2 tablespoons chili powder

1 teaspoon smoked paprika

1 teaspoon ground ancho chili

1 teaspoon dried oregano

2 (14.5-ounce) cans no-salt-added fire-roasted diced tomatoes

1 (15-ounce) can organic no-salt-added small red beans, drained and rinsed

½ ounce 85% dark chocolate, crumbled

¾ teaspoon sea salt

¼ teaspoon freshly ground black pepper

1 coconut wrap (see box, page 79)

Heat 1 tablespoon of the oil in a Dutch oven over medium-high heat. Add the onion, garlic, and bell pepper; cook, stirring occasionally, until the vegetables begin to soften, 2 to 3 minutes. Add the turkey and cook, breaking it into smaller pieces, until no longer pink, 5 to 6 minutes. Stir in the chili powder, paprika, ancho chili, and oregano and cook for 1 minute. Add the tomatoes, bring to a boil, and immediately reduce the heat to medium-low; cover and simmer, stirring occasionally, for 30 minutes, or until slightly thickened.

Meanwhile, preheat the oven to 400°F.

Stir the beans into the pot and cook for 5 minutes longer. Remove from the heat and stir in the chocolate, salt, and pepper; keep warm.

Place a large baking sheet in the oven and heat for 3 minutes. Remove from the oven and place the coconut wrap on the baking sheet. Place in the oven and cook until the wrap is lightly browned, about 1 minute. Remove from the oven and transfer the wrap to a cutting board. Cut the wrap in half, then cut each half crosswise into thin strips. Divide the chili among four bowls and top each with some of the wrap strips.

Nutrient Content per Serving

Calories:	380	Fat:	16 grams	Protein:	27 grams
Fiber:	8 grams	Saturated Fat:	5 grams	Carbs:	31 grams
Sodium:	925 mg	Sugars:	9 grams		

Chicken Soup with Parsnips

Grandma was right—chicken soup is good for the soul! There's nothing better on a cold, blustery day, when all you can think about is getting back under the covers. This American favorite is satisfying and savory, with just a hint of sweetness. Keep it at the ready in your freezer for up to 6 months.

Makes 6 servings

6 cups Homemade Chicken Stock (page 194) or low-sodium store-bought chicken broth
1 (12-ounce) bone-in skin-on chicken breast half
2 (6-ounce) bone-in skin-on chicken thighs
1 tablespoon olive oil
2 medium onions, chopped
3 celery stalks, cut into ½-inch-thick slices
3 carrots, cut into ½-inch-thick slices
2 parsnips, peeled and cut into ½-inch-thick slices
8 sprigs fresh parsley
2 sprigs fresh thyme
1 bay leaf
3 cups baby kale
1 teaspoon sea salt
¼ teaspoon freshly ground black pepper

Combine the stock, chicken breast, and chicken thighs in a Dutch oven over medium-high heat. Bring the liquid to a boil, cover, reduce the heat to medium-low, and simmer until the chicken is cooked through, 20 minutes. Transfer the chicken to a bowl and let cool for 10 minutes; reserve the stock in the Dutch oven. When cool enough to handle, discard the skin and shred the chicken; set aside.

Heat the oil in a large nonstick skillet over medium heat. Add the onions, celery, carrots, and parsnips; cook, stirring occasionally, until slightly softened, 6 to 7 minutes. Transfer the mixture to the Dutch oven with the stock, then stir in the parsley, thyme, and bay leaf. Bring to a boil over medium-high heat; cover, reduce the heat to medium-low, and simmer for 20 minutes. Remove the parsley, thyme, and bay leaf, then add the chicken meat and cook until heated through, about 2 minutes. Stir in the kale and cook for 5 minutes. Remove from the heat and season with the salt and pepper.

Nutrient Content per Serving

Calories:	160	**Fat:**	5 grams	**Protein:**	14 grams
Fiber:	4 grams	**Saturated Fat:**	1 gram	**Carbs:**	16 grams
Sodium:	500 mg	**Sugars:**	4 grams		

Yellow Split Pea Soup

Creamy, versatile, and easy to prepare, this soup spotlights the mellow-flavored cousin of the green pea. Peas are loaded with protein, so you can count on this soup to hold you over until your next meal. If a thinner soup is desired, add an additional cup of vegetable broth or water to the finished soup.

Makes 4 servings

1 tablespoon olive oil
2 medium onions, chopped
2 celery stalks, chopped
2 carrots, chopped
3 garlic cloves, minced
2 teaspoons fresh thyme leaves
1 bay leaf
¾ teaspoon ground cumin
½ teaspoon dried basil
8 ounces yellow split peas (about 1 cup)
5 cups Homemade Vegetable Stock (page 191) or low-sodium store-bought vegetable broth
½ cup water
¾ teaspoon sea salt
¼ teaspoon freshly ground black pepper

Heat the oil in a Dutch oven over medium heat. Add the onions, celery, carrots, garlic, thyme, bay leaf, cumin, and basil; cook, stirring occasionally, until tender, 9 to 10 minutes. Increase the heat to medium-high and stir in the split peas, stock, and water. Bring to a boil, reduce the heat to medium-low, cover, and simmer until tender, about 1 hour. Remove from the heat and let cool for 10 minutes. Remove the bay leaf, if desired, but it is not necessary. Working in batches, transfer the soup to a blender and puree. Return the pureed soup to the pot and stir in the salt and pepper.

Nutrient Content per Serving

Calories:	320	**Fat:**	9 grams	**Protein:**	14 grams
Fiber:	21 grams	**Saturated Fat:**	1 gram	**Carbs:**	48 grams
Sodium:	490 mg	**Sugars:**	6 grams		

Manhattan Clam Chowder

New Englander purists may not approve of this variation on a classic, but there's no denying that it's found its zesty place on menus everywhere. No need to hit the beach for a clam dig—fresh from the grocer is perfect; otherwise, substitute 2 (6.5-ounce) cans chopped clams (drain the juice). Manhattan clam chowder, unlike its New England cousin, is made without cream or butter, so it's significantly lighter, but no less satisfying.

Makes 4 servings

> 6 slices nitrate-free uncured bacon, chopped
> 3 celery stalks, finely chopped
> 3 medium carrots, finely chopped
> 3 garlic cloves, minced
> 1 onion, finely chopped
> 1 teaspoon dried oregano
> ½ teaspoon dried thyme
> 1½ cups diced butternut squash
> 1 bay leaf
> 1 (8-ounce) bottle clam juice
> 1 (14.5-ounce) can organic no-salt-added petite diced tomatoes
> 1 cup chopped fresh clams

Heat a Dutch oven over medium heat. Add the bacon and cook, stirring occasionally, until starting to brown, 4 to 5 minutes. Add the celery, carrots, garlic, onion, oregano, and thyme; cook, stirring occasionally, until the vegetables are starting to soften, 4 to 5 minutes. Add the butternut squash, bay leaf, clam juice, and tomatoes; bring to a simmer, cover, and reduce the heat to medium-low. Cook until the vegetables are tender, 18 to 20 minutes. Stir in the clams and cook for 5 minutes longer. Remove the bay leaf from the soup. Ladle into four bowls and serve.

Nutrient Content per Serving

Calories:	140	**Fat:**	4 grams	**Protein:**	7 grams
Fiber:	5 grams	**Saturated Fat:**	1.5 grams	**Carbs:**	19 grams
Sodium:	510 mg	**Sugars:**	5 grams		

Roasted Chicken and Vegetable Soup

There's chicken soup, and there's *chicken soup*. This is clearly the latter. Roasting the chicken and vegetables give this soup a deeper, richer flavor than regular chicken soup.

Makes 4 servings

1 tablespoon olive oil, plus more for the pan

2 medium onions, chopped

3 carrots, chopped

3 celery stalks, chopped

3 leeks, white and light green parts only, chopped

1½ pounds bone-in skin-on chicken thighs

6 cups Homemade Chicken Stock (page 194) or low-sodium store-bought chicken broth

5 sprigs fresh parsley

5 sprigs fresh dill

1 bay leaf

¾ teaspoon sea salt

¼ teaspoon freshly ground black pepper

Preheat the oven to 425°F. Lightly dampen a paper towel with olive oil and wipe two rimmed baking sheets with it.

Combine the tablespoon of oil, onions, carrots, celery, and leeks in a large bowl. Spread the vegetables on one of the prepared baking sheets. Place the chicken on the second baking sheet. Set the baking sheets in the oven; roast the chicken until a thermometer inserted into the thickest portion registers 165°F, about 25 minutes. Remove the chicken from the oven and set aside. Continue to roast the vegetables, stirring occasionally, until browned, about 10 minutes longer. Transfer the vegetables to a Dutch oven. Pour 1 cup of the chicken stock onto the baking sheet used to roast the vegetables and scrape up any browned bits; add the stock to the Dutch oven. Add the remaining 5 cups stock, the parsley, dill, and bay leaf. Bring to a boil over medium-high heat; reduce the heat to medium-low, cover, and simmer for 35 minutes. Discard the parsley, dill, and bay leaf.

Meanwhile, remove the skin from the chicken and discard all but one. Remove the chicken meat from the bones and coarsely chop. Stir the meat, salt, and pepper into the Dutch oven and cook until hot, 3 to 4 minutes longer. Ladle the soup into serving bowls. Cut the reserved chicken skin into thin strips and top each bowl with some of the skin.

Nutrient Content per Serving

Calories:	370	**Fat:**	20 grams	**Protein:**	27 grams
Fiber:	5 grams	**Saturated Fat:**	5 grams	**Carbs:**	22 grams
Sodium:	600 mg	**Sugars:**	6 grams		

Creamy Cauliflower Soup

This is comfort food, plain and simple—delicious and soothing. Cauliflower is often overlooked, but it's packed with B vitamins and antioxidants. For more of a pure, milder cauliflower-flavored soup, use all water instead of the vegetable broth.

Makes 4 servings

- 2 tablespoons olive oil
- 1 medium onion, chopped
- 2 celery stalks, chopped
- 1 carrot, chopped
- 1 teaspoon fresh thyme leaves
- 1 (2¼- to 2½-pound) head cauliflower, cut into florets
- 4 cups Homemade Vegetable Stock (page 191) or low-sodium store-bought vegetable broth
- 1½ cups water
- ¾ teaspoon sea salt

Heat the oil in a large pot over medium heat. Add the onion, celery, carrot, and thyme; cook, stirring occasionally, until tender but not browned, 12 to 14 minutes. Add the cauliflower, vegetable stock, and water; increase the heat to medium-high and bring to a boil. Reduce the heat to medium-low, cover, and simmer until the cauliflower is tender, 18 to 20 minutes. Uncover the pot; increase the heat to medium and simmer for 10 minutes longer. Remove from the heat and let cool for 10 minutes.

Working in batches, if necessary, transfer the soup to a blender and puree. Return the soup to the pot and let stand for 15 minutes. Reheat the soup over medium heat, 3 to 4 minutes. Season with the salt.

Nutrient Content per Serving

Calories:	190	**Fat:**	11 grams	**Protein:**	6 grams
Fiber:	8 grams	**Saturated Fat:**	1.5 grams	**Carbs:**	21 grams
Sodium:	560 mg	**Sugars:**	8 grams		

Onion-Mushroom Soup

Traditionally made with beef broth, I've transformed this hearty soup into a vegan-friendly bowl of goodness by using vegetable broth instead. And just like icing on a cake, the mushrooms add a good dose of umami to this classic.

Makes 4 servings

1 tablespoon Malaysian red palm fruit oil

1½ pounds onions, thinly sliced

1 pound white mushrooms, sliced

½ teaspoon monk fruit extract

1 tablespoon arrowroot powder

5 cups Homemade Vegetable Stock (page 191) or low-sodium store-bought vegetable broth

1 tablespoon low-sodium wheat-free tamari or coconut aminos

1 teaspoon chopped fresh thyme

1 bay leaf

½ teaspoon sea salt

¼ teaspoon freshly ground black pepper

Heat the oil in a large pot over medium heat. Add the onions, mushrooms, and monk fruit extract; cook, stirring occasionally, until the onions are soft and golden and the mushrooms are browned, 35 to 40 minutes. Add the arrowroot and cook for 1 minute. Stir in the stock, tamari, thyme, and bay leaf. Increase the heat to medium-high and bring to a boil. Reduce the heat to medium and simmer, uncovered, for 30 minutes. Remove the bay leaf and season with the salt and pepper.

Nutrient Content per Serving

Calories:	170	**Fat:**	8 grams	**Protein:**	4 grams
Fiber:	3 grams	**Saturated Fat:**	2.5 grams	**Carbs:**	23 grams
Sodium:	490 mg	**Sugars:**	8 grams		

Beans and Greens Stew

Beans and greens are a classic culinary dynamic duo (and it's fun to say!). This stew is warming and nutrient rich, but to make it even heartier, serve it over red quinoa or wild rice.

Makes 4 servings

- 2 tablespoons olive oil
- 2 medium onions, chopped
- 3 celery stalks, cut into ¾-inch pieces
- 2 medium leeks, white and light green parts only, chopped
- 6 garlic cloves, minced
- 1 tablespoon chopped fresh oregano
- 1 teaspoon ground coriander
- 1 (14.5-ounce) can no-salt-added fire-roasted diced tomatoes
- 3 cups Homemade Vegetable Stock (page 191) or low-sodium store-bought vegetable broth
- 2 (15-ounce) cans organic no-salt-added cannellini beans, drained and rinsed
- 6 cups baby spinach
- ½ cup sliced fresh basil leaves
- ¾ teaspoon sea salt
- ¼ teaspoon freshly ground black pepper

Heat the oil in a Dutch oven over medium-high heat. Add the onions, celery, leeks, garlic, oregano, and coriander; cook, stirring occasionally, until the vegetables are slightly softened, 5 to 6 minutes. Stir in the tomatoes and cook for 5 minutes. Add the stock and beans and bring to a boil. Reduce the heat to medium-low, cover, and simmer for 20 minutes. Stir in the spinach until wilted, about 2 minutes. Remove from the heat and stir in the basil, salt, and pepper.

Nutrient Content per Serving

Calories:	290	**Fat:**	11 grams	**Protein:**	9 grams
Fiber:	11 grams	**Saturated Fat:**	1.5 grams	**Carbs:**	43 grams
Sodium:	725 mg	**Sugars:**	8 grams		

Beef Bourguignon (Cycles 1/3)

Most Americans have Julia Child to thank for introducing us to beef bourguignon (thank you, Julia!). I hope you have as much fun making this traditional French stew as the master did in her iconic kitchen. For the best flavor, use a full-bodied red wine such as Cabernet Sauvignon, Merlot, or Syrah.

Makes 4 servings

1 pound chuck roast, trimmed and cut into 1-inch cubes

¾ teaspoon sea salt

½ teaspoon freshly ground black pepper

2 tablespoons olive oil

1 large onion, coarsely chopped (about 1½ cups)

8 ounces white mushrooms, sliced

1 tablespoon fresh thyme leaves

2 celery stalks, cut into 1-inch pieces

2 carrots, cut into ¾-inch pieces

5 garlic cloves, minced

¾ cup dry red wine

¼ cup tomato paste

2 cups Homemade Chicken Stock (page 194) or low-sodium store-bought chicken broth

2 cups butternut squash cubes (about 8 ounces)

Season the beef with ¼ teaspoon of the salt and ¼ teaspoon of the pepper in a medium bowl.

Heat 1 tablespoon of the oil in a Dutch oven over medium-high heat. Add the beef and cook, turning occasionally, until browned, 5 to 6 minutes. Transfer to a plate.

Return the Dutch oven to the stove and heat the remaining 1 tablespoon oil over medium heat. Add the onion, mushrooms, and thyme and cook, stirring occasionally, until slightly browned, 8 to 9 minutes. Stir in the celery, carrots, and garlic; cook until starting to soften, 4 to 5 minutes. Stir in the wine and tomato paste and bring to a boil; cook for 1 minute. Add the broth and browned beef; return to a boil, immediately reduce the heat to medium-low, cover, and gently simmer for 40 minutes, until the beef is nearly tender. Stir in the butternut squash, return to a gentle simmer, and cook until the beef and squash are tender, 18 to 20 minutes longer. Remove from the heat and stir in the remaining ½ teaspoon salt and ¼ teaspoon pepper.

Nutrient Content per Serving

Calories:	520	**Fat:**	29 grams	**Protein:**	37 grams
Fiber:	4 grams	**Saturated Fat:**	10 grams	**Carbs:**	22 grams
Sodium:	570 mg	**Sugars:**	9 grams		

Chicken and Okra Stew over Quinoa

If you're like me, okra makes you think of the South, and those old-timey Southern comfort foods. Okra is versatile and takes on the characteristics of whatever it's cooked with, so you can imagine how tasty and soothing it is when it's stewed with tomatoes!

Makes 4 servings

- 1 cup dry quinoa, rinsed
- 5 teaspoons coconut oil
- 1 pound boneless skinless chicken thighs, cut into 1-inch pieces
- ¾ teaspoon sea salt
- ¼ teaspoon freshly ground black pepper
- 1 medium onion, chopped
- 2 celery stalks, chopped
- 1 orange bell pepper, chopped
- 4 garlic cloves, minced
- 1 jalapeño pepper, finely chopped
- 1 teaspoon chopped fresh thyme
- 1 teaspoon dried oregano
- 12 ounces okra, cut into 1-inch pieces
- 1 (14.5-ounce) can no-salt-added diced tomatoes
- 2 cups Homemade Chicken Stock (page 194) or low-sodium store-bought chicken broth

Cook the quinoa according to the package directions.

Heat 2 teaspoons of the oil in a Dutch oven over medium-high heat. Season the chicken with ¼ teaspoon of the salt and ⅛ teaspoon of the black pepper; add half of the chicken to the Dutch oven and cook until browned, 4 minutes. Transfer to a plate. Repeat with 1 teaspoon of the oil and the remaining chicken.

Heat the remaining 2 teaspoons oil in the Dutch oven over medium-high heat. Add the onion, celery, bell pepper, garlic, jalapeño, thyme, and oregano; cook, stirring occasionally, until slightly softened, 3 to 4 minutes. Add the okra and cook for 1 minute. Add the tomatoes and cook for 5 minutes. Pour in the stock, bring to a boil, cover, reduce the heat to medium-low, and simmer until the okra is tender and the chicken is cooked through, 20 to 22 minutes. Season with the remaining ½ teaspoon salt and ⅛ teaspoon black pepper. Serve over the quinoa.

Nutrient Content per Serving

Calories:	450	**Fat:**	18 grams	**Protein:**	37 grams
Fiber:	6 grams	**Saturated Fat:**	8 grams	**Carbs:**	35 grams
Sodium:	540 mg	**Sugars:**	1 gram		

Indian-Style Lentil Soup

Lentil soup (or dal) is a humble, nurturing Indian staple. But don't let its appearance fool you—it's a great source of protein, fiber, B vitamins, iron, and zinc. This soup is also brimming with aromatic and flavorful spices like Madras curry powder, which is a spicy-hot curry. For a milder soup, use a generic curry powder.

Makes 6 servings

- 1 tablespoon coconut oil
- 2 medium onions, chopped
- 2 carrots, chopped
- 2 celery stalks, chopped
- 1 tablespoon minced fresh ginger
- 3 garlic cloves, minced
- 1 tablespoon Madras curry powder
- ½ teaspoon ground coriander
- 2 cups red split lentils
- 6 cups Homemade Vegetable Stock (page 191) or low-sodium store-bought vegetable broth
- 1 tablespoon lime juice
- ¾ teaspoon sea salt

Heat the oil in a Dutch oven over medium heat. Add the onions, carrots, celery, ginger, and garlic; cook until softened, 8 to 9 minutes. Add the curry powder and coriander; cook, stirring, until fragrant, 30 seconds. Stir in the lentils and cook for 30 seconds. Add the stock and increase the heat to medium-high; bring to a boil, cover, and reduce the heat to medium-low. Simmer until the soup has thickened and the lentils are very tender, 23 to 25 minutes. Remove from the heat and stir in the lime juice and salt.

Nutrient Content per Serving

Calories:	310	**Fat:**	7 grams	**Protein:**	18 grams
Fiber:	12 grams	**Saturated Fat:**	2.5 grams	**Carbs:**	46 grams
Sodium:	340 mg	**Sugars:**	5 grams		

Pork and Mushroom Stew with Sweet Potatoes (Cycles 1/3)

Pork tenderloin is high in protein, low in fat, and is packed with more B vitamins than many other types of meat. It's also very lean, so be careful not to cook the stew longer than specified, or the meat will be tough.

Makes 4 servings

> 2 tablespoons olive oil
>
> 1½ pounds pork tenderloin, trimmed and cut into 1-inch pieces
>
> ¾ teaspoon sea salt
>
> ½ teaspoon freshly ground black pepper
>
> 4 teaspoons arrowroot powder
>
> 2 medium red onions, chopped
>
> 8 ounces white mushrooms, sliced
>
> 1 teaspoon dried basil
>
> 4 garlic cloves, minced
>
> 2 celery stalks, cut into ¾-inch pieces
>
> 2 carrots, cut into ¾-inch pieces
>
> 3 cups Homemade Chicken Stock (page 194) or low-sodium store-bought chicken broth
>
> 3 tablespoons tomato paste
>
> 12 ounces sweet potatoes, peeled and cut into ½-inch pieces

Heat 2 teaspoons of the oil in a Dutch oven over medium-high heat. Combine the pork with ¼ teaspoon of the salt and ¼ teaspoon of the pepper in a large bowl. Add the arrowroot and toss well to coat. Add half of the pork to the Dutch oven and cook until browned, turning occasionally, 5 to 6 minutes; transfer to a plate. Repeat with 2 teaspoons oil and the remaining pork.

Heat the remaining 2 teaspoons oil in the Dutch oven over medium-high heat. Add the onions, mushrooms, basil, and ¼ teaspoon of the salt; cook, stirring occasionally, until the mushrooms are tender, 6 to 7 minutes. Add the garlic and cook for 2 minutes. Stir in the celery and carrots; cook until the vegetables are starting to soften slightly, 3 to 4 minutes. Add the stock and tomato paste; bring to a boil and cook for 2 minutes. Stir in the pork and any juices that have accumulated on the plate. Return to a boil, cover, reduce the heat to medium-low, and simmer for 10 minutes. Add the sweet potatoes and simmer until tender, 8 to 10 minutes longer. Season with the remaining ¼ teaspoon salt and ¼ teaspoon pepper.

Nutrient Content per Serving

Calories:	400	**Fat:**	11 grams	**Protein:**	40 grams
Fiber:	6 grams	**Saturated Fat:**	2 grams	**Carbs:**	36 grams
Sodium:	670 mg	**Sugars:**	9 grams		

Roasted Onion Gazpacho with Shrimp

Don't let cold soup scare you! This popular tomato-based Spanish soup is really refreshing, especially on hot, humid summer afternoons. Roasting the onions gives it a deep, rich flavor.

Serves 4

3 teaspoons olive oil, plus more for the pan

1 large red onion, chopped

1 pound extra-large shrimp, peeled and deveined

¾ teaspoon sea salt

1¼ pounds plum tomatoes, seeded and chopped

1 seedless cucumber, peeled and finely chopped

1 medium red bell pepper, finely chopped

1 garlic clove, minced

1 jalapeño pepper, finely chopped

1½ cups ice water

1½ tablespoons lemon juice

1 tablespoon extra-virgin olive oil

¼ cup chopped fresh basil, plus additional whole leaves, for garnish

2 teaspoons red wine vinegar

¼ teaspoon freshly ground black pepper

Preheat the oven to 425°F. Lightly dampen a paper towel with olive oil and wipe a rimmed baking sheet with it.

Combine the onion with 1 teaspoon of the olive oil in a small bowl. Transfer to the prepared baking sheet; bake until lightly browned, stirring occasionally, 18 to 20 minutes. Remove from the oven.

Meanwhile, heat the remaining 2 teaspoons olive oil in a large nonstick skillet over medium-high heat. Season the shrimp with ¼ teaspoon of the salt and add to the skillet; cook, turning once, until lightly browned and opaque, 2 to 2½ minutes per side. Transfer to a plate and let cool. Cover with plastic wrap and refrigerate until ready to serve.

Combine the roasted onion, tomatoes, cucumber, bell pepper, garlic, jalapeño, ice water, and lemon juice in a large bowl. Transfer 3 cups of the mixture to a blender and puree. Pour the pureed soup back into the bowl and combine with the unpureed vegetables. Stir in the extra-virgin olive oil, basil, vinegar, remaining ½ teaspoon salt, and the black pepper. Cover with plastic wrap and chill for at least 2 hours.

Remove the soup from the refrigerator and ladle it into four large bowls. Top each bowl with one-quarter of the shrimp, garnish with basil leaves, and serve immediately.

Nutrient Content per Serving

Calories:	190	**Fat:**	8 grams	**Protein:**	14 grams
Fiber:	4 grams	**Saturated Fat:**	1 gram	**Carbs:**	16 grams
Sodium:	930 mg	**Sugars:**	6 grams		

Salmon Bouillabaisse

Bouillabaisse is a traditional stew originally made by fishermen in Marseille, in the south of France. Recipes for bouillabaisse vary, but the two key elements are always saffron and tomatoes.

Makes 4 servings

2 tablespoons olive oil
1 large onion, chopped (about 1½ cups)
2 garlic cloves, minced
1 medium fennel bulb, cored and chopped
3 large plum tomatoes, seeded and chopped
¼ teaspoon saffron threads, lightly crushed
2 cups Homemade Chicken Stock (page 194) or low-sodium store-bought chicken broth
1 (8-ounce) bottle clam juice
1 (1-pound) skinless salmon fillet, cut into 12 pieces
12 ounces extra-large shrimp, peeled and deveined

Heat the oil in a Dutch oven over medium heat. Add the onion and garlic; cook, stirring occasionally, until the onion starts to soften, 2 to 3 minutes. Add the fennel, tomatoes, and saffron; cook until the vegetables have softened, 8 to 9 minutes. Increase the heat to medium-high and add the stock and clam juice. Bring the mixture to a boil, reduce the heat to medium, and simmer, uncovered, for 20 minutes. Add the salmon and shrimp and cook until the fish flakes easily with a fork and the shrimp are opaque, 6 to 7 minutes. Divide among four bowls and serve.

Nutrient Content per Serving

Calories:	390	**Fat:**	21 grams	**Protein:**	37 grams
Fiber:	3 grams	**Saturated Fat:**	3 grams	**Carbs:**	13 grams
Sodium:	690 mg	**Sugars:**	4 grams		

Winter Vegetable Minestrone

The beauty of this thick Italian soup is that it's like a soup canvas—it has no standard recipe. But this version is so flavorful, you may never want to make it any other way again. Freeze in individual portions for up to 6 months.

Makes 4 servings

2 tablespoons olive oil

1 medium onion, chopped

2 carrots, cut into ¾-inch pieces

2 celery stalks, cut into ¾-inch pieces

2 medium leeks, white and light green parts only, chopped

1 pound butternut squash, peeled, seeded, and cut into 1-inch pieces

3 garlic cloves, minced

1 tablespoon chopped fresh oregano

1 teaspoon chopped fresh thyme

4 cups Homemade Vegetable Stock (page 191) or low-sodium store-bought vegetable broth

1 (14.5-ounce) can no-salt-added diced tomatoes

4 cups coarsely chopped kale

1 (15-ounce) can organic no-salt-added cannellini beans, drained and rinsed

½ teaspoon sea salt

¼ teaspoon freshly ground black pepper

Heat the oil in a Dutch oven over medium-high heat. Add the onion, carrots, celery, leeks, squash, garlic, oregano, and thyme; cook, stirring occasionally, until the vegetables are starting to soften, 4 to 5 minutes. Stir in the stock, tomatoes, and kale; bring to a boil. Reduce the heat to medium-low, cover, and simmer until the vegetables are tender, 25 minutes. Add the beans, return to a simmer, and cook for 5 minutes longer. Remove from the heat and stir in the salt and pepper.

Nutrient Content per Serving

Calories:	300	**Fat:**	12 grams	**Protein:**	9 grams
Fiber:	11 grams	**Saturated Fat:**	1.5 grams	**Carbs:**	42 grams
Sodium:	440 mg	**Sugars:**	6 grams		

9

SIDES

Dismiss sides at your peril! They play a major role in your health and fast fat loss, and for a refresher on how highly I regard them, refer to the space I've given them on the Sugar Impact Plate.

In fact, nonstarchy veggie sides do so much to lower your SI and fuel your fat loss that you may recall I said you could have as many as you want (I dare you to try to OD on asparagus). Sides can also introduce elegant flavors and nutrients that offset the Main on your plate. I mean, chicken has its place, but Lemony Roasted Artichoke Hearts (page 170)? Come on!

VEGGIE SIDES

Sautéed Sugar Snaps and Radishes with Fresh Parsley and Orange Zest

Look for prepacked bags of "stringless" sugar snap peas—it will save you tons of time. Otherwise, you'll have to remove the tips and tough vein from each one (no thanks!). Serve these warm or at room temperature.

Makes 4 servings

1 tablespoon macadamia nut oil

1 medium red onion, thinly sliced

2 garlic cloves, minced

12 ounces stringless sugar snap peas

4 radishes, sliced

2 tablespoons chopped fresh parsley

2 teaspoons grated orange zest

¼ teaspoon sea salt

⅛ teaspoon freshly ground black pepper

Heat the oil in a large nonstick skillet over medium-high heat. Add the onion and cook until slightly softened, 2 to 3 minutes. Add the garlic and cook for 2 minutes longer. Stir in the sugar snap peas and cook until bright green, 3 minutes. Add the radishes and cook until just starting to soften, 2 minutes. Remove from the heat and stir in the parsley, orange zest, salt, and pepper.

Nutrient Content per Serving

Calories:	80	**Fat:**	3.5 grams	**Protein:**	2 grams
Fiber:	2 grams	**Saturated Fat:**	0 grams	**Carbs:**	9 grams
Sodium:	150 mg	**Sugars:**	3 grams		

Just Grilled Asparagus

Asparagus is packed with powerful anti-inflammatory nutrients and a wide variety of antioxidants, including vitamin C, beta-carotene, and vitamin E. It's also more perishable than other vegetables, which makes it more likely to lose water and wrinkle. When buying asparagus, look for firm, straight stalks and make sure the crowns have not gone to flower (gotten little bumps).

Makes 4 servings

1 pound asparagus, trimmed

1 tablespoon Malaysian red palm fruit oil

¼ teaspoon sea salt

⅛ teaspoon freshly ground black pepper

Preheat a grill pan over medium-high heat.

Toss the asparagus with the oil, salt, and pepper in a medium bowl. Place the asparagus on the grill pan and cook, turning occasionally, until marked and crisp-tender, 5 to 6 minutes. Serve warm or at room temperature.

Nutrient Content per Serving

Calories:	50	**Fat:**	3.5 grams	**Protein:**	3 grams
Fiber:	2 grams	**Saturated Fat:**	2 grams	**Carbs:**	4 grams
Sodium:	150 mg	**Sugars:**	2 grams		

Marjoram Seared Mushrooms

A truly delicious side. Common white mushrooms have a great flavor when they brown or "caramelize" in a skillet. The trick is to cook them long enough so they release their liquid; sprinkle them with a little salt when you add them to the skillet to speed up the process.

Makes 4 servings

>   2 tablespoons olive oil
>   1 medium onion, chopped
>   1 pound white mushrooms, sliced
>   1 tablespoon chopped fresh marjoram
>   ¼ teaspoon plus ⅛ teaspoon sea salt
>   ¼ teaspoon freshly ground black pepper

Heat the oil in a large nonstick skillet over medium-high heat. Add the onion and cook until starting to soften, 2 to 3 minutes. Stir in the mushrooms, marjoram, and ¼ teaspoon of the salt; cook, stirring occasionally, until the mushrooms are browned, 7 to 8 minutes. Remove from the heat and stir in the remaining ⅛ teaspoon salt and the pepper.

Nutrient Content per Serving

Calories:	100	**Fat:**	7 grams	**Protein:**	2 grams
Fiber:	1 gram	**Saturated Fat:**	1 gram	**Carbs:**	7 grams
Sodium:	230 mg	**Sugars:**	4 grams		

Shredded Brussels Sprouts with Easy Lemon Vinaigrette

Brussels sprouts are nutrient powerhouses that have the ability to help us detox, and they may even protect against cancer. Thinly slicing Brussels sprouts gives them a sweeter, nuttier flavor when they cook.

Makes 4 servings

  1 tablespoon olive oil

  1 medium red onion, thinly sliced

  4 garlic cloves, sliced

  1½ pounds Brussels sprouts, very thinly sliced

  2 tablespoons slow-roasted almonds (see page 97), chopped

  3 tablespoons Easy Lemon Vinaigrette (page 193)

  ¼ teaspoon sea salt

  ⅛ teaspoon freshly ground black pepper

Heat the oil in a large nonstick skillet over medium-high heat. Add the onion and garlic and cook, stirring occasionally, until slightly softened, 2 to 3 minutes. Add the Brussels sprouts and cook, stirring occasionally, until crisp-tender and lightly browned, 7 to 8 minutes. Add the almonds and cook for 1 minute longer. Remove from the heat and stir in the vinaigrette, salt, and pepper.

Nutrient Content per Serving

Calories:	210	**Fat:**	13 grams	**Protein:**	6 grams
Fiber:	7 grams	**Saturated Fat:**	1.5 grams	**Carbs:**	17 grams
Sodium:	310 mg	**Sugars:**	5 grams		

Steamed Broccoli with Garlic Oil Drizzle

You'll never dismiss this as boring ol' broccoli—the drizzle makes it sizzle! Plus, steaming the broccoli actually makes it more digestible. Whole stalks of broccoli (not just the florets) and broccoli rabe (rapini) make great substitutes, too.

Makes 4 servings

  8 cups broccoli florets

  2 tablespoons extra-virgin olive oil

  5 garlic cloves, thinly sliced

  ⅛ teaspoon red pepper flakes

  1 tablespoon grated lemon zest

  ¼ teaspoon sea salt

Bring a large pot of lightly salted water to a boil over high heat.

Add the broccoli to the pot, return to a boil, and cook for 1 minute. Drain in a colander, then transfer to a large bowl and set aside.

Heat the oil in a large nonstick skillet over medium heat. Add the garlic and red pepper flakes and cook until the garlic just starts to brown around the edges, 2 to 3 minutes. Pour the mixture over the broccoli and stir in the lemon zest and salt; toss well. Serve warm or at room temperature.

Nutrient Content per Serving

Calories:	110	**Fat:**	7 grams	**Protein:**	4 grams
Fiber:	5 grams	**Saturated Fat:**	1 gram	**Carbs:**	9 grams
Sodium:	180 mg	**Sugars:**	0 grams		

Braised Escarole with Pecorino

Escarole is slightly less bitter than other endives and can also be eaten raw. If you're dairy intolerant, omit the cheese and increase the salt by ⅛ teaspoon, if you so desire. As a vegan alternative, omit the cheese and use Homemade Vegetable Stock (page 191) or low-sodium store-bought vegetable broth.

Makes 4 servings

2 tablespoons extra-virgin olive oil
4 garlic cloves, thinly sliced
⅛ teaspoon red pepper flakes
1 head escarole (1½ pounds), trimmed and washed
½ cup Homemade Chicken Stock (page 194) or low-sodium store-bought chicken broth
1 tablespoon grated Pecorino Romano cheese
¼ teaspoon sea salt

Heat the oil in a large nonstick skillet over medium heat. Add the garlic and red pepper flakes; cook, stirring occasionally, until the garlic just starts to brown, 1½ to 2 minutes. Add the escarole and cook, stirring often, until it begins to wilt, 2 to 3 minutes. Pour in the stock, cover, and cook, stirring occasionally, until the escarole is tender, 7 to 8 minutes. Remove from the heat and stir in the cheese and salt.

Nutrient Content per Serving

Calories:	90	**Fat:**	8 grams	**Protein:**	2 grams
Fiber:	4 grams	**Saturated Fat:**	1.5 grams	**Carbs:**	5 grams
Sodium:	200 mg	**Sugars:**	0 grams		

Grilled Endive with Shallot-Bacon Vinaigrette

Grilling is a simple way to elevate the presence of the crispy endive, and the rich flavor of the vinaigrette helps counter its bitter flavor.

Makes 4 servings

2 slices nitrate-free uncured bacon
2 tablespoons chopped shallots
5 teaspoons walnut oil
2 teaspoons white wine vinegar
½ teaspoon Dijon mustard
¼ teaspoon sea salt
⅛ teaspoon freshly ground black pepper
1 teaspoon olive oil, plus more for the pan
6 endives, halved lengthwise

Heat a small nonstick skillet over medium heat. Add the bacon and cook, turning once, until crisp, 6 to 7 minutes. Transfer to a plate lined with a paper towel to drain. Return the skillet to the heat and add the shallots; cook, stirring, for 30 seconds. Remove the skillet from the heat and whisk in the walnut oil, vinegar, mustard, salt, and pepper. Immediately transfer to a small bowl and set aside.

Lightly brush the endives with the 1 teaspoon of olive oil. Lightly dampen a paper towel with a small amount of olive oil and wipe a grill pan with it; heat over medium-high heat. Add the endives and cook, turning once, until nicely marked and starting to wilt, 6 minutes. Transfer to a platter and spoon the reserved vinaigrette and bacon over the endive.

Nutrient Content per Serving

Calories:	100	**Fat:**	9 grams	**Protein:**	2 grams
Fiber:	2 grams	**Saturated Fat:**	1 gram	**Carbs:**	4 grams
Sodium:	200 mg	**Sugars:**	0 grams		

Italian-Style Peppers and Onion Sauté

Like most Italian food, this will make a flavorful statement on your plate. And it can certainly hold its own just as it is. But to make your dinner feel like a night out in the comfort of your own home, make it restaurant style by adding some sautéed sweet or hot Italian turkey sausage.

Makes 4 servings

- 2 tablespoons olive oil
- 1 medium onion, sliced
- 2 garlic cloves, minced
- ½ teaspoon dried basil
- ½ teaspoon dried oregano
- 2 red bell peppers, thinly sliced
- 1 green bell pepper, thinly sliced
- 1 tablespoon red wine vinegar
- ¼ teaspoon sea salt
- ⅛ teaspoon freshly ground black pepper

Heat the oil in a large nonstick skillet over medium-high heat. Add the onion and cook until slightly softened, 3 to 4 minutes. Stir in the garlic, basil, and oregano and cook for 1 minute. Add the bell peppers and vinegar and cook, stirring occasionally, until the onion has browned and the peppers are tender, 8 to 9 minutes. Remove from the heat and season with the salt and black pepper.

Nutrient Content per Serving

Calories:	100	**Fat:**	7 grams	**Protein:**	1 gram
Fiber:	3 grams	**Saturated Fat:**	1 gram	**Carbs:**	9 grams
Sodium:	160 mg	**Sugars:**	3 grams		

Lemony Roasted Artichoke Hearts

Artichokes are a rich source of fiber and the antioxidant vitamin C. After your artichoke hearts have thawed, pat them dry with paper towels before tossing with oil to help them brown a little better.

Makes 4 servings

- 2 tablespoons olive oil, plus more for the pan
- 2 (9-ounce) boxes frozen artichoke hearts, thawed
- ¼ teaspoon sea salt
- ⅛ teaspoon freshly ground black pepper
- 2 teaspoons grated lemon zest
- 1 teaspoon lemon juice

Preheat the oven to 450°F. Lightly dampen a paper towel with a small amount of olive oil and wipe a large rimmed baking sheet with it.

Combine the 2 tablespoons of oil, artichoke hearts, salt, and pepper in a large bowl and toss to coat. Place the artichoke hearts on the prepared baking sheet and roast, stirring occasionally, until browned and tender, 22 to 23 minutes. Transfer to a bowl and toss with the lemon zest and lemon juice.

Nutrient Content per Serving

Calories:	120	**Fat:**	8 grams	**Protein:**	3 grams
Fiber:	8 grams	**Saturated Fat:**	1 gram	**Carbs:**	11 grams
Sodium:	230 mg	**Sugars:**	0 grams		

Roasted Zucchini and Bell Pepper Medley

Who doesn't love a good medley? I have to say it—the colorful swirl of this nutritious side may just make you break into song. And here's a chef's tip: cutting the peppers into large triangle shapes helps them to cook in the same amount of time as the onion and zucchini. Now you know!

Makes 4 servings

Olive oil for the pan
2 medium zucchini, trimmed, halved lengthwise, and cut into 1-inch half-moons
1 medium red bell pepper, quartered lengthwise, each panel halved on a diagonal
1 medium yellow bell pepper, quartered lengthwise, each panel halved on a diagonal
1 medium orange bell pepper, quartered lengthwise, each panel halved on a diagonal
1 medium red onion, cut into 1½-inch pieces
1 tablespoon Malaysian red palm fruit oil
1 teaspoon dried oregano
½ teaspoon sea salt
¼ teaspoon freshly ground black pepper

Preheat the oven to 425°F. Lightly dampen a paper towel with a small amount of olive oil and wipe a large rimmed baking sheet with it.

Combine the zucchini, bell peppers, onion, palm fruit oil, oregano, salt, and pepper in a large bowl and toss well. Transfer the vegetables to the prepared baking sheet and roast, stirring occasionally, until tender and lightly browned, 28 to 30 minutes.

Nutrient Content per Serving

Calories:	90	**Fat:**	4 grams	**Protein:**	2 grams
Fiber:	5 grams	**Saturated Fat:**	2 grams	**Carbs:**	13 grams
Sodium:	320 mg	**Sugars:**	5 grams		

Sautéed Kale with Caramelized Onions

Kale is one of those nutrient-dense greens that makes you feel like you're getting healthier by the bite. But its stems are really tough and unpleasant to chew, so make sure you remove them completely before cooking.

Makes 4 servings

2 tablespoons olive oil

2 medium red onions, thinly sliced

2 garlic cloves, minced

1 teaspoon fresh thyme leaves

1 bunch kale (1¼ pounds), woody stems removed, leaves torn into smaller pieces, washed, and left damp

½ cup water

¼ teaspoon sea salt

⅛ teaspoon freshly ground black pepper.

Heat 1 tablespoon of the oil in a large nonstick skillet over medium heat. Add the onion, garlic, and thyme; cook, stirring occasionally, until the onion is golden, 18 to 20 minutes. Transfer to a bowl and set aside.

Return the skillet to the stove and heat the remaining 1 tablespoon of oil over medium-high heat. Add the kale and cook, stirring occasionally, until wilted, 2 to 3 minutes. Pour in the water and cook, stirring often, until tender, 3 to 4 minutes. Stir in the onion mixture, salt, and pepper; cook for 2 minutes, until heated through.

Nutrient Content per Serving

Calories:	140	**Fat:**	8 grams	**Protein:**	6 grams
Fiber:	3 grams	**Saturated Fat:**	1 gram	**Carbs:**	12 grams
Sodium:	190 mg	**Sugars:**	2 grams		

Spicy Ginger and Celery Stir-Fry

Ginger is aromatic and spicy, and it adds its typical zest to this stir-fry. It also offers medicinal benefits, so you may want to keep extra around—it can calm the tummy and is even effective in alleviating symptoms of gastrointestinal distress. To add some color to this dish, toss in a sliced carrot.

Makes 4 servings

    1 tablespoon toasted sesame oil
    1 medium onion, chopped (about 1 cup)
    1 tablespoon minced fresh ginger
    2 garlic cloves, minced
    ⅛ teaspoon red pepper flakes
    6 celery stalks, cut into ¼ x 2-inch sticks
    4 teaspoons low-sodium wheat-free tamari
    ¼ cup thinly sliced green onions

Heat the oil in a large nonstick skillet over medium-high heat. Add the onion, ginger, garlic, and red pepper flakes; cook, stirring often, until slightly softened, 3 minutes. Stir in the celery and cook, stirring occasionally, until crisp-tender, 4 to 5 minutes. Add the tamari and cook, stirring, for 10 seconds. Stir in green onions and cook for 30 seconds longer.

Nutrient Content per Serving

Calories:	70	**Fat:**	3.5 grams	**Protein:**	2 grams
Fiber:	2 grams	**Saturated Fat:**	0.5 grams	**Carbs:**	9 grams
Sodium:	310 mg	**Sugars:**	2 grams		

Spicy Okra with Ginger, Garlic, and Tomatoes

Okra is also known as "lady's fingers" in parts of the world—isn't that fun? The entire plant is edible and because of its high fiber content, it can be a useful digestive aid. If you can't find fresh okra, substitute an equal amount of frozen sliced okra and let it thaw.

Makes 4 servings

  2 tablespoons Malaysian red palm fruit oil

  1 medium onion, chopped

  1 tablespoon minced fresh ginger

  2 garlic cloves, minced

  ⅛ teaspoon red pepper flakes

  12 ounces okra, cut into ½-inch-thick slices

  2 plum tomatoes (about 10 ounces), seeded and chopped

  ½ cup water

  ¼ teaspoon sea salt

Heat the oil in a large nonstick skillet over medium heat. Add the onion and cook, stirring occasionally, until slightly softened, 4 minutes. Stir in the ginger, garlic, and red pepper flakes; cook for 2 minutes. Add the okra and tomatoes and cook for 5 minutes. Stir in the water, cover, reduce the heat to medium-low, and simmer until the okra is tender, 14 to 15 minutes. Remove from the heat and stir in the salt.

Nutrient Content per Serving

Calories:	110	**Fat:**	7 grams	**Protein:**	2 grams
Fiber:	4 grams	**Saturated Fat:**	3.5 grams	**Carbs:**	11 grams
Sodium:	150 mg	**Sugars:**	3 grams		

Warm Wax Bean and Green Bean Salad

I've mixed it up for presentation here, but you won't be robbed of taste or nutrition if your store doesn't have yellow wax beans (in fact, green beans have more vitamin A). All you have to do is double the amount of green beans you use, and all will be right with this salad.

Makes 4 servings

  6 ounces yellow wax beans, halved crosswise

  6 ounces green beans, halved crosswise

  1 carrot, thinly sliced

  1 celery stalk, thinly sliced

  2 tablespoons extra-virgin olive oil

  2 tablespoons sliced fresh basil leaves

  1 tablespoon red wine vinegar

  ¼ teaspoon sea salt

  ⅛ teaspoon freshly ground black pepper

Bring a large pot of lightly salted water to a boil over high heat.

Add the beans to the pot, cover, and return the water to a boil; cook for 2 minutes. Add the carrots to the pot and immediately drain. Transfer the vegetables to a large bowl and stir in the celery, oil, basil, vinegar, salt, and pepper. Toss well and serve warm or at room temperature.

Nutrient Content per Serving

Calories:	100	**Fat:**	7 grams	**Protein:**	2 grams
Fiber:	3 grams	**Saturated Fat:**	1 gram	**Carbs:**	8 grams
Sodium:	170 mg	**Sugars:**	3 grams		

Whole Roasted Cauliflower

As far as I'm concerned, you can't eat enough cruciferous veggies like cauliflower—but I'd like you to try! Pile them on your Sugar Impact Plate! Cauliflower is an excellent source of vitamins C and K, and will give you a serious bump in your daily fiber. For an added treat, you can serve the cauliflower under a little drizzle of the Caper Vinaigrette (page 192).

Makes 4 servings

   Olive oil for the pan
   1 (2- to 2¼-pound) head cauliflower
   1 tablespoon plus 1½ teaspoons extra-virgin olive oil
   ½ teaspoon sea salt
   ¼ teaspoon freshly ground black pepper

Preheat the oven to 400°F. Lightly dampen a paper towel with a small amount of olive oil and wipe a rimmed baking sheet with it.

With a sharp knife, trim the leaves from the cauliflower, then remove the woody core. Rub the cauliflower all over with 1 tablespoon of the extra-virgin olive oil, then season with the salt and pepper. Place the cauliflower head round-side up on the prepared baking sheet.

Roast the cauliflower until it is browned and easily pierced with a knife, 48 to 50 minutes. Transfer to a cutting board and cut the cauliflower into four wedges. Drizzle with the remaining 1½ teaspoons of the extra-virgin olive oil and serve.

Nutrient Content per Serving

Calories:	90	**Fat:**	5 grams	**Protein:**	3 grams
Fiber:	3 grams	**Saturated Fat:**	0.5 grams	**Carbs:**	9 grams
Sodium:	340 mg	**Sugars:**	3 grams		

Braised Leeks

The onion-like taste of leeks is delicate, not overpowering, and braising them in vegetable or chicken stock gives them a buttery richness.

Makes 4 servings

- 1 tablespoon extra-virgin olive oil
- 3 garlic cloves, minced
- 1 teaspoon fresh thyme leaves
- 1 cup Homemade Vegetable Stock (page 191) or low-sodium store-bought vegetable broth
- ¼ teaspoon sea salt
- ⅛ teaspoon freshly ground black pepper
- 6 leeks, white and light green parts only, halved lengthwise

Heat the oil in a nonstick skillet, large enough to hold the leeks in a single layer, over medium heat. Add the garlic and thyme; cook, stirring occasionally, until the garlic is starting to brown, 1 to 1½ minutes. Stir in the stock, salt, and pepper; bring the stock to a boil, reduce the heat to medium, and add the leeks in a single layer, cut-side down. Cover and simmer until the leeks are tender, 33 to 35 minutes. Uncover the skillet, increase the heat to medium-high, and bring to a boil. Cook until the liquid has reduced by one-third, 3 to 4 minutes.

This can be served with the broth spooned over or not, depending on your preference.

Nutrient Content per Serving

Calories:	120	**Fat:**	4.5 grams	**Protein:**	2 grams
Fiber:	3 grams	**Saturated Fat:**	0.5 grams	**Carbs:**	20 grams
Sodium:	170 mg	**Sugars:**	4 grams		

Roasted Eggplant with Fresh Basil Dressing

Eggplant is a vine-growing member of the nightshade family of vegetables. It belongs on your plate for lots of reasons, including its disease-fighting phytonutrients and high fiber content. When you buy an eggplant, it should be very firm. Softer eggplants are older and tend to have more seeds and be bitter.

Makes 4 servings

1 tablespoon olive oil, plus more for the pan

1 (1¼-pound) eggplant, trimmed and cut into ¾-inch cubes

½ teaspoon dried basil

¼ teaspoon sea salt

⅛ teaspoon freshly ground black pepper

3 tablespoons Basil Vinaigrette (page 197)

Preheat the oven to 450°F. Lightly dampen a paper towel with a small amount of olive oil and wipe a rimmed baking sheet with it.

Combine the eggplant, the 1 tablespoon of oil, basil, salt, and pepper in a large bowl and toss well to coat. Place the eggplant on the prepared baking sheet. Roast until lightly browned and tender, 20 to 22 minutes. Transfer the eggplant to a bowl; add the basil vinaigrette and toss well. Serve warm or at room temperature.

Nutrient Content per Serving

Calories:	130	Fat:	10 grams	Protein:	5 grams
Fiber:	4 grams	Saturated Fat:	1.5 grams	Carbs:	8 grams
Sodium:	230 mg	Sugars:	3 grams		

Roasted Brussels Sprouts with Prosciutto

The salty, smoky flavor of prosciutto is a worthy match for the sprouts' strong presence, but for a vegan-friendly version, you can just leave it out.

Makes 4 servings

2 tablespoons olive oil, plus more for the pan

1 pound Brussels sprouts, trimmed and halved

¼ teaspoon sea salt

⅛ teaspoon freshly ground black pepper

2 ounces nitrate-free deli-sliced prosciutto, chopped

Preheat the oven to 425°F. Lightly dampen a paper towel with a small amount of olive oil and wipe a baking sheet with it.

Combine the Brussels sprouts, 4 teaspoons of the oil, the salt, and the pepper in a large bowl. Transfer to the prepared baking sheet and bake, stirring occasionally, until the Brussels sprouts are browned and crisp-tender, 20 to 22 minutes. Transfer to a bowl.

Meanwhile, heat the remaining 2 teaspoons oil in a large nonstick skillet over medium-high heat. Add the prosciutto and cook, stirring occasionally, until lightly browned and crisp, 4 to 5 minutes. Transfer to the bowl with the Brussels sprouts and toss well to combine.

Nutrient Content per Serving

Calories:	140	**Fat:**	9 grams	**Protein:**	7 grams
Fiber:	4 grams	**Saturated Fat:**	1.5 grams	**Carbs:**	8 grams
Sodium:	560 mg	**Sugars:**	3 grams		

Stir-Fried Bok Choy

Bok choy is a dark-leafed, cruciferous vegetable that—in addition to being great stir-fried—also works well steamed, in soups and salads, and as a stir-in to other side dishes. Baby bok choy is sweeter and more delicate than adult varieties.

Makes 4 servings

- 1 tablespoon Malaysian red palm fruit oil
- 1 medium onion, chopped
- 2 garlic cloves, minced
- 1 tablespoon minced fresh ginger
- 1/8 teaspoon red pepper flakes
- 1½ pounds baby bok choy, cut into bite-size pieces
- 4 teaspoons low-sodium wheat-free tamari or coconut aminos

Heat the oil in a large nonstick skillet over medium-high heat. Add the onion, garlic, ginger, and red pepper flakes; cook until starting to soften, 2 to 3 minutes. Add the bok choy and cook, stirring often, until crisp-tender, 4 minutes. Stir in the tamari and cook for 1 minute longer.

Nutrient Content per Serving

Calories:	70	**Fat:**	4 grams	**Protein:**	4 grams
Fiber:	3 grams	**Saturated Fat:**	2 grams	**Carbs:**	8 grams
Sodium:	370 mg	**Sugars:**	4 grams		

Sesame Wilted Spinach

Popeye never stood a chance at keeping this elixir to himself. Look for flat-leaf spinach rather than curly (also known as savoy spinach, which tends to be tougher and has a slightly bitter flavor).

Makes 4 servings

- 2 pounds flat-leaf spinach, trimmed, washed, and spun dry
- 2 teaspoons Malaysian red palm fruit oil
- 1 tablespoon minced fresh ginger
- 2 garlic cloves, minced
- 4 green onions, chopped
- 2 teaspoons low-sodium wheat-free tamari or coconut aminos
- 2 teaspoons Asian sesame oil
- 2 teaspoons sesame seeds

Heat a large nonstick skillet over medium heat. Add the spinach and cook, stirring, until wilted, 2 to 3 minutes. Transfer to a strainer, let cool for 5 minutes, then squeeze out any excess liquid.

Return the skillet to the stove and heat the palm fruit oil over medium-high heat; add the ginger and garlic and cook, stirring, until fragrant, 30 seconds. Add the green onions and cook, stirring, until wilted, 1 minute. Add the spinach and cook until heated through, 1 minute. Add the tamari and sesame oil; cook for 1 minute and remove from the heat. Stir in the sesame seeds.

Nutrient Content per Serving

Calories:	110	**Fat:**	6 grams	**Protein:**	7 grams	
Fiber:	6 grams	**Saturated Fat:**	1.5 grams	**Carbs:**	10 grams	
Sodium:	300 mg	**Sugars:**	1 gram			

STARCHY SIDES

Tuscan White Beans with Roasted Grape Tomatoes and Parmesan

Tuscans are often referred to as *mangia fagioli*, or bean eaters, and this recipe will leave no doubt as to why. Grape tomatoes lend a little sweetness to this fresh side. If you have a dairy intolerance, leave off the Parmesan. If you don't and you prefer a sharper cheese, try using Pecorino Romano.

Makes 4 servings

    3 teaspoons olive oil, plus more for the pan
    1 pint grape tomatoes
    1 medium red onion, chopped
    3 garlic cloves, minced
    1 tablespoon chopped fresh oregano
    1 (15-ounce) can organic no-salt-added cannellini beans, drained and rinsed
    1 tablespoon red wine vinegar
    2 tablespoons grated Parmesan cheese
    1 tablespoon extra-virgin olive oil
    ¼ teaspoon sea salt
    ¼ teaspoon freshly ground black pepper

Preheat the oven to 425°F. Lightly dampen a paper towel with a small amount of olive oil and wipe a rimmed baking sheet with it.

Combine 1 teaspoon of the olive oil and the tomatoes in a medium bowl. Arrange the tomatoes on the prepared baking sheet. Roast the tomatoes until tender, wilted, and browned in spots, 18 to 20 minutes.

Heat the remaining 2 teaspoons olive oil in a large nonstick skillet over medium-high heat. Add the onion and cook until slightly softened, 2 to 3 minutes. Add the garlic and oregano and cook until fragrant, 1 minute. Stir in the tomatoes, beans, and vinegar and cook until hot, 2 minutes. Remove from the heat and add the cheese, extra-virgin olive oil, salt, and pepper.

Nutrient Content per Serving

Calories:	150	**Fat:**	8 grams	**Protein:**	5 grams
Fiber:	4 grams	**Saturated Fat:**	1.5 grams	**Carbs:**	15 grams
Sodium:	210 mg	**Sugars:**	4 grams		

Coconut Curry Butternut Squash Puree

Butternut squash oozes goodness and is so soothing to eat. When you add the exotic flavor of coconut curry, one bite will transport you out of this world. For a little flavor boost, use coconut oil on your baking sheet.

Makes 4 servings

> Olive oil for the pan
>
> 1 (2- to 2¼-pound) butternut squash, halved lengthwise and seeded
>
> 1 tablespoon coconut butter
>
> ¼ teaspoon curry powder
>
> ½ teaspoon sea salt

Preheat the oven to 375°F. Lightly dampen a paper towel with a small amount of olive oil and wipe a rimmed baking sheet with it.

Place the squash on the prepared baking sheet, cut-side down. Bake the squash until easily pierced with a fork, 43 to 45 minutes. Remove from the oven and let cool slightly, 3 minutes.

While the squash is still hot, scoop out the flesh and place it in a food processor. Add the coconut butter, curry powder, and salt; puree.

Nutrient Content per Serving

Calories:	120	**Fat:**	3 grams	**Protein:**	2 grams
Fiber:	5 grams	**Saturated Fat:**	2.5 grams	**Carbs:**	26 grams
Sodium:	300 mg	**Sugars:**	5 grams		

Raw Butternut Squash "Pappardelle" with Garlic and Oil

This side delivers all the creamy comfort of pappardelle without any of the assault on your blood sugar and waistline. All you need is a good vegetable peeler to make the thin strips of butternut squash "pasta"—then it's all about the treat to your taste buds.

Makes 4 servings

> 1 (1¾-pound) butternut squash, peeled, halved, and seeded
>
> ½ teaspoon plus ⅛ teaspoon sea salt
>
> 2 tablespoons extra-virgin olive oil
>
> 4 garlic cloves, thinly sliced
>
> ¼ cup thinly sliced fresh basil leaves

With a vegetable peeler, shave or "peel" the squash into 3½-inch-long by 1- to 1½-inch-wide strips. Toss the strips in a large bowl with ½ teaspoon of the salt and briefly rub the salt into the squash with your fingers; let stand for 20 minutes.

Rinse off the squash and drain well in a colander, then pat lightly with paper towels to dry slightly.

Combine the oil and garlic in a small skillet over low heat. Cook, stirring occasionally, until the garlic is translucent, 5 to 7 minutes. Remove from the heat and toss with the squash. Add the basil and remaining ⅛ teaspoon salt. Serve immediately.

Nutrient Content per Serving

Calories:	140	**Fat:**	7 grams	**Protein:**	2 grams
Fiber:	3 grams	**Saturated Fat:**	1 gram	**Carbs:**	21 grams
Sodium:	370 mg	**Sugars:**	4 grams		

Red Lentil Dal

This traditional Indian dish, which is essentially lentil soup, is rich and comforting. Red lentils tend to have a mushy texture and are perfect for dishes like dal. Available in most supermarkets and health food stores, red lentils are often labeled "masoor" in Asian markets.

Makes 4 servings

1 tablespoon coconut oil
1 medium onion, chopped
1 tablespoon minced fresh ginger
3 garlic cloves, minced
1 teaspoon curry powder
½ teaspoon ground cumin
⅛ teaspoon cayenne pepper
1 cup red lentils
2⅔ cups water
½ teaspoon sea salt

Heat the oil in a large saucepan over medium-high heat. Add the onion and cook, stirring occasionally, until starting to brown, 5 to 6 minutes. Add the ginger and garlic and cook, stirring, until fragrant, 30 seconds. Add the curry, cumin, and cayenne pepper and cook for 15 seconds. Pour in the lentils, water, and salt; bring to a boil, reduce the heat to medium-low, cover, and simmer until the lentils are tender, 15 minutes.

Nutrient Content per Serving

Calories:	220	**Fat:**	4.5 grams	**Protein:**	14 grams
Fiber:	8 grams	**Saturated Fat:**	3 grams	**Carbs:**	32 grams
Sodium:	300 mg	**Sugars:**	3 grams		

Red Quinoa with Slow-Roasted Almonds and Caramelized Shallots

It hardly seems fair to call this dish a side. The nutrient density of quinoa makes it a major player on your plate—it's a concentrated source of protein, iron, and fiber, and it's also high in antioxidants. Did I forget to say it's yummy, too? If there's excess liquid at the end of cooking, simply drain quinoa in a sieve.

Makes 6 servings

1 cup dry red quinoa, rinsed
½ teaspoon sea salt
2 tablespoons Malaysian red palm fruit oil
2 cups thinly sliced shallots
¼ teaspoon monk fruit extract
⅓ cup slow-roasted almonds (see page 97), coarsely chopped
2 teaspoons lemon juice
⅛ teaspoon freshly ground black pepper

Cook the quinoa with ¼ teaspoon of the salt according to the package directions.

Meanwhile, heat the oil in a medium nonstick skillet over medium-high heat. Add the shallots and monk fruit extract; cook, stirring occasionally, until the shallots are browned, 8 to 9 minutes. Stir in the almonds and cook for 1 minute. Transfer to a bowl and stir in the cooked quinoa, lemon juice, remaining ¼ teaspoon salt, and the pepper.

Nutrient Content per Serving

Calories:	220	**Fat:**	10 grams	**Protein:**	7 grams
Fiber:	4 grams	**Saturated Fat:**	2.5 grams	**Carbs:**	30 grams
Sodium:	240 mg	**Sugars:**	5 grams		

Chickpeas with Sautéed Greens

Chickpeas, also known as garbanzo beans, are legumes with a nutty flavor and buttery texture (they're the main ingredient in hummus). They're a great source of protein and fiber, which means they positively impact both your digestion and blood sugar control. To warm leftovers, heat them in a large skillet over medium heat and add a little Homemade Vegetable Stock (page 191) to help moisten them.

Makes 4 servings

- 1 bunch broccoli rabe (about 1 pound), woody stems trimmed
- 2 tablespoons extra-virgin olive oil
- 5 garlic cloves, thinly sliced
- ⅛ teaspoon red pepper flakes
- 1 (15-ounce) can organic no-salt-added chickpeas, drained and rinsed
- 2 teaspoons grated orange zest
- ½ teaspoon sea salt

Bring a large pot of lightly salted water to a boil. Add the broccoli rabe, return to a boil, and cook for 1 minute; drain, rinse under cold water, and drain again. Gently press or squeeze any excess water from the broccoli rabe.

Heat the oil in a large nonstick skillet over medium-high heat. Add the garlic and red pepper flakes and cook for 1 minute. Add the chickpeas and cook until the garlic starts to brown, 2 minutes. Stir in the broccoli rabe and cook, tossing, until hot, 2 minutes. Season with the orange zest and salt.

Nutrient Content per Serving

Calories:	160	**Fat:**	7 grams	**Protein:**	8 grams
Fiber:	3 grams	**Saturated Fat:**	1 gram	**Carbs:**	18 grams
Sodium:	340 mg	**Sugars:**	2 grams		

Peas with Onions, Garlic, and Bacon

Peas are just plain fun, but bacon lends a taste and texture that make this classic feel all grown up. As an alternative to regular bacon, try nitrate-free uncured bacon, which has a smokier, meatier flavor.

Makes 4 servings

- 1 teaspoon olive oil
- 4 slices nitrate-free bacon, chopped
- 2 medium onions, sliced (about 2 cups)
- 4 garlic cloves, thinly sliced
- ½ teaspoon fresh thyme leaves
- 1½ cups frozen peas
- ¼ teaspoon sea salt
- ⅛ teaspoon freshly ground black pepper

Heat the oil in a large nonstick skillet over medium-high heat. Add the bacon and cook, stirring occasionally, until starting to brown, 4 minutes. Stir in the onions, garlic, and thyme; cook until lightly browned, 5 to 6 minutes. Add the peas and cook, stirring occasionally, until bright green, 2 minutes. Remove from the heat and stir in the salt and pepper.

Nutrient Content per Serving

Calories:	70	**Fat:**	3 grams	**Protein:**	3 grams
Fiber:	2 grams	**Saturated Fat:**	1 gram	**Carbs:**	8 grams
Sodium:	290 mg	**Sugars:**	5 grams		

Spaghetti Squash with Capers, Onion, and Bell Pepper

Spaghetti squash is a swap I always recommend for pasta because you'll give up nothing in the trade except high Sugar Impact and lots of calories. You're getting a more colorful meal that's richer in nutrients and has a fiber content similar to pasta, so you'll be just as full (again, on fewer calories!). With all that in mind, my guess is that you'll like it even better. But don't let it hurt you—use a kitchen towel to hold the hot squash when scraping out the flesh.

Makes 4 servings

2 tablespoons olive oil, plus more for the pan
1 (2- to 2¼-pound) spaghetti squash, halved lengthwise and seeded
1 large onion, thinly sliced
1 teaspoon chopped fresh thyme
1 medium red bell pepper, thinly sliced
1 tablespoon drained capers
½ teaspoon sea salt
¼ teaspoon freshly ground black pepper

Preheat the oven to 350°F. Lightly dampen a paper towel with a small amount of olive oil and wipe a rimmed baking sheet with it.

Place the squash, cut-sides down, on the prepared baking sheet. Prick all over with the tip of a knife. Bake until very tender, 28 to 30 minutes. Remove from the oven and let cool for 5 minutes. Turn the squash over and using the tines of a fork, scrape out the flesh—it will come out in long, thin, spaghetti-like strands.

Heat the 2 tablespoons of oil in a large nonstick skillet over medium-high heat. Add the onion and thyme; cook, stirring occasionally, until softened and starting to brown, 6 to 7 minutes. Add the bell pepper and cook until tender, 4 minutes. Add the capers and cook for 1 minute. Stir in the squash and cook, tossing, until hot and well mixed, 1 to 2 minutes. Remove from the heat and season with the salt and black pepper.

Nutrient Content per Serving

Calories:	130	**Fat:**	8 grams	**Protein:**	2 grams
Fiber:	4 grams	**Saturated Fat:**	1 gram	**Carbs:**	15 grams
Sodium:	410 mg	**Sugars:**	5 grams		

Lima Beans with Lemon and Spinach

The two most popular types of lima beans in the United States are baby limas and Fordhook limas (also known as butterbeans). Baby limas are smaller, thinner, and less flavorful than their larger cousin. That means Fordhook lima beans are not "adult" baby limas—they're a different variety that's plumper and has a deeper flavor than baby limas. The good news is that both types will work in this recipe!

Makes 4 servings

1 (10-ounce) package frozen Fordhook lima beans, thawed
1 tablespoon olive oil
3 garlic cloves, minced
¼ cup chopped shallots
5 cups baby spinach
2 teaspoons grated lemon zest
½ teaspoon sea salt
¼ teaspoon freshly ground black pepper

Bring a medium saucepan of lightly salted water to a boil over high heat. Add the lima beans and return the water to a boil. Cook until the lima beans are tender, 7 minutes; drain and set aside.

Heat the oil in a large nonstick skillet over medium-high heat. Add the garlic and shallots; cook, stirring often, until starting to soften, 2 to 3 minutes. Add the lima beans and cook for 2 minutes. Stir in the spinach and cook until wilted, about 2 minutes. Remove from the heat and stir in the lemon zest, salt, and pepper.

Nutrient Content per Serving

Calories:	130	**Fat:**	3.5 grams	**Protein:**	1 gram
Fiber:	5 grams	**Saturated Fat:**	0 grams	**Carbs:**	20 grams
Sodium:	340 mg	**Sugars:**	1 gram		

Quinoa with Celery and Mushrooms

You may end up wishing this were the main dish! Quinoa is closely related to spinach and is packed with high-quality protein and fiber. Mushrooms are no nutritional slouches, either, but make sure you buy them whole and slice your own to make the most of their nutrient density. Water can be substituted for the stock, which will result in a lighter-flavored dish.

Makes 4 servings

1 cup dry quinoa, rinsed
2½ cups Homemade Vegetable Stock (page 191) or low-sodium store-bought vegetable broth
2 tablespoons olive oil
1 medium onion, chopped
8 ounces white mushrooms, sliced
1 teaspoon dried marjoram
2 celery stalks, finely chopped
¼ cup chopped fresh parsley
½ teaspoon sea salt
¼ teaspoon freshly ground black pepper

Cook the quinoa according to the package directions, using the stock instead of water.

Heat the oil in a large nonstick skillet over medium-high heat. Add the onion, mushrooms, and marjoram; cook, stirring occasionally, until the mushrooms start to brown slightly, 6 to 7 minutes. Add the celery and cook until starting to soften, 3 to 4 minutes. Add the cooked quinoa and cook, stirring, for 1 minute. Remove from the heat and stir in the parsley, salt, and pepper.

Nutrient Content per Serving

Calories:	270	**Fat:**	12 grams	**Protein:**	8 grams
Fiber:	5 grams	**Saturated Fat:**	1.5 grams	**Carbs:**	35 grams
Sodium:	330 mg	**Sugars:**	3 grams		

Roasted Butternut Squash with Thyme

I'd choose the sweet, nutty taste of roasted butternut squash over a regular (less nutritious) side of mashed potatoes every day of the week and twice on Sundays. When you're buying butternut squash, look for even cream-colored skin. It should feel heavy for its size and be firm and fairly smooth.

Makes 4 servings

  1 tablespoon olive oil, plus more for the pan
  1 (1½-pound) butternut squash, peeled, seeded, and cut into 1-inch pieces
  1½ teaspoons chopped fresh thyme
  ½ teaspoon ground cinnamon
  ½ teaspoon sea salt
  ¼ teaspoon freshly ground black pepper

Preheat the oven to 425°F. Position a rack in the center. Lightly dampen a paper towel with a small amount of olive oil and wipe a rimmed baking sheet with it.

   Combine the squash, the 1 tablespoon of oil, thyme, cinnamon, salt, and pepper in a large bowl. Arrange the squash on the baking sheet in a single layer. Bake, stirring occasionally, until the squash is light brown and tender, 28 to 30 minutes.

Nutrient Content per Serving

Calories:	110	**Fat:**	3.5 grams	**Protein:**	2 grams
Fiber:	4 grams	**Saturated Fat:**	0.5 grams	**Carbs:**	20 grams
Sodium:	300 mg	**Sugars:**	4 grams		

Spiced Sweet Potato "Fries" (Cycles 1/3)

"Sugar" and spice and everything nice...that's what these sweet potato "fries" are made of! They're gobble-up good, with a little heat to make them extra sassy. For best results, make sure the sweet potatoes are cut evenly so that all of the fries are the same size.

Makes 4 servings

  Olive oil for the pan
  1 pound sweet potatoes, peeled and cut lengthwise into ¼-inch-thick wedges
  1 tablespoon Malaysian red palm fruit oil
  ½ teaspoon ground coriander
  ¼ teaspoon ground cinnamon
  ¼ teaspoon sea salt
  ¼ teaspoon cayenne pepper

Preheat the oven to 450°F. Position racks in the center and upper third of the oven. Lightly dampen a paper towel with a small amount of olive oil and wipe two rimmed baking sheets with it.

Combine the sweet potatoes and palm fruit oil in a large bowl. Combine the coriander, cinnamon, salt, and cayenne pepper in a separate small bowl. Add the spice mixture to the potatoes and toss well to coat. Arrange the potatoes in a single layer on the prepared baking sheets, being mindful not to overcrowd the pans.

Bake, turning the potatoes once and switching the upper and lower pans about halfway through cooking, until browned and crisp, 20 to 22 minutes.

Nutrient Content per Serving

Calories:	130	**Fat:**	3.5 grams	**Protein:**	2 grams
Fiber:	4 grams	**Saturated Fat:**	2 grams	**Carbs:**	23 grams
Sodium:	210 mg	**Sugars:**	5 grams		

Wild Rice and Vegetable Pilaf

Wild rice is not rice at all—it's grass! Adding vegetables to this pilaf ratchets up the flavor and helps it do double duty on your Sugar Impact Plate. Cooking directions for wild rice can vary from brand to brand, so make sure to read them carefully before you start cooking.

Makes 4 servings

1 cup dry wild rice
½ teaspoon sea salt
1 tablespoon olive oil
1 medium red onion, chopped
2 garlic cloves, minced
1 small zucchini, cut into ¼-inch dice
1 small yellow squash, cut into ¼-inch dice
¼ teaspoon freshly ground black pepper

Cook the wild rice according to the package directions with ¼ teaspoon of the salt.

Heat the oil in a large nonstick skillet over medium-high heat. Add the onion and garlic; cook, stirring occasionally, until starting to soften, 1 to 2 minutes. Add the zucchini and squash and cook until lightly browned and tender, 7 to 8 minutes. Stir in the cooked rice and cook until hot, 1 to 2 minutes. Stir in the remaining ¼ teaspoon salt and the pepper.

Nutrient Content per Serving

Calories:	180	**Fat:**	2 grams	**Protein:**	7 grams
Fiber:	4 grams	**Saturated Fat:**	0 grams	**Carbs:**	35 grams
Sodium:	300 mg	**Sugars:**	4 grams		

10

SAUCES, STOCKS, RUBS, AND DRESSINGS

Sauces, rubs, and dressings are usually high–Sugar Impact, diet-killing saboteurs. They're vehicles for hidden sugars and gluten to sneak into your diet and send your blood sugar off the rails, not to mention the long-term hit they give your health and waistline.

These recipes will let you slather and rub to your heart's content, knowing you've dodged the high-SI bullet delivered in store-bought bottles. They'll bring the party to your taste buds and actually help support your fast fat-loss goals and health. Yes, that kind of turnabout is fair play!

Chimichurri Sauce

Argentina gets credit for gifting this delicious, versatile sauce to the world. Bright green color adds beauty as well as a great herbaceous flavor to your dish.

Makes about ⅔ cup (1 tablespoon per serving)

½ cup chopped fresh cilantro

½ cup chopped fresh basil

¼ cup chopped fresh parsley

1 garlic clove, minced

3 tablespoons white wine vinegar

½ teaspoon ground cumin

¼ cup extra-virgin olive oil

¾ teaspoon sea salt

¼ teaspoon freshly ground black pepper

Combine the cilantro, basil, parsley, garlic, vinegar, cumin, oil, salt, and pepper in a small bowl. Store the chimichurri sauce in an airtight container in the refrigerator for up to 1 week.

Nutrient Content per Serving

Calories:	70	**Fat:**	7 grams	**Protein:**	1 gram
Fiber:	1 gram	**Saturated Fat:**	1 gram	**Carbs:**	2 grams
Sodium:	230 mg	**Sugars:**	0 grams		

Homemade Vegetable Stock

So good! Roasting the vegetables beforehand brings out their flavors and adds richness to the stock, so there's no worry about the sodium, high-fructose corn syrup, and MSG some store-bought brands rely on for flavor. Freeze in 1- to 2-cup portions to have on hand for sauces or soups.

Makes 4 cups

   1 tablespoon olive oil, plus more for the pan
   1¾ pounds onions, chopped
   2 medium leeks, trimmed, washed, and chopped
   4 carrots, chopped
   3 celery stalks, chopped
   1 medium fennel bulb, chopped
   10 cups water
   4 plum tomatoes, seeded and chopped
   6 sprigs fresh parsley
   4 sprigs fresh thyme
   12 whole black peppercorns
   6 garlic cloves
   1 bay leaf

Preheat the oven to 400°F. Lightly dampen a paper towel with a small amount of olive oil and wipe two rimmed baking sheets with it.

Combine the onions, leeks, carrots, celery, fennel, and the tablespoon of oil in a large bowl. Transfer to the prepared baking sheets. Roast the vegetables, stirring occasionally, until browned, 35 to 38 minutes.

Transfer the vegetables to a large pot. Pour 1 cup of the water onto each of the baking sheets and scrape up any browned bits, then add the water to the pot with the vegetables. Add the remaining 8 cups water, the tomatoes, parsley, thyme, peppercorns, garlic, and bay leaf. Bring to a boil over high heat. Reduce the heat to medium-low and simmer for 1½ hours.

Strain the stock through a colander set over a bowl; discard the solids in the colander. Return the liquid to the pot and bring to a simmer over medium heat. Cook until reduced to 4 cups, 35 to 40 minutes. Remove from the heat and let cool to room temperature before refrigerating or freezing.

Nutrient Content per Serving

Calories:	35	**Fat:**	3.5 grams	**Protein:**	0 grams
Fiber:	0 grams	**Saturated Fat:**	0 grams	**Carbs:**	1 gram
Sodium:	5 mg	**Sugars:**	0 grams		

Caper Vinaigrette

The flavors in this tangy dressing make it a perfect pairing with a Mediterranean-style salad, or drizzle it over freshly sliced summer tomatoes for an easy and delicious snack.

Makes ¾ cup (2 tablespoons per serving)

2 tablespoons lemon juice
2 teaspoons red wine vinegar
1 tablespoon drained capers, chopped
1 tablespoon chopped shallots
1 teaspoon Dijon mustard
½ teaspoon sea salt
¼ teaspoon freshly ground black pepper
½ cup macadamia nut oil

Combine the lemon juice, vinegar, capers, shallots, mustard, salt, and pepper in a small bowl. Slowly whisk in the oil until well combined. Store in an airtight container in the refrigerator for up to 2 weeks.

Nutrient Content per Serving

Calories:	90	**Fat:**	1 gram	**Protein:**	0 grams
Fiber:	0 grams	**Saturated Fat:**	0 grams	**Carbs:**	0 grams
Sodium:	135 mg	**Sugars:**	0 grams		

Dijon Vinaigrette

Not only does this simple dressing take a scrumptious salad to the next level (check out the recipe for my BLT Wedge Salad with Avocado and Dijon Vinaigrette on page 89), it also makes a great quick marinade.

Makes ¾ cup (2 tablespoons per serving)

2½ tablespoons sherry vinegar

5 teaspoons Dijon mustard

½ teaspoon sea salt

¼ teaspoon freshly ground black pepper

½ cup walnut oil

Combine the vinegar, mustard, salt, and pepper in a small bowl. Slowly whisk in the oil until well combined. Store in an airtight container in the refrigerator for up to 2 weeks.

Nutrient Content per Serving

Calories:	80	**Fat:**	9 grams	**Protein:**	0 grams
Fiber:	0 grams	**Saturated Fat:**	1 gram	**Carbs:**	0 grams
Sodium:	150 mg	**Sugars:**	0 grams		

Easy Lemon Vinaigrette

It's no accident "easy" is in the name of this vinaigrette. I hope simple, tasty recipes like this one encourage you to make your own dressings and avoid the sugar bombs sitting in jars on grocery store shelves.

Makes ¾ cup (2 tablespoons per serving)

1½ teaspoons grated lemon zest

3 tablespoons lemon juice

2 teaspoons Dijon mustard

½ teaspoon sea salt

¼ teaspoon freshly ground black pepper

½ cup extra-virgin olive oil

Combine the lemon zest, lemon juice, mustard, salt, and pepper in a small bowl. Slowly whisk in the oil until well combined. Store in an airtight container in the refrigerator for up to 10 days.

Nutrient Content per Serving

Calories:	80	**Fat:**	9 grams	**Protein:**	0 grams
Fiber:	0 grams	**Saturated Fat:**	1 gram	**Carbs:**	0 grams
Sodium:	115 mg	**Sugars:**	0 grams		

Homemade Chicken Stock

It will come as no surprise that this homemade stock is better tasting than store-bought brands, and has less sodium. Freeze it in 1- or 2-cup containers so you have it on hand when you go to make one of my comforting chicken soups, like the Roasted Chicken and Vegetable Soup on page 153.

Makes 20 cups

    9 pounds chicken backs, trimmed of excess fat
    5 onions, coarsely chopped
    5 carrots, cut into 1½-inch pieces
    5 celery stalks, cut into 1½-inch pieces
    10 whole garlic cloves
    20 whole black peppercorns
    15 sprigs fresh parsley
    10 sprigs fresh thyme
    5 bay leaves
    5 quarts water

Combine the chicken, onions, carrots, celery, garlic, peppercorns, parsley, thyme, bay leaves, and water in a large stockpot. Bring to a boil over medium-high heat. Reduce the heat to medium and gently simmer for 4 hours. Strain through a wire-mesh sieve into another pot and discard the solids in the sieve. Let cool, then cover and refrigerate for 6 hours to allow any fat to congeal. Skim the fat from the surface of the stock and discard. Store in an airtight container in the refrigerator for up to 3 days or freeze for up to 1 year.

Nutrient Content per Serving

Calories:	20	**Fat:**	0 grams	**Protein:**	2 grams
Fiber:	0 grams	**Saturated Fat:**	0 grams	**Carbs:**	1 gram
Sodium:	10 mg	**Sugars:**	0 grams		

Smoky BBQ Spice Rub

Prepare for grilling greatness. My smoky BBQ spice rub is excellent on beef, pork, lamb, poultry, and fish like tuna and salmon. You'll be happy to know it can be easily scaled up.

Makes about rounded ⅓ cup

3 tablespoons smoked paprika

1½ tablespoons chili powder

1 tablespoon ground cumin

1 teaspoon garlic powder

1 teaspoon monk fruit extract

1 teaspoon sea salt

¼ teaspoon ground chipotle pepper

Combine the paprika, chili powder, cumin, garlic powder, monk fruit extract, salt, and chipotle pepper in a small bowl; mix well. Store in an airtight container for up to 6 months.

Nutrient Content per Serving

Calories:	15	**Fat:**	0.5 grams	**Protein:**	1 gram
Fiber:	1 gram	**Saturated Fat:**	0 grams	**Carbs:**	2 grams
Sodium:	390 mg	**Sugars:**	0 grams		

Jerk Rub

A great take on a Jamaican classic. Put on some reggae music while mixing it up and let the islands come to you! It's great on beef, pork, lamb, chicken, fish, shellfish, vegetables, and…well, just about anything!

Makes ⅔ cup

⅓ cup paprika

2 tablespoons ground allspice

1 tablespoon dried thyme

1 tablespoon sea salt

2 teaspoons freshly ground black pepper

1 teaspoon ground nutmeg

1 teaspoon ground cinnamon

1 teaspoon monk fruit extract

1 to 1½ teaspoons cayenne pepper

Combine the paprika, allspice, thyme, salt, black pepper, nutmeg, cinnamon, monk fruit extract, and cayenne pepper to taste in a small bowl; mix well. Store in an airtight container for up to 6 months.

Nutrient Content per Serving

Calories:	20	**Fat:**	0.5 grams	**Protein:**	1 gram
Fiber:	2 grams	**Saturated Fat:**	0 grams	**Carbs:**	4 grams
Sodium:	700 mg	**Sugars:**	0 grams		

Cilantro Pesto

And you didn't think pesto could get any better! Cilantro pesto is mild and less expensive than the basil version. It can be wonderful on pasta, bread, or meat.

Makes about 1 cup

> 3 cups tightly packed fresh cilantro
> 1 garlic clove
> ¼ cup slow-roasted almonds (see page 97)
> 1 teaspoon grated lime zest
> ½ jalapeño pepper, seeded
> ¼ teaspoon sea salt
> ⅓ cup olive oil

Combine the cilantro, garlic, almonds, lime zest, jalapeño pepper, and salt in a food processor. Process until the cilantro mixture is finely chopped. With the machine running, add the oil in a steady stream until a thick puree forms. Store in an airtight container in the refrigerator for up to 2 weeks or freeze for up to 2 months.

Nutrient Content per Serving

Calories:	70	**Fat:**	7 grams	**Protein:**	1 gram
Fiber:	0 grams	**Saturated Fat:**	1 gram	**Carbs:**	1 gram
Sodium:	65 mg	**Sugars:**	0 grams		

Sugar Impact Mayonnaise

Store-bought mayo can contain damaging oils, added sugar, and something called "natural flavors." Hmmm. Make this fresh, flavorful, homemade version and feel good about your effort with every spoonful.

Makes 1 cup (1 tablespoon per serving)

> ¼ cup unsweetened coconut milk
>
> ½ cup raw cashews
>
> 4 teaspoons lemon juice
>
> 1 tablespoon Dijon mustard
>
> ½ teaspoon sea salt
>
> ½ cup macadamia nut oil

Combine the coconut milk, cashews, lemon juice, mustard, and salt in a blender and puree. With the blender running, add the oil in a slow, steady stream until the mixture is thick and creamy. Store in an airtight container in the refrigerator for up to 3 weeks.

Nutrient Content per Serving

Calories:	90	**Fat:**	9 grams	**Protein:**	1 gram
Fiber:	0 grams	**Saturated Fat:**	1 gram	**Carbs:**	2 grams
Sodium:	105 mg	**Sugars:**	0 grams		

Basil Vinaigrette

Head down to your local farmers' market for the freshest basil, or better yet, grow your own in a kitchen herb garden. Now *that's* fresh! Using a sharp knife to chop the basil will keep it from bruising and help the leaves stay green.

Makes ¾ cup (2 tablespoons per serving)

3 tablespoons white wine vinegar

3 tablespoons chopped fresh basil

1 teaspoon Dijon mustard

½ teaspoon monk fruit extract

½ teaspoon sea salt

¼ teaspoon freshly ground black pepper

½ cup extra-virgin olive oil

Combine the vinegar, basil, mustard, monk fruit extract, salt, and pepper in a small bowl. Slowly whisk in the oil until well combined. Store in an airtight container in the refrigerator for up to 2 weeks.

Nutrient Content per Serving

Calories:	80	**Fat:**	9 grams	**Protein:**	0 grams
Fiber:	0 grams	**Saturated Fat:**	1 gram	**Carbs:**	0 grams
Sodium:	105 mg	**Sugars:**	0 grams		

11

DESSERTS

The first thing most diets do is try to cut the heart out of your sugar addiction by taking dessert off the table. Well, if that won't send you into cold sweats, what will?

The very name of the Sugar Impact Diet tells you that I'm taking aim at damaging sugars—sugars that hit your health and midsection harder than others. I have intentionally not called it the No Sugar Diet. Not only is that unrealistic, but it's unnecessary.

The Sugar Impact Diet is not about deprivation. These sensational desserts will satisfy your sweet tooth, but they won't spike your blood sugar or derail your weight loss goals. You'll notice that they even have some nutritional value, so indulge guilt free. Have your cake, and eat your cake (I'm a giver, not a taker!).

Grilled Peaches (Cycles 1/3)

The secret to succulent grilled peaches is to start with peaches that are firm and ripe, not overly soft and juicy. They'll be saccharine enough—the grilling helps coax out their natural sweetness.

Makes 4 servings

4 medium peaches, halved and pitted
2 teaspoons coconut oil, melted
⅛ teaspoon ground nutmeg
⅛ teaspoon ground cinnamon
Olive oil for the pan

Brush the peaches with the coconut oil, then sprinkle with the nutmeg and cinnamon.

Lightly dampen a paper towel with a small amount of olive oil and wipe a grill pan with it; heat over medium heat. Add the peaches and cook until well-marked, warmed through, and slightly tender, 3 minutes per side.

Nutrient Content per Serving

Calories:	80	**Fat:**	2.5 grams	**Protein:**	1 gram
Fiber:	2 grams	**Saturated Fat:**	2 grams	**Carbs:**	14 grams
Sodium:	0 mg	**Sugars:**	12 grams		

Pumpkin Bread Pudding

You're going to love this so much I'm going to give you an excuse to have it more often. Sure, it's a decadent dessert, but it can pass as a great brunch dish, too. You're welcome!

Makes 12 servings

Olive oil for the pan
1 loaf Coconut-Pumpkin Bread (page 74), preferably 1 to 2 days old, cubed
4 large eggs
2 cups lite culinary coconut milk (see box, page 132)
2 teaspoons monk fruit extract
1 teaspoon vanilla extract
¾ teaspoon ground cinnamon
¼ teaspoon ground nutmeg

Preheat the oven to 350°F. Position a rack in the center. Lightly dampen a paper towel with a small amount of olive oil and wipe a 9-inch square baking pan with it.

Place the bread cubes in the prepared pan. Whisk together the eggs, coconut milk, monk fruit extract, vanilla, cinnamon, and nutmeg in a medium bowl. Pour the egg mixture over the bread cubes, pressing down on the bread to make sure all of it gets wet, and let stand for 20 minutes.

Bake until puffed and the custard has set, 38 to 40 minutes. Let cool for 10 minutes before cutting and serving.

Nutrient Content per Serving

Calories:	210	**Fat:**	18 grams	**Protein:**	6 grams
Fiber:	4 grams	**Saturated Fat:**	11 grams	**Carbs:**	7 grams
Sodium:	250 mg	**Sugars:**	1 gram		

Chocolate–Almond Butter Protein Popsicles

Plain old Popsicles will never darken the door of your fridge again. These are just as easy to make, and so much more flavorful.

Makes 6 servings

2 scoops chocolate protein blend

10 ounces unsweetened coconut milk

2 tablespoons almond butter

1 teaspoon ground cinnamon

¼ teaspoon almond extract

Whisk together the protein, coconut milk, almond butter, cinnamon, and almond extract in a medium bowl until well blended. Pour the mixture into six Popsicle molds and freeze overnight.

Dip the bottoms of the molds into warm water to remove the Popsicles. Store in a resealable plastic container in the freezer.

Nutrient Content per Serving

Calories:	70	**Fat:**	4 grams	**Protein:**	5 grams
Fiber:	2 grams	**Saturated Fat:**	1.5 grams	**Carbs:**	3 grams
Sodium:	35 mg	**Sugars:**	1 gram		

Coconut-Avocado Mousse

Creamy, rich coconut has never been so luscious. Go ahead, say *mmm* by the spoonful. Make sure to buy unsweetened flaked coconut to keep the SI low.

Makes 4 servings

1 ripe avocado, halved, pitted, peeled, and mashed

¾ cup unsweetened cultured coconut milk (such as So Delicious brand)

1½ teaspoons monk fruit extract

1 teaspoon grated lime zest

¼ teaspoon coconut extract

¼ cup unsweetened coconut flakes

Combine the avocado, coconut milk, monk fruit extract, lime zest, and coconut extract in a medium bowl. Beat with a handheld electric mixer on the highest setting until light and fluffy. Gently fold in the coconut flakes. Divide among four bowls and refrigerate for at least 1 hour before serving.

Nutrient Content per Serving

Calories:	110	**Fat:**	10 grams	**Protein:**	2 grams
Fiber:	2 grams	**Saturated Fat:**	4.5 grams	**Carbs:**	6 grams
Sodium:	15 mg	**Sugars:**	0 grams		

Vanilla-Coconut "Yogurt" Pudding Pops

Being dairy-free does not mean being deprived of deliciousness. Cultured coconut milk stands in for Greek-style yogurt in this refreshing, dairy-free treat.

Makes 5 servings

1 (16-ounce) container unsweetened vanilla cultured coconut milk
1 teaspoon vanilla extract
2 teaspoons monk fruit extract

Whisk together the coconut milk, vanilla extract, and monk fruit extract in a medium bowl. Pour the mixture into five Popsicle molds and freeze overnight.

Dip the bottoms of the molds into warm water to remove the pops. Store in a resealable plastic container in the freezer.

Nutrient Content per Serving

Calories:	20	**Fat:**	2 grams	**Protein:**	0 grams
Fiber:	0 grams	**Saturated Fat:**	1.5 grams	**Carbs:**	1 gram
Sodium:	25 mg	**Sugars:**	0 grams		

Strawberry Ice Cream (Cycles 1/3)

Fresh, juicy strawberries just scream "sweet treat," and since we all scream for ice cream...you see where I'm going with this? Put your feet up and savor every dreamy spoonful. If your strawberries are not very sweet, you may want to increase the sweetener by a teaspoon or two.

Makes 10 servings (about ⅓ cup per serving)

2 (11-ounce) boxes original culinary coconut milk (see box, page 132)
1½ pounds strawberries, hulled and chopped
2 tablespoons erythritol
½ teaspoon vanilla extract

Combine the coconut milk and strawberries in a medium saucepan over medium heat. Bring to a simmer and cook until the strawberries are tender, 10 to 12 minutes. Remove from the heat and let stand for 10 minutes. Transfer to a blender and puree. Pour into a bowl and stir in the erythritol and vanilla extract. Cover and chill for 2 hours.

Pour the mixture through a sieve to remove any seeds and transfer to an ice cream maker. Churn according to the manufacturer's directions. Transfer to a covered container and freeze for at least 1 hour to harden. Let stand at room temperature for 10 to 15 minutes to soften before serving.

Nutrient Content per Serving

Calories:	35	**Fat:**	1.5 grams	**Protein:**	0 grams
Fiber:	2 grams	**Saturated Fat:**	1 gram	**Carbs:**	9 grams
Sodium:	20 mg	**Sugars:**	3 grams		

Lemon Cookies

The essence of what a good cookie should be—irresistible! Grated lemon and orange zest give these treats their great citrus flavor. Happy crunching!

Makes 24 cookies (12 servings)

2 cups almond flour
2 tablespoons erythritol
½ teaspoon baking powder
¼ teaspoon baking soda
⅛ teaspoon sea salt
⅓ cup coconut butter
2 large eggs
1 teaspoon grated lemon zest
1 teaspoon grated orange zest

Preheat the oven to 350°F. Line a large baking sheet with parchment paper.

Combine the almond flour, erythritol, baking powder, baking soda, and salt in a medium bowl. Transfer the flour mixture to a food processor and pulse in the coconut butter, eggs, lemon zest, and orange zest.

Form level tablespoons of batter into 24 balls and place them on the baking sheet. Press each ball down to a thickness of ½ inch.

Bake until lightly browned, 16 to 18 minutes. Remove from the oven and let cool completely, 30 minutes.

Nutrient Content per Serving

Calories:	170	**Fat:**	15 grams	**Protein:**	5 grams
Fiber:	3 grams	**Saturated Fat:**	5 grams	**Carbs:**	8 grams
Sodium:	95 mg	**Sugars:**	1 gram		

PART III

THE SUGAR IMPACT DIET MEAL PLANS

This is where it all begins. You'll look back on the moment you start the Sugar Impact Diet as one of the big turning points in your life, so take a good look around!

I've included seven of the most popular meal plans in this cookbook to help you fine-tune the Sugar Impact Diet for your specific needs. But if you don't see yourself in these meal plans, there are many more at http://sugarimpact.com/resources. They target conditions like high blood pressure and menopause, and offer support for everything from being on a budget to throwing a low-SI bash. More than one may apply—if you're an athlete dealing with food intolerance, you may want to incorporate the Virgin Diet while you're lowering your Sugar Impact. Or you may be paleo and trying to feed a finicky family. Mix and match to suit!

Also, I've built these meal plans to give you a lot of variety each week. If you prefer to repeat meals and keep it simple or you're cooking for one or two, you can opt to have your leftovers from dinner for lunch the next day, or repeat your evening meal two days in a row. These meal plans are meant to be a starting guide, not an absolute.

I think you'll be surprised by how quickly you'll kick your sugar habit. Your sensitivity to it could reset in just a few days, which means super energy, stable moods, and weight loss will follow, fast. You'll be eating foods that shift you from burning sugar to burning fat and begin to heal you (you may even see a dramatic reduction in your symptoms right away). On average, my clients lose 10 pounds in the 2 weeks of Cycle 2—and you can, too, just by following the recipes and meal plans in this cookbook. That's why you're here, right? To lose weight and feel better fast? You'll get there soon, and you'll never want to leave.

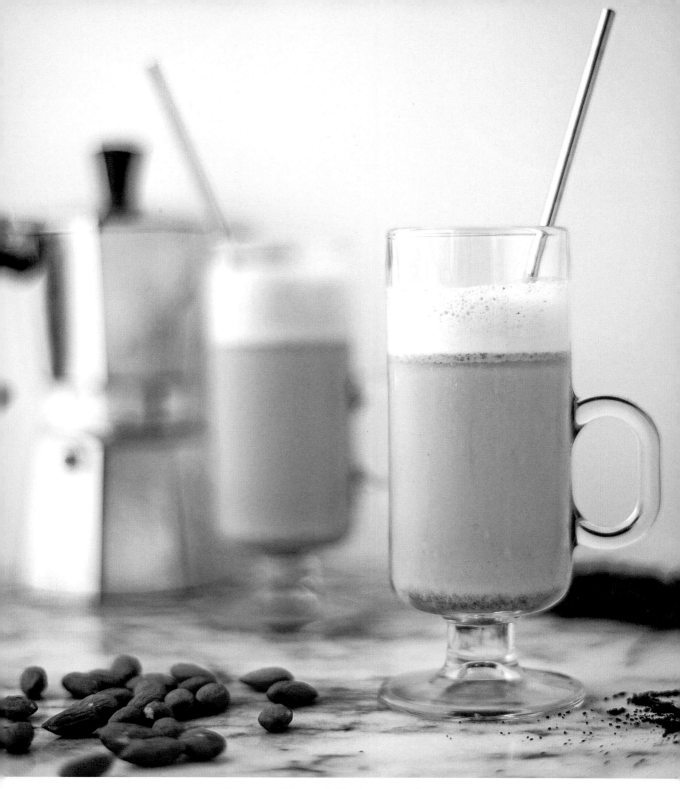

Espresso-Almond Shake, page 67

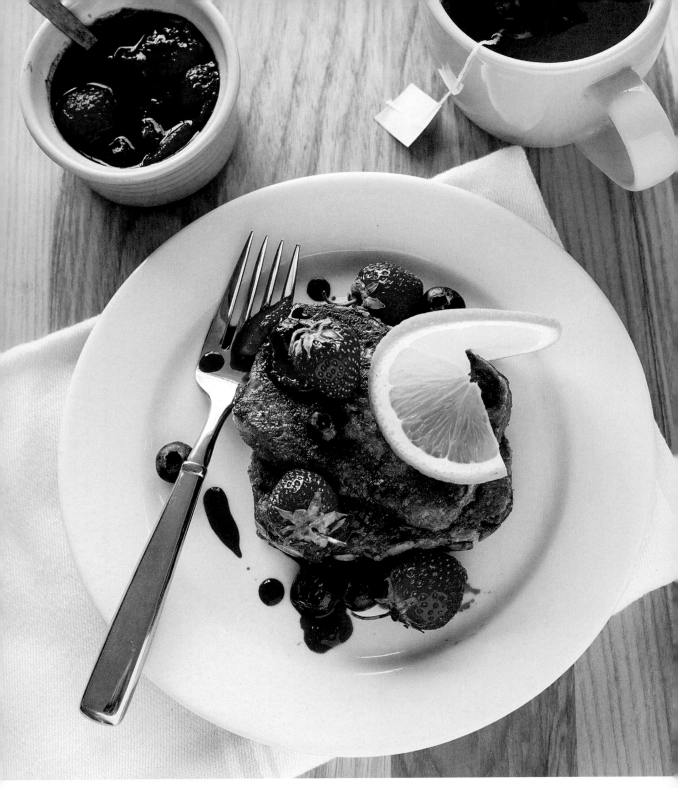

Pumpkin Bread French Toast with Berry Compote, page 72

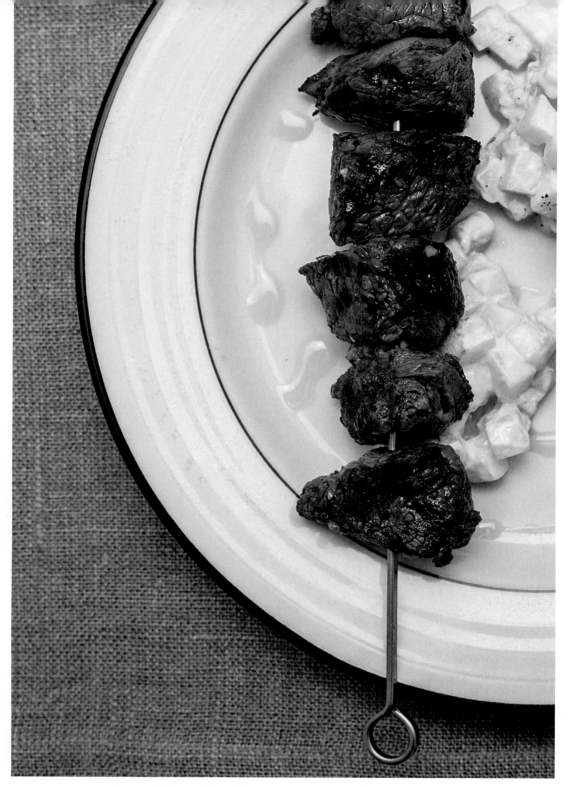

Lamb Souvlaki with Cultured Coconut Milk Tzatziki, page 87

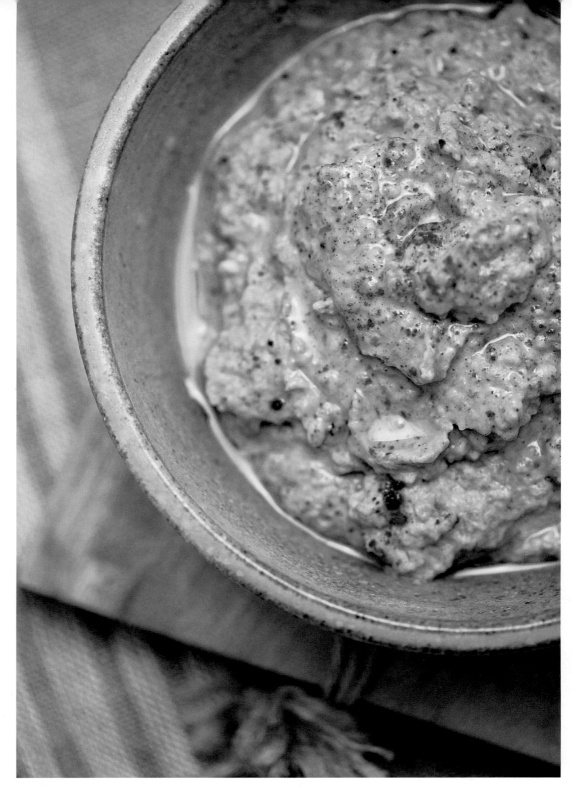

Smoky Baba Ghanoush, page 96

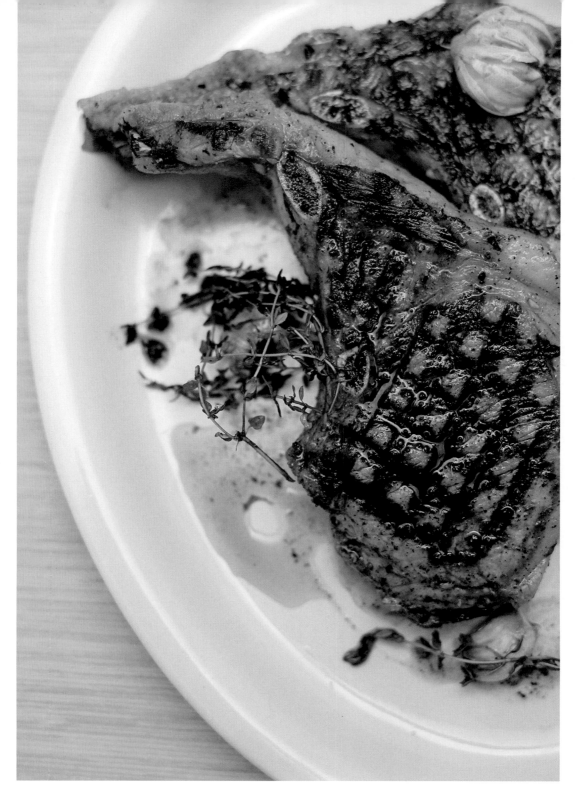

Mustard and Garlic–Marinated Pork Chops, page 107

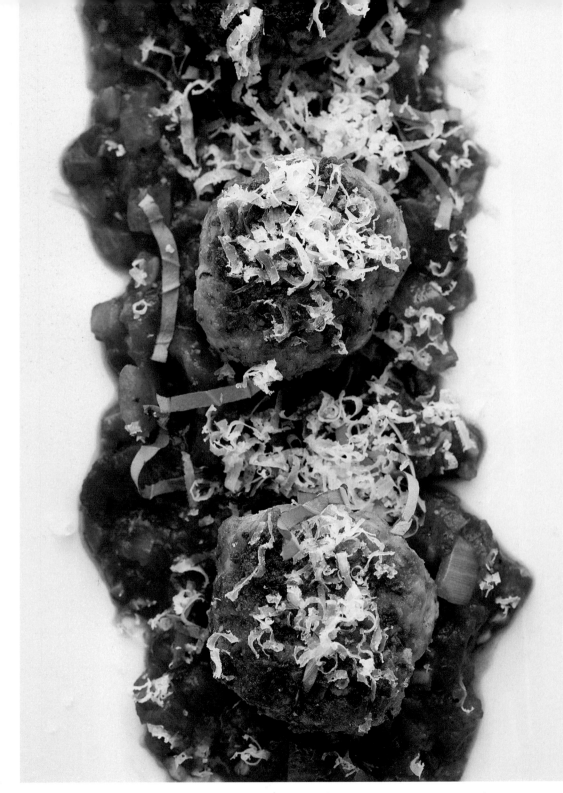

Turkey Meatballs with Parmesan and Tomato Sauce, page 126

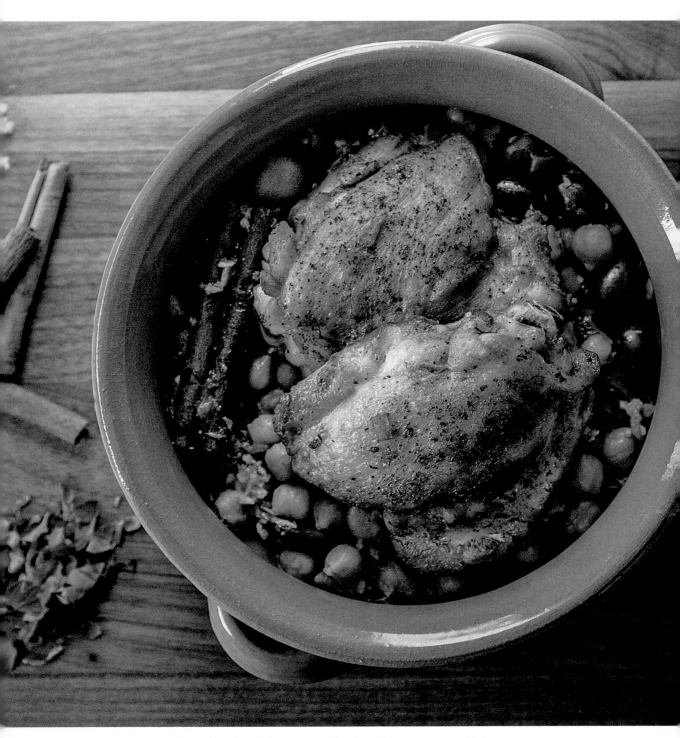

Slow Cooker Moroccan Chicken Tagine, page 128

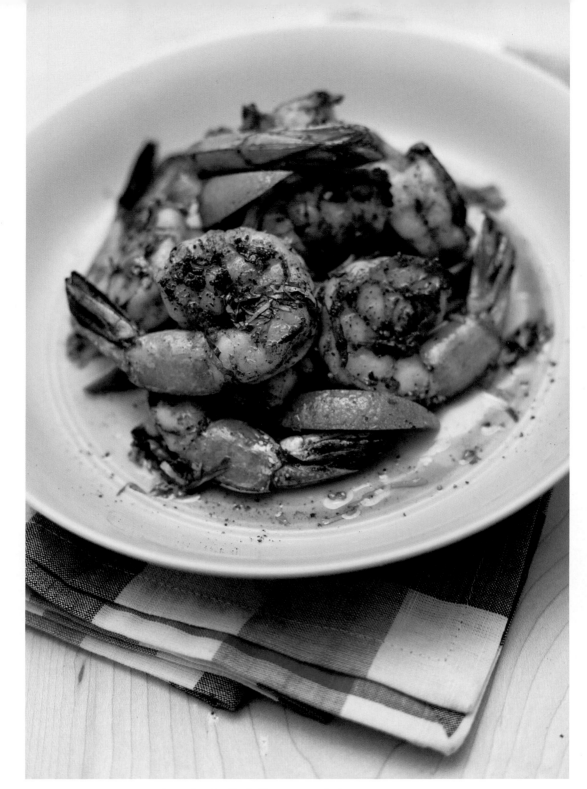

Simply Grilled Shrimp with Lime, page 133

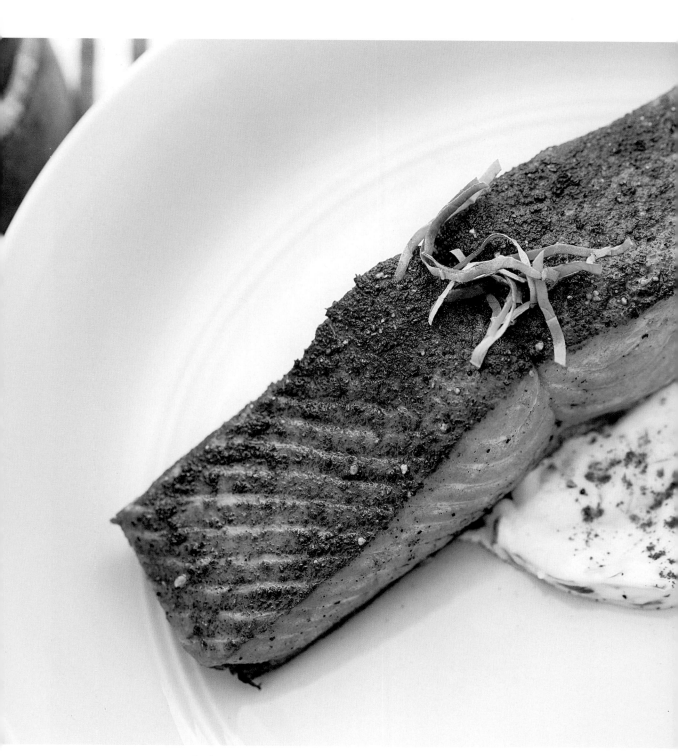

Blackened Salmon with Basil Aioli, page 135

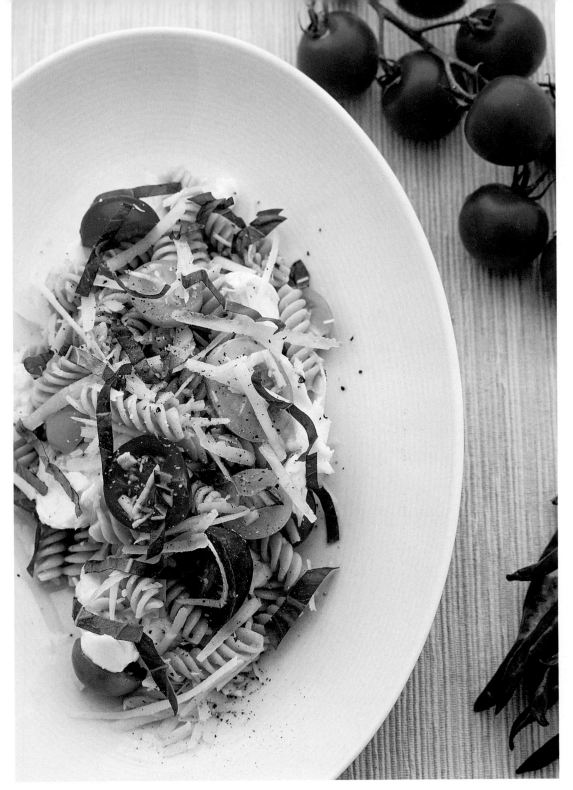

Quinoa Pasta alla Checca, page 144

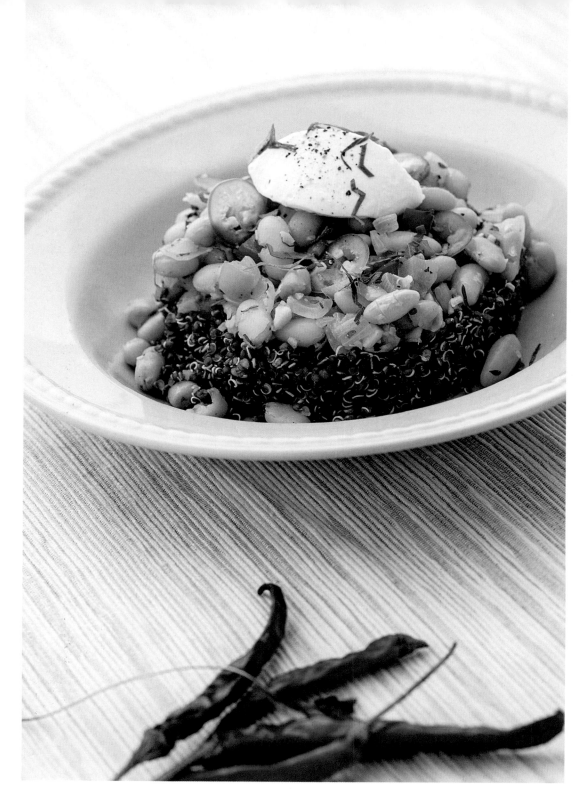

Easy Vegetarian White Chili, page 144

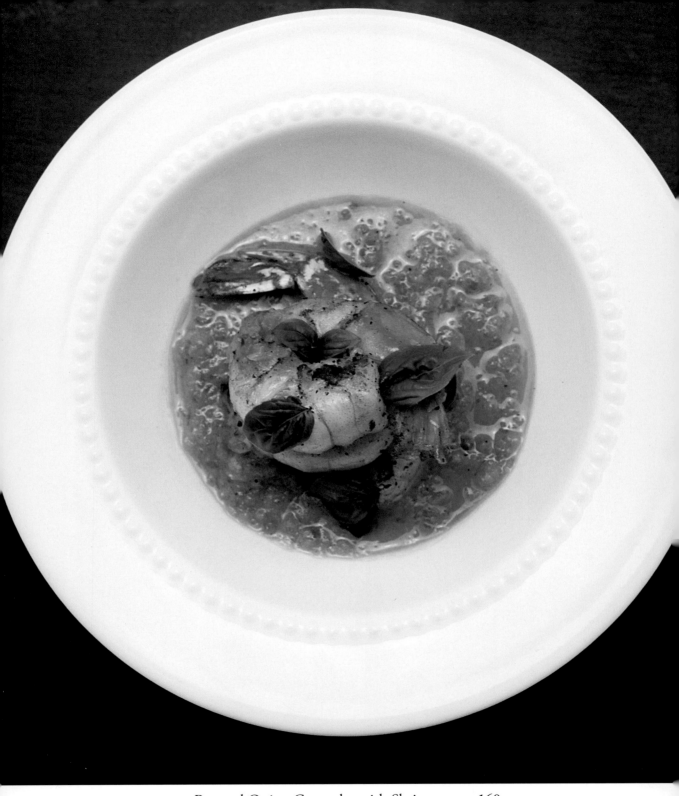

Roasted Onion Gazpacho with Shrimp, page 160

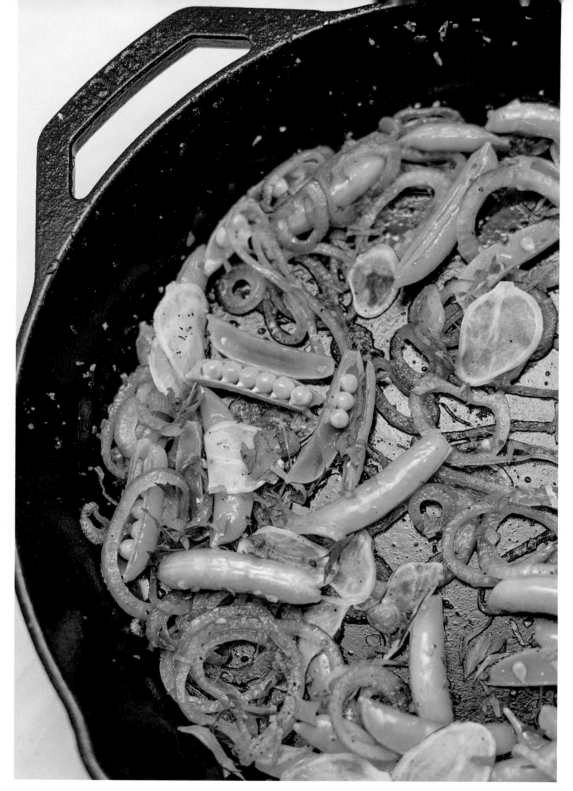

Sautéed Sugar Snaps and Radishes with Fresh Parsley and Orange Zest, page 164

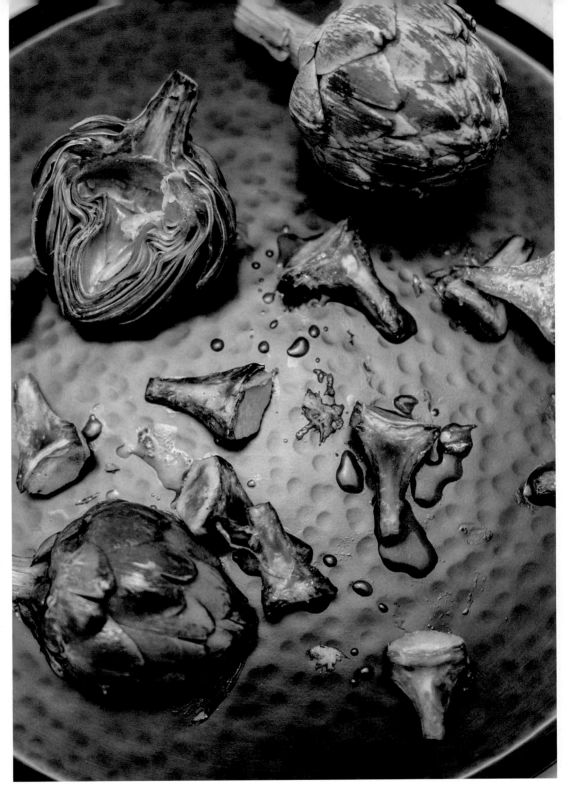

Lemony Roasted Artichoke Hearts, page 170

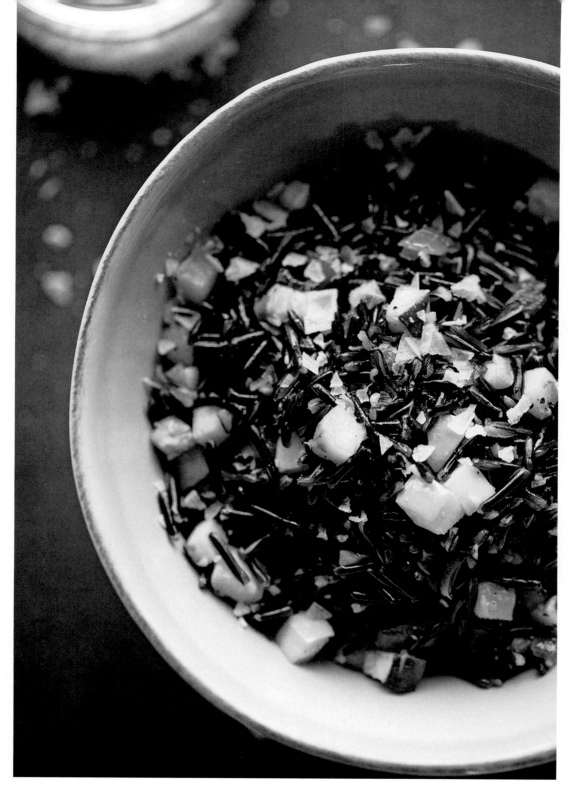

Wild Rice and Vegetable Pilaf, page 189

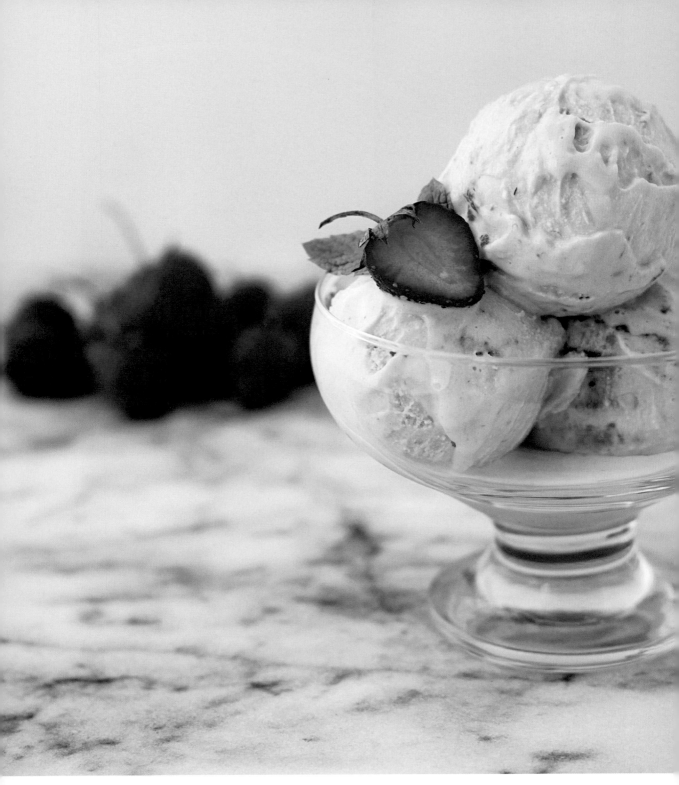

Strawberry Ice Cream, page 202

12

THE BASICS

Who doesn't want to lose up to 10 pounds in 2 weeks and feel better than ever? No one I know! That's why the Sugar Impact Diet is for everyone, because no matter where you start, it will rev your metabolism, boost your energy, and soothe your achy self. This Basic Plan is your broad-strokes guide to learning how to easily and effortlessly shift to a low-SI way of life and reap all its rewards.

So start here if you're not dealing with any specific conditions (if you are, there are detailed meal plans just for you) and if you're the kind of person who says "Just tell me what to do and I'll do it." You know the sooner you get started, the faster you'll get where you want to be.

BASIC MEAL PLAN

This basic meal plan will guide you effortlessly through the three cycles of the Sugar Impact Diet meal by meal, day by day. Each italicized recipe is detailed in Part II of this book, in its category (Salad, Mains, etc.), so refer to the indicated page numbers for step-by-step instructions on how to make each dish.

Cycle 1

DAY 1

BREAKFAST

Sugar Impact Shake (page 65) with 1 serving low- or medium-SI fruit

LUNCH

Southwest Grilled Steak Salad on Crisped Rice Tortillas (page 83)

DINNER

Simply Grilled Shrimp with Lime (page 133) over brown rice
Stir-Fried Bok Choy (page 178)

OPTIONAL SNACK

Cinnamon Almond Butter (page 104) with apple slices

DAY 2

BREAKFAST

Pumpkin Bread French Toast with Berry Compote (page 72)

LUNCH

Super Greens Shake (page 66) with an apple added

DINNER

Turkey Meatballs with Parmesan and Tomato Sauce (page 126)
Spaghetti Squash with Capers, Onion, and Bell Pepper (page 185)

OPTIONAL SNACK

Smoky Baba Ghanoush (page 96) with bean chips

DAY 3

BREAKFAST

Blueberry-Peach Shake (page 70)

LUNCH

Turkey, Spinach, and Strawberry Wrap (page 78)

DINNER

Pork and Mushroom Stew with Sweet Potatoes (page 159)

Mixed green salad with *Basil Vinaigrette* (page 197)

OPTIONAL SNACK

Lime and Jalapeño Hummus (page 95) with rice chips

DAY 4

BREAKFAST

Tex-Mex Scrambled Eggs with Avocado and Salsa (page 71) in a rice wrap

LUNCH

Pumpkin Spice Shake (page 67) with an apple added

DINNER

Herbed Salmon Cakes with Tartar Sauce (page 134)

Spiced Sweet Potato "Fries" (page 188)

Mixed green salad with *Easy Lemon Vinaigrette* (page 193)

OPTIONAL SNACK

Spicy Black Bean Dip with Celery (page 101) with rice chips

DAY 5

BREAKFAST

Espresso-Almond Shake (page 67) with ½ banana

LUNCH

Chicken Soup with Parsnips (page 150)

Mixed green salad with *Dijon Vinaigrette* (page 193)

DINNER

Jerk-Spiced Chicken Thighs with Roasted Pineapple Chutney (page 123)

½ baked sweet potato

Steamed Broccoli with Garlic Oil Drizzle (page 167)

OPTIONAL SNACK

Garlic Hummus with Lentil Chips (page 100)

DAY 6

BREAKFAST

Old-Fashioned Oatmeal with Cinnamon, Blueberries, and Raspberries (page 73) with a side of nitrate-free bacon or chicken breakfast sausage

LUNCH

Chocolate, Flax, and Avocado Shake (page 69) with 1 serving blackberries

DINNER

Slow-Cooker Tomato-Braised Lamb Shanks (page 105)
Chickpeas with Sautéed Greens (page 183)
Mixed green salad with *Dijon Vinaigrette* (page 193)

OPTIONAL SNACK

White and Red Bean Salsa with White Onion, Tomato, and Cilantro (page 93) with rice chips

DAY 7

BREAKFAST

Coconut-Vanilla Shake (page 68) with 1 serving low- or medium-SI fruit

LUNCH

Mediterranean Salmon Wrap with Caper Dressing (page 88) with the coconut wrap swapped out for a rice wrap

DINNER

Quinoa Pasta alla Checca (page 144) with a grilled chicken breast
Shredded Brussels Sprouts with Easy Lemon Vinaigrette (page 166)

OPTIONAL SNACK

Cucumber Chips with Guacamole (page 101) with the cucumber chips swapped out for rice chips

Cycle 2

DAY 1

BREAKFAST

Pumpkin Spice Shake (page 67)

LUNCH

Flank Steak and Vegetable Wrap with Chimichurri Sauce (page 81)

DINNER

BBQ-Rubbed Whole Roasted Chicken (page 123)

Beans and Greens Stew (page 155)

OPTIONAL SNACK

Vanilla-Coconut "Yogurt" Pudding Pops (page 202)

DAY 2

BREAKFAST

Tex-Mex Scrambled Eggs with Avocado and Salsa (page 71)

LUNCH

Easy Vegetarian White Chili (page 144)

Mixed green salad with *Dijon Vinaigrette* (page 193)

DINNER

Roasted Pork Tenderloin with Basil Vinaigrette (page 106)

Wild Rice and Vegetable Pilaf (page 189)

OPTIONAL SNACK

Lemon-Chili Roasted Almonds (page 95)

DAY 3

BREAKFAST

Cappuccino Protein Shake (page 69)

LUNCH

Warm Chicken Salad with Pecans, Basil, and Caper Vinaigrette (page 132)

DINNER

Beef and Pork Meat Loaf (page 114)

Roasted Butternut Squash with Thyme (page 187)

Sautéed Kale with Caramelized Onions (page 172)

OPTIONAL SNACK

Smoky Baba Ghanoush (page 96) with crudités

DAY 4

BREAKFAST

Goat Cheese and Vegetable Omelet (page 74)

LUNCH

Espresso-Almond Shake (page 67)

DINNER

Seared Halibut with Lemon-Basil Gremolata (page 140)

Lima Beans with Lemon and Spinach (page 186)

Mixed green salad with Easy Lemon Vinaigrette (page 193)

OPTIONAL SNACK

Roasted Spiced Chickpeas (page 98)

DAY 5

BREAKFAST

Sugar Impact Shake (page 65)

LUNCH

Mediterranean Salmon Wrap with Caper Dressing (page 88)

DINNER

Pepper-Crusted Turkey Paillards over Spinach with Dijon Vinaigrette (page 120)

Red Quinoa with Slow-Roasted Almonds and Caramelized Shallots (page 183)

OPTIONAL SNACK

Chocolate–Almond Butter Protein Popsicles (page 201)

DAY 6

BREAKFAST

Coconut-Pumpkin Bread (page 74) with a side of nitrate-free bacon or chicken breakfast sausage

LUNCH

Super Greens Shake (page 66)

DINNER

Simply Grilled Shrimp with Lime (page 133)
Asian Confetti Quinoa Salad with Almonds (page 85)

OPTIONAL SNACK

Lime and Jalapeño Hummus (page 95) with crudités

DAY 7

BREAKFAST

Chocolate, Flax, and Avocado Shake (page 69)

LUNCH

Chicken, Shirataki Noodle, and Snap Pea Salad (page 80)

DINNER

Blackened Salmon with Basil Aioli (page 135)
Spicy Okra with Ginger, Garlic, and Tomatoes (page 173)

OPTIONAL SNACK

Spicy Black Bean Dip with Celery (page 101)

DAY 8

BREAKFAST

Tex-Mex Scrambled Eggs with Avocado and Salsa (page 71)

LUNCH

Pumpkin Spice Shake (page 67)

DINNER

BLT Wedge Salad with Avocado and Dijon Vinaigrette (page 89)

Strip Steaks with Tomatoes, Olives, and Parsley (page 109)

Marjoram Seared Mushrooms (page 166)

OPTIONAL SNACK

Coconut-Avocado Mousse (page 201)

DAY 9

BREAKFAST

Sugar Impact Shake (page 65)

LUNCH

Roasted Chicken and Vegetable Soup (page 153)

DINNER

Thai Coconut Steamed Mussels (page 136)

Coconut Curry Butternut Squash Puree (page 180)

Mixed green salad with *Basil Vinaigrette* (page 197)

OPTIONAL SNACK

White and Red Bean Salsa with White Onion, Tomato, and Cilantro (page 93) with crudités

DAY 10

BREAKFAST

Coconut-Pumpkin Bread (page 74) with a side of nitrate-free bacon or chicken breakfast sausage

LUNCH

Super Greens Shake (page 66)

DINNER

Fillet of Sole Piccata (page 140)
Lemony Roasted Artichoke Hearts (page 170)
Wild Rice and Vegetable Pilaf (page 189)

OPTIONAL SNACK

Chipotle Kale Chips (page 103)

DAY 11

BREAKFAST

Cappuccino Protein Shake (page 69)

LUNCH

Classic Greek Salad with Pan-Grilled Chicken and Feta Cheese (page 91)

DINNER

Turkey-Bean Chili with Crispy Coconut Wrap Strips (page 148)
Mixed green salad with *Dijon Vinaigrette* (page 193)

OPTIONAL SNACK

Cucumber Chips with Guacamole (page 101)

DAY 12

BREAKFAST

Chocolate, Flax, and Avocado Shake (page 69)

LUNCH

Lamb Souvlaki with Cultured Coconut Milk Tzatziki (page 87)

DINNER

Tandoori Chicken (page 129)
Red Lentil Dal (page 182)
Steamed Broccoli with Garlic Oil Drizzle (page 167)

OPTIONAL SNACK

Fresh-Baked Gluten-Free Sesame "Pretzels" (page 94)

DAY 13

BREAKFAST
Coconut-Vanilla Shake (page 68)

LUNCH
Goat Cheese Burger Wrap (page 86)
Crudités

DINNER
Spicy Black Bean Burgers with Goat Cheese and Wilted Tomato Salsa (page 146)
Warm Wax Bean and Green Bean Salad (page 174)

OPTIONAL SNACK
Cinnamon Almond Butter (page 104) with celery

DAY 14

BREAKFAST
Individual Baked Breakfast Frittatas (page 75)

LUNCH
Espresso-Almond Shake (page 67)

DINNER
Slow Cooker–Braised Chicken Legs with Rosemary, Onions, and Celery (page 125)
Winter Vegetable Minestrone (page 162)

OPTIONAL SNACK
Slow-Roasted Nuts (page 97)

Cycle 3

DAY 1

BREAKFAST
Sugar Impact Shake (page 65) with 1 serving low- or medium–SI fruit

LUNCH

Southwest Grilled Steak Salad on Crisped Rice Tortillas (page 83)

DINNER

Simply Grilled Shrimp with Lime (page 133) over brown rice

Stir-Fried Bok Choy (page 178)

OPTIONAL SNACK

Cinnamon Almond Butter (page 104) with apple slices

DAY 2

BREAKFAST

Pumpkin Bread French Toast with Berry Compote (page 72)

LUNCH

Super Greens Shake (page 66) with an apple added

DINNER

Turkey Meatballs with Parmesan and Tomato Sauce (page 126)

Spaghetti Squash with Capers, Onion, and Bell Pepper (page 185)

OPTIONAL SNACK

Smoky Baba Ghanoush (page 96) with bean chips

DAY 3

BREAKFAST

Blueberry-Peach Shake (page 70)

LUNCH

Turkey, Spinach, and Strawberry Wrap (page 78)

DINNER

Pork and Mushroom Stew with Sweet Potatoes (page 159)

Mixed green salad with Basil Vinaigrette (page 197)

OPTIONAL SNACK

Lime and Jalapeño Hummus (page 95) with rice chips

DAY 4

BREAKFAST

Tex-Mex Scrambled Eggs with Avocado and Salsa (page 71) in a rice wrap

LUNCH

Pumpkin Spice Shake (page 67) with an apple added

DINNER

Herbed Salmon Cakes with Tartar Sauce (page 134)

Spiced Sweet Potato "Fries" (page 188)

Mixed green salad with *Easy Lemon Vinaigrette* (page 193)

OPTIONAL SNACK

Spicy Black Bean Dip with Celery (page 101) with rice chips

DAY 5

BREAKFAST

Espresso-Almond Shake (page 67) with ½ banana

LUNCH

Chicken Soup with Parsnips (page 150)

Mixed green salad with *Dijon Vinaigrette* (page 193)

DINNER

Jerk-Spiced Chicken Thighs with Roasted Pineapple Chutney (page 123)

½ baked sweet potato

Steamed Broccoli with Garlic Oil Drizzle (page 167)

OPTIONAL SNACK

Garlic Hummus with Lentil Chips (page 100)

DAY 6

BREAKFAST

Old-Fashioned Oatmeal with Cinnamon, Blueberries, and Raspberries (page 73) with a side of nitrate-free bacon or chicken breakfast sausage

LUNCH

Chocolate, Flax, and Avocado Shake (page 69) with 1 serving blackberries

DINNER

Slow-Cooker Tomato-Braised Lamb Shanks (page 105)

Baked potato (high–SI challenge)

Mixed green salad with *Dijon Vinaigrette* (page 193)

OPTIONAL SNACK

White and Red Bean Salsa with White Onion, Tomato, and Cilantro (page 93) with rice chips

DAY 7

BREAKFAST

Coconut-Vanilla Shake (page 68) with 1 serving low- or medium-SI fruit

LUNCH

Mediterranean Salmon Wrap with Caper Dressing (page 88) with the coconut wrap swapped for a rice wrap

DINNER

Quinoa Pasta alla Checca (page 144) with a grilled chicken breast

Shredded Brussels Sprouts with Easy Lemon Vinaigrette (page 166)

OPTIONAL SNACK

Cucumber Chips with Guacamole (page 101) with the cucumber chips swapped out for rice chips

13

DIABETES AND INSULIN RESISTANCE

Diabetes doesn't happen overnight. But when your metabolic machinery finally breaks, it wreaks havoc and the consequences can be deadly.

When you eat, you bump up your blood sugar. Every food raises blood sugar, but high–Sugar Impact foods can send it soaring. More than about a teaspoon of sugar (or glucose) in your bloodstream can create serious problems, so your pancreas releases a hormone called insulin to get blood sugar back in check.

Insulin shuttles glucose out of your blood into your cells, which can use that sugar as a quick energy hit or store it as glycogen to use later. That's the plan, anyway. But you know how plans go!

If your blood sugar stays elevated because of a steady stream of high-SI foods, your overworked pancreas keeps cranking out insulin to stabilize that blood sugar. Eventually your cells stop "hearing" its call. Your liver and muscles, where excess sugar is stored, declare "No vacancy." But that excess glucose has to go somewhere. It can't just hang out in your bloodstream or you'll have a very big problem.

One of the things your body does to avoid that is repackage glucose as fat, which makes itself at home around your midsection. Believe it or not, that's the least of your problems, as chronically high blood sugar levels eventually morph into full-blown diabetes and all its wicked complications.

INSULIN RESISTANCE: HERE COMES TROUBLE

When you hang out with your friends at a bar, you learn to tune out that obnoxiously drunk guy who keeps hitting on you. Eventually, insulin becomes "that guy." Your cells get burned out from the insulin barrage related to chronically high sugar levels and stop responding to it, leading to a condition called insulin resistance.

Insulin resistance doesn't happen all at once. Your muscle and liver cells are the first to stop "hearing" insulin's call, but you know which cells are last in line to stop responding? Yep: your fat cells. They're shouting, "Plenty of room here, come on in!"

Insulin resistance also doesn't occur in a vacuum. The risks associated with it include:

- Coronary disease
- Diabetes
- High triglycerides
- Hyperinsulinemia (excessive amounts of insulin)
- Hypertension (high blood pressure)
- Inflammation
- Obesity
- Stroke
- Weight loss resistance

FRUCTOSE: THE WORST OFFENDER

Insulin resistance is a direct result of eating too many high-SI foods for too long. Other substances like trans fats have been implicated, but high-SI foods are the head honchos. Of the sugar in those foods, it's not glucose that does the most damage (although it *can* create insulin resistance). There's a much nastier sugar: fructose.

You know high-fructose corn syrup is a giant sugar offender, but even when you cut processed foods and sugary drinks out of your diet, you might still be getting pounded with fructose if you overdo fruit, salad dressings, and other higher-fructose foods.

In the echelon of sugar, fructose takes the prize for being the worst. It can:

- Elevate blood pressure.
- Elevate uric acid, leading to gout.
- Contribute to small intestine bacterial overgrowth (SIBO), leaky gut, intestinal yeast overgrowth, insulin resistance, and kidney disease.
- Create liver inflammation—100% of fructose goes to your liver, which converts that fructose into triglycerides.
- Create leptin resistance—leptin is a hormone that tells your brain to stop eating. Even when you eat excessive amounts of fructose, your brain never gets the message to stop eating.

I could go on, but you get the very ugly point.

In some cases, the impact of fructose can be offset, as it is in fruit. All fruit contains fructose to one degree or another, but some fruits have perks that outweigh the heavy fructose load. Take berries: raspberries are high in fiber, and blueberries are antioxidant powerhouses. Avocados (actually a berry) are all-around rock stars that are very low in sugar and high in fiber and nutrients. If you do eat fruit, stick with low–Sugar Impact choices.

Even then, I don't want you going overboard. And if you have any type of blood sugar imbalance, I want you to severely limit or eliminate higher-fructose fruits like apples or pears beyond Cycle 2 of the program.

HOW DO I KNOW IF I'M ON THE ROAD TO DIABETES?

Eventually, insulin resistance morphs into prediabetes and later, full-blown type 2 diabetes. You don't always get there in a straight line, though. First, you might deal with symptoms like these:

- Feeling lousy after meals
- Fuzzy thinking
- Weight loss resistance
- Low libido
- Feeling anxious, fatigued, or stressed out
- Discolored skin or tags on the back of the neck and underarms

- A waist circumference greater than 34 inches for a woman or 40 inches for a man
- High blood pressure (at or above 140/90 mmHg)
- Prediabetes (fasting plasma glucose level from 5.6 mmol/L or 100 mg/dL to 6.9 mmol/L or 125 mg/dL)
- High triglycerides (TG) (150 and up is considered above normal; high is 200 and up)
- Low HDL cholesterol (<40 for men; <50 for women)

  Note: A better predictor for heart disease and other issues is your TG/HDL Ratio:

  - 5 or above—problematic
  - 3 to 4—good
  - 2 or lower—optimal
- Women: irregular periods, acne, and facial hair

Any one of those conditions puts your health at risk, but having more than one means you might need to make balancing your blood sugar a priority.

THE OUTCOME IS UP TO YOU

Your doctor can run tests, including a hemoglobin A1C test, to officially diagnose prediabetes or diabetes. He or she might also suggest a pharmaceutical drug to normalize your blood sugar.

I'm here to let you know there's another way to control insulin resistance, and I recommend you talk with your doctor about it. Diabetes is often completely preventable and even reversible with a few simple but powerfully effective natural action steps that don't involve drugs or crazy diets. The path you choose is entirely up to you.

When you take control of your blood sugar, you get some pretty sweet bonuses: your blood pressure goes down, your lipid profile improves, you look and feel (so much) better, and you lose fat fast.

How can you make that happen? Work with your doctor to make food your medicine. The recipes in this book are your ticket. They combine clean, lean protein, healthy fats, and low-glycemic, high-fiber carbs, and I've recommended the best sources for each. The meal timing laid out by the Sugar Impact Clock makes sure the protein, fats, and fiber work to keep your blood sugar stable, your fat burning machinery in high gear, and inflammation at bay. Simply put: incorporating the right foods and following these 7 strategies can help you naturally control blood sugar to reduce the devastating impact of insulin resistance.

Eat More Fiber

High-fiber foods should get major play in your diet, especially if you struggle with insulin resistance or diabetes. Fiber helps stabilize blood sugar, increase satiety, and prevent the spike-and-crash roller coaster that hits you after high-SI meals. Eat more fiber and you'll feel fuller longer, have fewer cravings for dessert, and won't feel like a slug an hour after you eat. What's not to love?

I want you to target 50 grams of fiber a day from high-fiber powerhouses like avocados, legumes, nuts, and seeds. Getting that much from food can become a challenge, so use a fiber-blend supplement powder whenever possible, too.

Up Your Omega-3s

The essential fatty acids in fish and fish oil, also called omega-3 fatty acids, can lower high blood pressure, triglycerides, and inflammation—three serious complications related to insulin resistance and diabetes. Omega-3s also offset the effects of pro-inflammatory omega-6 fatty acids, which feature heavily in a typical American diet.

In an ideal world, you'd get all the omega-3s you need by eating wild-caught salmon and other fish three or four times each week, adding freshly ground flaxseeds or chia seeds to your shakes, and making walnuts your snack of choice. But even if you're eating those foods, I highly recommend supplementing with an essential fatty acids formula.

If you're vegan or vegetarian and are against taking fish oil, you'll want to focus on ALA-rich foods like flaxseeds and chia seeds, as well as walnuts. You can also find a vegan (algae-derived) DHA supplement to meet your omega-3 needs.

Increase Your Vitamin D

Studies show vitamin D deficiencies contribute to or exacerbate insulin resistance. A few foods like mushrooms and wild-caught fish contain vitamin D, and 10 or 15 minutes of unprotected sun exposure can help your body make this crucial vitamin. Unless you're lucky enough to live somewhere like Honolulu, though, you'll still benefit from supplementing.

Take a 25-hydroxy vitamin D test and aim to keep your levels between 50 and 80 ng/ml. Supplementing with 2,000 to 5,000 IUs once you hit that mark will be enough for maintenance.

Step Up Your Protein

You'll get major blood sugar–balancing benefits from choosing foods like protein, good fats, and high-fiber starchy carbs over higher-carbohydrate (high-SI) foods. One study found that increasing protein helped people with diabetes have better control over their blood sugar levels. Other studies show healthy fats like raw nuts did the same.

Increasing your protein is easy when you use a plant-based non-soy powder for your morning shake and then fill the protein section of your Sugar Impact Plate with wild-caught fish, grass-fed beef, free-range poultry, or barnyard eggs (if you can tolerate them) at every meal.

Vegans and vegetarians—you probably already know you really need to tune in and make sure you're getting enough protein. Smart plant-based proteins include quinoa, legumes, and nuts and seeds.

Burst to Balance Blood Sugar in Just Minutes a Day

Burst training, also known as high-intensity interval training (HIIT), is the most efficient, effective exercise for balancing blood sugar levels.

Studies show burst training can reduce diabetes-related complications, and the good news is that you can get a complete, intense workout in just minutes a day. Whoops, there went that excuse! Best of all, you can do burst training almost anywhere, from the stairs in your house to your hotel room. You can learn more about burst training at www.jjvirgin .com.

Sleep Deeply

Just one night of poor sleep can knock insulin and other blood sugar–related hormones out of whack. And that can have serious consequences. One study determined that not getting enough sleep can actually pave the way for insulin resistance and obesity! Wow!

Aim for 7 to 9 hours of quality, uninterrupted sleep every night to optimize insulin and other hormone levels. Sleep doesn't just happen. You need to prepare for it. Curb the caffeine by noon (especially if you're a slow metabolizer), do some deep breathing, or take a hot bath to help you unwind and slowly drift into sleep.

Reduce Your Stress

Chronic stress elevates cortisol, a hormone that should be highest in the morning and gradually taper off throughout the day. Keeping cortisol cranked up past its sell-by date elevates blood sugar, breaks down muscle, and stores fat. That's an anti–weight loss trifecta if there ever was one.

If you have any degree of insulin resistance, it's critical that you make stress management a priority and not an indulgence. Figure out what "de-stress" means for you. It might be a yoga class or meditation. Maybe it's a good book and a cup of chamomile tea, or a walk around the block with your pooch. Even if you have to schedule it, make downtime *that* important.

DIABETES AND INSULIN RESISTANCE MEAL PLAN

Cycle 1

DAY 1

BREAKFAST
   Sugar Impact Shake (page 65) with low- or medium-SI fruit

LUNCH
   Mediterranean Salmon Wrap with Caper Dressing (page 88) with the coconut wrap
      swapped out for a rice wrap
   Smoky Baba Ghanoush (page 96) with crudités

DINNER
   Pork and Mushroom Stew with Sweet Potatoes (page 159)
   Mixed green salad with *Dijon Vinaigrette* (page 193)

OPTIONAL SNACK
   Lime and Jalapeño Hummus (page 95) with rice chips

DAY 2

BREAKFAST

Coconut-Vanilla Shake (page 68) with low- or medium-SI fruit

LUNCH

Turkey, Spinach, and Strawberry Wrap (page 78)

DINNER

Slow-Cooker Tomato-Braised Lamb Shanks (page 105)
Roasted Zucchini and Bell Pepper Medley (page 171)

OPTIONAL SNACK

Spicy Black Bean Dip with Celery (page 101) with rice chips

DAY 3

BREAKFAST

Pumpkin Bread French Toast with Berry Compote (page 72) with a side of nitrate-free
   bacon or chicken breakfast sausage

LUNCH

Super Greens Shake (page 66) with an apple added

DINNER

Turkey Meatballs with Parmesan and Tomato Sauce (page 126)
Raw Butternut Squash "Pappardelle" with Garlic and Oil (page 181)
Mixed green salad with Basil Vinaigrette (page 197)

OPTIONAL SNACK

Slow-Roasted Nuts (page 97) with fresh berries

DAY 4

BREAKFAST

Blueberry-Peach Shake (page 70)

LUNCH

Spicy Black Bean Burgers with Goat Cheese and Wilted Tomato Salsa (page 146) with a rice wrap

Mixed green salad with *Easy Lemon Vinaigrette* (page 193)

DINNER

Simply Grilled Shrimp with Lime (page 133) over brown rice

Stir-Fried Bok Choy (page 178)

OPTIONAL SNACK

White and Red Bean Salsa with White Onion, Tomato, and Cilantro (page 93) with rice chips

DAY 5

BREAKFAST

Tex-Mex Scrambled Eggs with Avocado and Salsa (page 71) with a rice wrap

LUNCH

Super Greens Shake (page 66) with an apple added

DINNER

Chinese Black Bean, Turkey, and Almond Stir-Fry (page 118) over brown rice

Steamed Broccoli with Garlic Oil Drizzle (page 167)

OPTIONAL SNACK

Garlic Hummus with Lentil Chips (page 100)

DAY 6

BREAKFAST

Coconut-Vanilla Shake (page 68) with low- or medium-SI fruit

LUNCH

Southwest Grilled Steak Salad on Crisped Rice Tortillas (page 83)

DINNER

Quinoa Pasta alla Checca (page 144) with a grilled chicken breast

Warm Wax Bean and Green Bean Salad (page 174)

OPTIONAL SNACK

Cinnamon Almond Butter (page 104) with apple slices

DAY 7

BREAKFAST

Old-Fashioned Oatmeal with Cinnamon, Blueberries, and Raspberries (page 73) with a side of nitrate-free bacon or chicken breakfast sausage

LUNCH

Pumpkin Spice Shake (page 67) with an apple added

DINNER

Fillet of Sole Piccata (page 140)
Lemony Roasted Artichoke Hearts (page 170)
½ cup brown rice

OPTIONAL SNACK

Slow-Roasted Nuts (page 97) with fresh berries

Cycle 2

DAY 1

BREAKFAST

Sugar Impact Shake (page 65)

LUNCH

Lamb Souvlaki with Cultured Coconut Milk Tzatziki (page 87)
Roasted Spiced Chickpeas (page 98)

DINNER

Seared Halibut with Lemon-Basil Gremolata (page 140)
Lima Beans with Lemon and Spinach (page 186)

OPTIONAL SNACK

Chocolate–Almond Butter Protein Popsicles (page 201)

DAY 2

BREAKFAST
Individual Baked Breakfast Frittatas (page 75)

LUNCH
Super Greens Shake (page 66)

DINNER
Pounded Chicken Breasts with Roasted Peppers and Capers (page 120)
Red Quinoa with Slow-Roasted Almonds and Caramelized Shallots (page 183)
Mixed green salad with *Caper Vinaigrette* (page 192)

OPTIONAL SNACK
Lemon-Chili Roasted Almonds (page 95)

DAY 3

BREAKFAST
Pumpkin Spice Shake (page 67)

LUNCH
Simply Grilled Shrimp with Lime (page 133)
Asian Confetti Quinoa Salad with Almonds (page 85)

DINNER
Pepper-Crusted Turkey Paillards over Spinach with Dijon Vinaigrette (page 120)
Tuscan White Beans with Roasted Grape Tomatoes and Parmesan (page 179)

OPTIONAL SNACK
Smoky Baba Ghanoush (page 96) with crudités

DAY 4

BREAKFAST
Chocolate, Flax, and Avocado Shake (page 69)

LUNCH

Classic Greek Salad with Pan-Grilled Chicken and Feta Cheese (page 91)

DINNER

Beef and Pork Meat Loaf (page 114)

Roasted Butternut Squash with Thyme (page 187)

Steamed Broccoli with Garlic Oil Drizzle (page 167)

OPTIONAL SNACK

Roasted Spiced Chickpeas (page 98)

DAY 5

BREAKFAST

Goat Cheese and Vegetable Omelet (page 74)

LUNCH

Pumpkin Spice Shake (page 67)

DINNER

Plank-Roasted Salmon (page 137)

Wild Rice and Vegetable Pilaf (page 189)

Mixed green salad with Easy Lemon Vinaigrette (page 193)

OPTIONAL SNACK

Lime and Jalapeño Hummus (page 95) with crudités

DAY 6

BREAKFAST

Espresso-Almond Shake (page 67)

LUNCH

Mediterranean Salmon Wrap with Caper Dressing (page 88)

Smoky Baba Ghanoush (page 96) with crudités

DINNER

Roasted Pork Tenderloin with Basil Vinaigrette (page 106)

Chickpeas with Sautéed Greens (page 183)

OPTIONAL SNACK

Coconut-Avocado Mousse (page 201)

DAY 7

BREAKFAST

Coconut-Vanilla Shake (page 68)

LUNCH

Mushroom, Cashew, Spinach, and Lentil Skillet (page 142)

DINNER

Chinese Black Bean, Turkey, and Almond Stir-Fry (page 118)

Stir-Fried Bok Choy (page 178)

OPTIONAL SNACK

Spicy Black Bean Dip with Celery (page 101)

DAY 8

BREAKFAST

Tex-Mex Scrambled Eggs with Avocado and Salsa (page 71)

LUNCH

Super Greens Shake (page 66)

DINNER

Tandoori Chicken (page 129)

Indian-Style Lentil Soup (page 159)

Whole Roasted Cauliflower (page 175)

OPTIONAL SNACK

White and Red Bean Salsa with White Onion, Tomato, and Cilantro (page 93) with crudités

DAY 9

BREAKFAST
Cappuccino Protein Shake (page 69)

LUNCH
Flank Steak and Vegetable Wrap with Chimichurri Sauce (page 81)
Lime and Jalapeño Hummus (page 95) with crudités

DINNER
Salmon Bouillabaisse (page 162)
Garlic Hummus (page 100) with crudités in the place of the lentil chips

OPTIONAL SNACK
Slow-Roasted Nuts (page 97)

DAY 10

BREAKFAST
Coconut-Pumpkin Bread (page 74) with side of nitrate-free bacon or chicken breakfast sausage

LUNCH
Espresso-Almond Shake (page 67)

DINNER
Spicy Black Bean Burgers with Goat Cheese and Wilted Tomato Salsa (page 146)
Mixed green salad with *Easy Lemon Vinaigrette* (page 193)

OPTIONAL SNACK
Cucumber Chips with Guacamole (page 101)

DAY 11

BREAKFAST
Coconut-Vanilla Shake (page 68)

LUNCH

Classic Greek Salad with Pan-Grilled Chicken and Feta Cheese (page 91)

DINNER

Seared Halibut with Lemon-Basil Gremolata (page 140)

Quinoa with Celery and Mushrooms (page 187)

Lemony Roasted Artichoke Hearts (page 170)

OPTIONAL SNACK

Vanilla-Coconut "Yogurt" Pudding Pops (page 202)

DAY 12

BREAKFAST

Espresso-Almond Shake (page 67)

LUNCH

Mediterranean Salmon Wrap with Caper Dressing (page 88)

Smoky Baba Ghanoush (page 96) with crudités

DINNER

Broiled Herb and Pepper–Crusted Lamb Chops (page 113)

Raw Butternut Squash "Pappardelle" with Garlic and Oil (page 181)

Just Grilled Asparagus (page 165)

OPTIONAL SNACK

Cinnamon Almond Butter (page 104) with celery

DAY 13

BREAKFAST

Cappuccino Protein Shake (page 69)

LUNCH

Turkey-Bean Chili with Crispy Coconut Wrap Strips (page 148)

Mixed green salad with *Easy Lemon Vinaigrette* (page 193)

DINNER

Seared Halibut with Lemon-Basil Gremolata (page 140)

Lima Beans with Lemon and Spinach (page 186)

OPTIONAL SNACK

Fresh-Baked Gluten-Free Sesame "Pretzels" (page 94)

DAY 14

BREAKFAST

Goat Cheese and Vegetable Omelet (page 74)

LUNCH

Sugar Impact Shake (page 65)

DINNER

Chinese Black Bean, Turkey, and Almond Stir-Fry (page 118)

Stir-Fried Bok Choy (page 178)

OPTIONAL SNACK

Chipotle Kale Chips (page 103)

Cycle 3

DAY 1

BREAKFAST

Sugar Impact Shake (page 65) with low- or medium-SI fruit

LUNCH

Mediterranean Salmon Wrap with Caper Dressing (page 88) with the coconut wrap swapped out for a rice wrap

Smoky Baba Ghanoush (page 96) with crudités

DINNER

Pork and Mushroom Stew with Sweet Potatoes (page 159)

Mixed green salad with *Dijon Vinaigrette* (page 193)

OPTIONAL SNACK

Lime and Jalapeño Hummus (page 95) with rice chips

DAY 2

BREAKFAST

Coconut-Vanilla Shake (page 68) with low- or medium-SI fruit

LUNCH

Turkey, Spinach, and Strawberry Wrap (page 78)

DINNER

Slow-Cooker Tomato-Braised Lamb Shanks (page 105)
Roasted Zucchini and Bell Pepper Medley (page 171)

OPTIONAL SNACK

Spicy Black Bean Dip with Celery (page 101) with rice chips

DAY 3

BREAKFAST

Pumpkin Bread French Toast with Berry Compote (page 72) with a side of nitrate-free
  bacon or chicken breakfast sausage

LUNCH

Super Greens Shake (page 66) with an apple added

DINNER

Turkey Meatballs with Parmesan and Tomato Sauce (page 126)
Raw Butternut Squash "Pappardelle" with Garlic and Oil (page 181)
Mixed green salad with *Basil Vinaigrette* (page 197)

OPTIONAL SNACK

Slow-Roasted Nuts (page 97) with fresh berries

DAY 4

BREAKFAST

Blueberry-Peach Shake (page 70)

LUNCH

Spicy Black Bean Burgers with Goat Cheese and Wilted Tomato Salsa (page 146) with a rice wrap

Mixed green salad with Easy Lemon Vinaigrette (page 193)

DINNER

Simply Grilled Shrimp with Lime (page 133) over brown rice

Stir-Fried Bok Choy (page 178)

OPTIONAL SNACK

White and Red Bean Salsa with White Onion, Tomato, and Cilantro (page 93) with rice chips

DAY 5

BREAKFAST

Tex-Mex Scrambled Eggs with Avocado and Salsa (page 71) with a rice wrap

LUNCH

Super Greens Shake (page 66) with an apple added

DINNER

Chinese Black Bean, Turkey, and Almond Stir-Fry (page 118) over brown rice

Steamed Broccoli with Garlic Oil Drizzle (page 167)

OPTIONAL SNACK

Garlic Hummus with Lentil Chips (page 100)

DAY 6

BREAKFAST

Coconut-Vanilla Shake (page 68) with low- or medium-SI fruit

LUNCH

Southwest Grilled Steak Salad on Crisped Rice Tortillas (page 83)

DINNER

Quinoa Pasta alla Checca (page 144) with a grilled chicken breast

Warm Wax Bean and Green Bean Salad (page 174)

OPTIONAL SNACK

Cinnamon Almond Butter (page 104) with apple slices

DAY 7

BREAKFAST

Old-Fashioned Oatmeal with Cinnamon, Blueberries, and Raspberries (page 73) with a side
of nitrate-free bacon or chicken breakfast sausage

LUNCH

Pumpkin Spice Shake (page 67) with an apple added

DINNER

Herbed Salmon Cakes with Tartar Sauce (page 134)

French fries (high-SI challenge)

OPTIONAL SNACK

Slow-Roasted Nuts (page 97) with fresh berries

14

GASTROINTESTINAL HEALING

Imagine living in a polluted, filthy environment surrounded by criminals and other unsavory types. From the air you breathe to the water you drink, everything is riddled with toxins. It's not a place you'd want to call home, is it?

The environment in your gut, called a microbiome, can be a lot like that. If most of your microbiome's inhabitants—called microbiota—include nasty characters (or bad bacteria), that highly unpleasant environment can eventually wreak havoc on your entire body.

Running to the bathroom 20 minutes after you eat isn't normal. Neither are gas, bloating, belching, cramping, or any other sign of post-meal misery. They could be not-so-subtle clues that you have an unbalanced microbiome rearing its ugly head as leaky gut and other gastrointestinal issues.

Gut dysbiosis or imbalances come in different forms, but they often manifest similarly: besides the aforementioned problems, diarrhea, constipation, fatigue, and nutrient malabsorption frequently occur.

Because about two-thirds of your immune system resides in your gut, you're more prone to colds and viruses. Chronic inflammation is another hallmark of dysbiosis, creating insulin resistance, fluid retention, digestive issues, and weight loss resistance. Overall, it's a recipe for disaster that extends far beyond your gut.

I can't address every gastrointestinal-related issue in this chapter, but I frequently see these three:

- **Leaky Gut**—a compromised gut wall allows particles of partly digested food, microbes, waste, and toxins into your bloodstream. Your body treats these things as foreign invaders and your immune system releases a cascade of inflammatory chemicals designed to neutralize the threat, which can also wreak havoc on your intestinal lining. If you've read *The Virgin Diet*, you're likely familiar with intestinal permeability (also called leaky gut) and the most common foods that trigger it.

- **Small Intestine Bacterial Overgrowth (SIBO)**—SIBO is essentially bacteria in revolt. You need a balance of good and bad gut bacteria, though the good should prevail. SIBO occurs when bad bacteria usurp the scene, paving the way for other gut imbalances. Experts like Mark Pimentel, M.D., author of *A New IBS Solution*, believe that irritable bowel syndrome (IBS) is actually a group of symptoms triggered by SIBO.

- **Candida**—your gut contains small amounts of the yeast *Candida albicans*, which your beneficial bacteria normally keep in check. When they don't, candida can grow out of control and what should be a harmless fungus can become an opportunistic pathogen. Left unchecked, candida overgrowth can become systemic candidiasis, meaning it can spread throughout your body and contribute to chronic fatigue syndrome, IBS, and a host of other conditions. Candida overgrowth can also weaken your immune system and increase toxins and free radicals, which stresses your detoxification machinery.

So you see, it's never just a gut issue: SIBO and other gastrointestinal problems eventually affect your entire body, creating discomfort, toxicity, and weight loss resistance.

WHAT TRIGGERS DYSBIOSIS?

SIBO, candida, leaky gut, and other gut issues don't happen overnight, and rarely does one clear culprit emerge. Most forms of dysbiosis result from years of being stressed out, eating a crappy diet, not sleeping well, popping antacids, and taking prescription drugs or antibiotics.

Food-wise, gluten and artificial sweeteners are big gut offenders. No contest: high–Sugar Impact foods play a huge role in dysbiosis. High–Sugar Impact foods can:

- Raise blood sugar, which raises insulin, which leads to inflammation.
- Feed yeast, which contributes to yeast overgrowth and sugar cravings.
- Feed bad bacteria with conditions like SIBO, forcing your body to extract more calories from the food you eat, store those calories as fat, and create digestive problems including gas and bloating.
- Dampen your immune system and deplete nutrients, setting the stage for more food intolerances.

HEALING YOUR GUT NATURALLY

If you suspect dysbiosis, an integrative practitioner can test for and then help eliminate gut imbalances. My rule is to test, not guess, and I don't want you to waste time, money, and effort determining potential gastrointestinal issues. Visit a specialist, get appropriate testing, and work with him or her to develop an effective strategy to eliminate the problem and heal your gut.

Having said that, you can implement a number of simple, effective strategies to heal your gut and minimize symptoms. Eliminating high–Sugar Impact foods is a given. Especially with conditions like candida that *love* sugar, you need to go the extra mile and confirm that no hidden sugars are slipping into your meals.

You will also want to remove vinegar (except apple cider vinegar), all fruits (except avocados and tomatoes), and high–Sugar Impact starchy carbs during Cycle 1. You can add these back later, but for now we want to pull out all the stops to improve your gut health.

The good news is that when you incorporate these strategies to heal your gut, you create fat loss and lasting health in the bargain.

Make Breakfast a Protein Shake

Start your day with a high-SI muffin or other dessert and the repercussions will land along your waistline—plus, you'll feed bad bacteria and worsen your gut health.

Avoid that disastrous path with a protein shake, which helps balance blood sugar, gives your digestive system a break, provides gut-healing nutrients like glutamine, and keeps you full, focused, and burning fat for hours.

Blend non-soy plant-based or defatted beef protein powder with avocado, kale or other leafy greens, freshly ground flaxseed, and unsweetened coconut or almond milk for the perfect low–Sugar Impact breakfast that helps balance blood sugar and gut bacteria.

Pull the Offenders

Gluten, dairy, soy, eggs, peanuts, corn, sugar, and artificial sweeteners can wreak havoc on your gut, creating leaky gut, metabolic issues, and other problems.

I provide detailed instructions in *The Virgin Diet* about how to eliminate and then challenge these foods. Whether you struggle with leaky gut or other gut issues, removing food intolerances should be a huge focus for gut healing.

Incorporate These Gut-Healing Herbs

Garlic and ginger offer unique gut-healing properties. Besides being anti-inflammatory and promoting healthy bacterial growth, they reduce bloating and other gut-related problems. Steam your green veggies with freshly sliced garlic, which can liven up most any food (but is not recommended for first dates!). A little—emphasis on *little*—crushed ginger in your protein shake can give your gut an anti-inflammatory boost.

Unwind with Therapeutic Teas

Enjoy your morning java and then switch over to decaffeinated teas. Ginger tea with lemon can provide therapeutic amounts of this "universal remedy." Peppermint tea also does the job: one study found that peppermint oil offers antimicrobial benefits to reduce IBS-like symptoms in SIBO. You can also get peppermint oil in a coated-capsule form. Reducing stress is a nice added bonus to drinking herbal teas.

Repopulate Correctly

Prebiotics and probiotics help replenish your good bacteria. Incorporate onions, asparagus, chicory, dandelion root, Jerusalem artichoke, and cruciferous veggies, which provide good amounts of the prebiotics inulin and fructo-oligosaccharides (FOS), into your meals. Fermented foods like unpasteurized sauerkraut and kimchi also help repopulate good gut flora.

A 2006 study in the journal *Gastroenterology* from the National University of Ireland showed that, at least in animal studies, probiotics provide antibacterial, anti-inflammatory, and immune benefits for SIBO and intestinal failure.

Even if you eat plenty of fermented foods, consider a multistrain, professional-quality probiotic supplement.

De-stress

Stress and gut problems go hand in hand. Chronic stress erodes your gut wall, significantly contributing to leaky gut and other problems. Gut issues, in turn, adversely impact digestion and can decrease hydrochloric acid needed to break down protein.

Your adrenals also play a significant role here. Increased levels of the stress hormone cortisol exacerbate gut and systemic inflammation. Excess adrenaline can also disrupt digestion.

We all have to make peace with some level of stress, and that involves finding effective strategies to reduce its impact. I like music, a hot bath, and deep breathing, but what works for me may not work for you, so make finding your personal de-stressor a priority.

Increase Fiber

Insoluble fiber is the only carbohydrate that gut bacteria don't feed on. Fiber benefits SIBO and other gut conditions by balancing your blood sugar, reducing gastric emptying, and preventing constipation. As an added bonus, it promotes satiety and reduces cravings, so you're less tempted for seconds or to have a big slice of apple pie after dinner.

Aim for 50 grams of fiber a day from berries, nuts and seeds, avocados, and leafy greens. Look for a fiber-blend supplement powder—ideally one with prebiotics and probiotics— to complement these and other fiber-rich foods.

Take a Digestive Enzyme

As you get older, you're probably making fewer digestive enzymes, which could further decrease your body's ability to break down and absorb foods. A professional-quality supplement can help your digestive system better digest and absorb nutrients. Look for a full-spectrum digestive enzyme with betaine HCl, which helps your stomach break down protein and absorb B12 more efficiently.

Use Gut-Healing Nutrients

Ideally, you'll work with an integrative practitioner to include these and other supplements that address your condition:

- **Berberine**—Among this plant extract's multitasking functions are blood sugar metabolism and gut support. One study showed berberine could positively impact gut microbiota to improve obesity and type 2 diabetes.
- **Aged garlic extract**—An anti-inflammatory, antiviral, antifungal, and antimicrobial powerhouse that's especially beneficial if eating garlic isn't your thing.
- **Glutamine**—My number-one gut healer that also helps sugar cravings. Available in capsules, but to get therapeutic amounts I prefer more efficient powder that blends easily into your shake or water.
- **Ginger**—An antioxidant that reduces inflammation and supports gut healing. If you aren't adding ginger to shakes and meals, consider supplementing.
- **Quercetin**—A natural antihistamine and antioxidant that boosts immunity.

GI HEALING: CANDIDA, SIBO, AND LEAKY GUT MEAL PLAN

Cycle 1

Have ¼ cup of cultured veggies with breakfast and lunch. For a video on how to prepare these, go to http://sugarimpact.com/resources. Drink 8 ounces of a cultured or probiotic coconut drink daily—I like KeVita or CocoBiotic. Replace any vinegar in recipes with apple cider vinegar.

DAY 1

BREAKFAST
> *Sugar Impact Shake* (page 65) with low-SI fruit

LUNCH
> *Mediterranean Salmon Wrap with Caper Dressing* (page 88) with the coconut wrap
> swapped out for a rice wrap

DINNER
> *Chinese Black Bean, Turkey, and Almond Stir-Fry* (page 118) over brown rice
> *Sesame Wilted Spinach* (page 179)

OPTIONAL SNACK

Cultured coconut milk or Greek-style yogurt (if not dairy sensitive) with low-SI fruit

DAY 2

BREAKFAST

Coconut-Vanilla Shake (page 68) with low-SI fruit

LUNCH

Chicken Soup with Parsnips (page 150)

Mixed green salad with *Easy Lemon Vinaigrette* (page 193)

DINNER

Jerk-Spiced Chicken Thighs with Roasted Pineapple Chutney (page 123)

½ sweet potato

Sautéed Kale with Caramelized Onions (page 172)

OPTIONAL SNACK

Cultured coconut milk or Greek-style yogurt (if not dairy sensitive) with low-SI fruit

DAY 3

BREAKFAST

Blueberry-Peach Shake (page 70)

LUNCH

Turkey, Spinach, and Strawberry Wrap (page 78)

DINNER

Pork and Mushroom Stew with Sweet Potatoes (page 159)

Roasted Zucchini and Bell Pepper Medley (page 171)

OPTIONAL SNACK

Cultured coconut milk or Greek-style yogurt (if not dairy sensitive) with low-SI fruit

DAY 4

BREAKFAST

Super Greens Shake (page 66) with an apple added

LUNCH

Pan-Seared Seafood Salad with Tomatoes and Fennel (page 85) with rice crackers
on the side

DINNER

Slow-Cooker Tomato-Braised Lamb Shanks (page 105)
Whole Roasted Cauliflower (page 175)
Brown rice

OPTIONAL SNACK

Cultured coconut milk or Greek-style yogurt (if not dairy sensitive) with low-SI fruit

DAY 5

BREAKFAST

Sugar Impact Shake (page 65) with low-SI fruit

LUNCH

Southwest Grilled Steak Salad on Crisped Rice Tortillas (page 83)

DINNER

Quinoa Pasta alla Checca (page 144) with a grilled chicken breast
Steamed Broccoli with Garlic Oil Drizzle (page 167)

OPTIONAL SNACK

Cultured coconut milk or Greek-style yogurt (if not dairy sensitive) with low-SI fruit

DAY 6

BREAKFAST

Coconut-Vanilla Shake (page 68) with low-SI fruit

LUNCH

Roasted Beet and Arugula Salad with Shallots and Lemon (page 81) with added
roasted chicken, served with rice or lentil chips

DINNER

Simply Grilled Shrimp with Lime (page 133) over brown rice
Stir-Fried Bok Choy (page 178)

OPTIONAL SNACK

Cultured coconut milk or Greek-style yogurt (if not dairy sensitive) with low–SI fruit

DAY 7

BREAKFAST

Blueberry-Peach Shake (page 70)

LUNCH

Chicken Soup with Parsnips (page 150) with quinoa pasta
Crudités

DINNER

Beef Pepper Steak–Broccolini Stir-Fry (page 115) with brown rice
Mixed green salad with Basil Vinaigrette (page 197)

OPTIONAL SNACK

Cultured coconut milk or Greek-style yogurt (if not dairy sensitive) with low–SI fruit

Cycle 2

DAY 1

BREAKFAST

Sugar Impact Shake (page 65)

LUNCH

Lamb Souvlaki with Cultured Coconut Milk Tzatziki (page 87) with ¼ cup
chickpeas

DINNER
   Tandoori Chicken (page 129)
   Indian-Style Lentil Soup (page 159)
   Whole Roasted Cauliflower (page 175)

OPTIONAL SNACK
   Cultured coconut milk or Greek-style yogurt (if not dairy sensitive) with crudités

DAY 2

BREAKFAST
   Cappuccino Protein Shake (page 69)

LUNCH
   Mediterranean Salmon Wrap with Caper Dressing (page 88)
   Garlic Hummus (page 100) with crudités in the place of the lentil chips

DINNER
   Turkey and Vegetable Skillet (page 122)
   Quinoa with Celery and Mushrooms (page 187)

OPTIONAL SNACK
   Cultured coconut milk or Greek-style yogurt (if not dairy sensitive) with crudités

DAY 3

BREAKFAST
   Super Greens Shake (page 66)

LUNCH
   Mushroom, Cashew, Spinach, and Lentil Skillet (page 142)

DINNER
   Thai Coconut Steamed Mussels (page 136)
   Coconut Curry Butternut Squash Puree (page 180)
   Sesame Wilted Spinach (page 179)

OPTIONAL SNACK

Cultured coconut milk or Greek-style yogurt (if not dairy sensitive) with crudités

DAY 4

BREAKFAST

Espresso-Almond Shake (page 67)

LUNCH

Pan-Seared Seafood Salad with Tomatoes and Fennel (page 85)
Cup of *Yellow Split Pea Soup* (page 151)

DINNER

Beef and Pork Meat Loaf (page 114)
Roasted Butternut Squash with Thyme (page 187)
Just Grilled Asparagus (page 165)

OPTIONAL SNACK

Cultured coconut milk or Greek-style yogurt (if not dairy sensitive) with crudités

DAY 5

BREAKFAST

Coconut-Vanilla Shake (page 68)

LUNCH

Classic Greek Salad with Pan-Grilled Chicken and Feta Cheese (page 91)

DINNER

Mustard and Garlic–Marinated Pork Chops (page 107)
Lemony Roasted Artichoke Hearts (page 170)
Winter Vegetable Minestrone (page 162)

OPTIONAL SNACK

Cultured coconut milk or Greek-style yogurt (if not dairy sensitive) with crudités

DAY 6

BREAKFAST

Pumpkin Spice Shake (page 67)

LUNCH

Goat Cheese Burger Wrap (page 86)
Roasted Spiced Chickpeas (page 98)

DINNER

Slow Cooker–Braised Chicken Legs with Rosemary, Onions, and Celery (page 125)
Quinoa with Celery and Mushrooms (page 187)

OPTIONAL SNACK

Cultured coconut milk or Greek-style yogurt (if not dairy sensitive) with crudités

DAY 7

BREAKFAST

Chocolate, Flax, and Avocado Shake (page 69)

LUNCH

Simply Grilled Shrimp with Lime (page 133)
Asian Confetti Quinoa Salad with Almonds (page 85)

DINNER

Broiled Herb and Pepper–Crusted Lamb Chops (page 113)
Chickpeas with Sautéed Greens (page 183)

OPTIONAL SNACK

Cultured coconut milk or Greek-style yogurt (if not dairy sensitive) with crudités

DAY 8

BREAKFAST

Pumpkin Spice Shake (page 67)

LUNCH

Chicken and Okra Stew over Quinoa (page 158)
Smoky Baba Ghanoush (page 96) with crudités

DINNER

Pepper-Crusted Turkey Paillards over Spinach with Dijon Vinaigrette (page 120)
Wild Rice and Vegetable Pilaf (page 189)

OPTIONAL SNACK

Cultured coconut milk or Greek-style yogurt (if not dairy sensitive) with crudités

DAY 9

BREAKFAST

Super Greens Shake (page 66)

LUNCH

BLT Wedge Salad with Avocado and Dijon Vinaigrette (page 89)

DINNER

Fillet of Sole Piccata (page 140)
Red Quinoa with Slow-Roasted Almonds and Caramelized Shallots (page 183)
Shredded Brussels Sprouts with Easy Lemon Vinaigrette (page 166)

OPTIONAL SNACK

Cultured coconut milk or Greek-style yogurt (if not dairy sensitive) with crudités

DAY 10

BREAKFAST

Cappuccino Protein Shake (page 69)

LUNCH

Chinese Black Bean, Turkey, and Almond Stir-Fry (page 118)

DINNER

Seared Halibut with Lemon-Basil Gremolata (page 140)
Lima Beans with Lemon and Spinach (page 186)

OPTIONAL SNACK

Cultured coconut milk or Greek-style yogurt (if not dairy sensitive) with crudités

DAY 11

BREAKFAST

Espresso-Almond Shake (page 67)

LUNCH

Mediterranean Salmon Wrap with Caper Dressing (page 88)

Garlic Hummus (page 100) with crudités in the place of the lentil chips

DINNER

Turkey and Vegetable Skillet (page 122)

Quinoa with Celery and Mushrooms (page 187)

OPTIONAL SNACK

Cultured coconut milk or Greek-style yogurt (if not dairy sensitive) with crudités

DAY 12

BREAKFAST

Coconut-Vanilla Shake (page 68)

LUNCH

Warm Chicken Salad with Pecans, Basil, and Caper Vinaigrette (page 132)

Cup of *Yellow Split Pea Soup* (page 151)

DINNER

BBQ-Rubbed Whole Roasted Chicken (page 123)

Raw Butternut Squash "Pappardelle" with Garlic and Oil (page 181)

Steamed Broccoli with Garlic Oil Drizzle (page 167)

OPTIONAL SNACK

Cultured coconut milk or Greek-style yogurt (if not dairy sensitive) with crudités

DAY 13

BREAKFAST

Sugar Impact Shake (page 65)

LUNCH

Classic Greek Salad with Pan-Grilled Chicken and Feta Cheese (page 91)

DINNER

Beef and Pork Meat Loaf (page 114)

Roasted Butternut Squash with Thyme (page 187)

Just Grilled Asparagus (page 165)

OPTIONAL SNACK

Cultured coconut milk or Greek-style yogurt (if not dairy sensitive) with crudités

DAY 14

BREAKFAST

Chocolate, Flax, and Avocado Shake (page 69)

LUNCH

Goat Cheese Burger Wrap (page 86)

Roasted Spiced Chickpeas (page 98)

DINNER

Pounded Chicken Breasts with Roasted Peppers and Capers (page 120)

Spaghetti Squash with Capers, Onion, and Bell Pepper (page 185)

Mixed green salad with Caper Vinaigrette (page 192)

OPTIONAL SNACK

Cultured coconut milk or Greek-style yogurt (if not dairy sensitive) with crudités

Cycle 3

DAY 1

BREAKFAST

Sugar Impact Shake (page 65) with low-SI fruit

LUNCH

Mediterranean Salmon Wrap with Caper Dressing (page 88) with the coconut wrap swapped out for a rice wrap

DINNER

Chinese Black Bean, Turkey, and Almond Stir-Fry (page 118) over brown rice
Sesame Wilted Spinach (page 179)

OPTIONAL SNACK

Cultured coconut milk or Greek-style yogurt (if not dairy sensitive) with low-SI fruit

DAY 2

BREAKFAST

Coconut-Vanilla Shake (page 68) with low-SI fruit

LUNCH

Chicken Soup with Parsnips (page 150)
Mixed green salad with *Easy Lemon Vinaigrette* (page 193)

DINNER

Jerk-Spiced Chicken Thighs with Roasted Pineapple Chutney (page 123)
½ sweet potato
Sautéed Kale with Caramelized Onions (page 172)

OPTIONAL SNACK

Cultured coconut milk or Greek-style yogurt (if not dairy sensitive) with low-SI fruit

DAY 3

BREAKFAST

Blueberry-Peach Shake (page 70)

LUNCH

Turkey, Spinach, and Strawberry Wrap (page 78)

DINNER

Pork and Mushroom Stew with Sweet Potatoes (page 159)
Roasted Zucchini and Bell Pepper Medley (page 171)

OPTIONAL SNACK

Cultured coconut milk or Greek-style yogurt (if not dairy sensitive) with low–SI fruit

DAY 4

BREAKFAST

Super Greens Shake (page 66) with an apple added

LUNCH

Pan-Seared Seafood Salad with Tomatoes and Fennel (page 85) with rice crackers on the side

DINNER

Slow-Cooker Tomato-Braised Lamb Shanks (page 105)
Whole Roasted Cauliflower (page 175)
Brown rice

OPTIONAL SNACK

Cultured coconut milk or Greek-style yogurt (if not dairy sensitive) with
low–SI fruit

DAY 5

BREAKFAST

Sugar Impact Shake (page 65) with low–SI fruit

LUNCH

Southwest Grilled Steak Salad on Crisped Rice Tortillas (page 83)

DINNER

Quinoa Pasta alla Checca (page 144) with a grilled chicken breast
Steamed Broccoli with Garlic Oil Drizzle (page 167)

OPTIONAL SNACK

Cultured coconut milk or Greek-style yogurt (if not dairy sensitive) with low-SI fruit

DAY 6

BREAKFAST

Coconut-Vanilla Shake (page 68) with low-SI fruit

LUNCH

Warm Chicken Salad with Pecans, Basil, and Caper Vinaigrette (page 132) with julienned roasted beets

DINNER

Simply Grilled Shrimp with Lime (page 133) over brown rice
Stir-Fried Bok Choy (page 178)

OPTIONAL SNACK

Cultured coconut milk or Greek-style yogurt (if not dairy sensitive) with low-SI fruit

DAY 7

BREAKFAST

Blueberry-Peach Shake (page 70)

LUNCH

Chicken Soup with Parsnips (page 150) with quinoa pasta
Crudités

DINNER

Beef Pepper Steak–Broccolini Stir-Fry (page 115) with brown rice

Mixed green salad with *Basil Vinaigrette* (page 197)

OPTIONAL SNACK

Cultured coconut milk or Greek-style yogurt (if not dairy sensitive)

Rice cakes with apple butter (high-SI challenge)

15

PALEO AND LOW CARB

Ah, the 1980s. The era of acid-washed jeans, crimping irons, and low-fat diets.

Until about a decade ago, fat remained vilified as the evildoer in our war against weight. Simply lose the fat to lose fat. Duh!

Except that didn't work so well, because our bodies aren't that simple. They require certain fats to function. What our bodies *don't* require are carbohydrates; certainly not the high–Sugar Impact foods that populate the standard American diet. During the past decade, a seismic shift has occurred. Fat was finally let off the hook and it became clear that sugar was public enemy #1, at least among more enlightened health experts.

Classifying macronutrients as good or bad really isn't fair. Some carbs—like processed grains and sugars—*are* clearly bad, but carbohydrate-rich foods like leafy greens and squashes are full of important nutrients and have very low SI. So let's not throw the baby out with the bathwater. Focus on low-SI carbs; don't eliminate carbs altogether.

A low-carb diet is not nearly as controversial as it once was. It's an excellent way to balance blood sugar as well as reverse insulin resistance and its many complications. A study at the University of North Carolina published in 2011 in the journal *Nutrition in Clinical Practice* declared it was "time to embrace [low-carb] diets as a viable option to aid in reversing diabetes mellitus, risk factors for heart disease, and the epidemic of obesity."

If you've done a low-carb diet, you probably know it has a lot of benefits. You get to improve your health and eat satisfying foods while curbing hunger and cravings. It's a win-win.

There's really no one definition of "low carb." Some folks count carb grams, while others stick with a whole foods, Paleolithic diet. There are some differences between the two—Paleo doesn't include dairy or soy, though low carb may—but they share a similar approach to removing high-SI foods.

Regardless of what you call your plan, high protein, high fiber, and healthy fats are trademarks of Paleo and low-carb diets. They emphasize the whole-foods approach people thrived on *thousands* of years ago. Paleo and low-carb diets focus on foods our ancestors (from the Paleolithic era, naturally) could have plucked, hunted, fished, or otherwise caught in the wild.

But a common complaint about low-carb and Paleo plans is that they can be boring, because most people end up eating the same foods over and over. The delicious, easy-to-prepare, low–Sugar Impact recipes in this book will help you change that tune! They burst with flavor and will bring some fun back to mealtime.

Whether you've been doing low carb since Dr. Robert Atkins put out his first book in the early 1970s or just recently started flirting with a Paleo diet, these strategies can help you thrive on your plan and overcome any hurdles you might encounter along the way.

PALEO OR LOW CARB DOESN'T MEAN ALL-YOU-CAN-EAT

Thanks to a hormone called cholecystokinin (CCK), when you eat protein and good fats, your brain gets the message to put the fork down, so you're less likely to overeat. High–Sugar Impact foods don't create that same signaling, which explains why you can eat a dozen chocolate chip cookies but not a dozen chicken breasts—even though they have the same calories!

Regardless, too much of even the healthiest foods can stall fat loss. Yes, I know we're not counting calories on the Sugar Impact Diet—and if you eat by the Plate and follow my guidelines, you don't have to count, period. Calories often take a backseat in low-carb and Paleo plans (the source of calories is more important than counting them). But the truth is, they still matter, since those excess calories have to go somewhere.

We can agree that you're probably not going to eat a dozen chicken breasts, but overdoing nuts, avocado, cheese, or unsweetened Greek yogurt (staples on many low-carb and Paleo diets) can derail your hard work and slam you into a fat-loss plateau. Know yourself and keep the enemies—even healthy ones—out of your house.

MAKE AN OIL CHANGE

Coconut has become quite the star in Paleo and low-carb diets, but I still see too many folks cooking with vegetable oils or pouring on salad dressings loaded with low-quality oils.

Inflammation plays a part in nearly every modern disease, from obesity to diabetes to cancer. Our Paleo ancestors got about a 4:1 omega-6/omega-3 ratio. Today, we're more like 20:1 in favor of pro-inflammatory fats.

A few tweaks can make a huge difference:

- For high-heat cooking, swap vegetable oils for coconut or Malaysian red palm fruit oils.
- Drizzle salads with extra-virgin olive oil and vinegar.
- Incorporate healthy fats like olives, avocado, and nuts and seeds.
- Load flaxseeds or chia seeds into your protein shakes.
- Snack on walnuts.
- Supplement with an essential fatty acids formula.

STEP UP HIGH-FIBER, LOW-SI FOODS

Can we stop it with the all-meat diets already? Low carb was never code for plates of bacon and eggs, and Paleo doesn't suddenly mean you get a pass on eating a gargantuan grass-fed steak.

Keep your grass-fed steak and nitrate-free bacon, but also fill your plate with plenty of high-fiber, low-SI foods. A study published in 2005 in the journal *Nutrition* found that while most people consume less than half of the recommended fiber in their diets, low-carb dieters get even less than that. Fiber's benefits include increased satiety, balanced blood sugar, and staying "regular." Make sure you get enough!

Incorporating high-fiber foods into your Paleo or low-carb diet is easy when you use these tips:

- Toss sliced avocado onto your grass-fed burger or salad.
- Throw frozen raspberries (when you are through Cycle 2) and flaxseeds or chia seeds into your protein shakes.

- Snack on almonds and other nuts and seeds.
- Have one or two nonstarchy veggies and a salad at your meals.

Your goal is 50 grams of fiber every day. If you're not meeting that quota, add a fiber blend to your morning Sugar Impact Shake (page 65) and try stirring a fiber-blend supplement powder into a tall glass of water to drink 30 to 60 minutes before meals to help with satiety.

STAY AWAY FROM THE PROCESSED STUFF

I did a double take the other day, but what I saw was real: low-carb versions of candy. Seriously? That *totally* misses the low-carb/Paleo whole-foods point.

When you ditch the high-SI foods, manufacturers realize you're desperate for "legal" versions of old favorites, which is why you're bombarded with Paleo bread, low-carb granola bars, and "low-net-carb" chocolate chip cookies.

Many of these foods come loaded with very un-Paleo ingredients like soy protein isolate, gluten, preservatives, artificial sweeteners, trans fats, and lots of other stuff your ancestors wouldn't recognize.

Steer clear of the middle aisles at the grocery store and most foods with a bar code. If you're craving something sweet, have a few squares of low-sugar, 85% or higher dark chocolate. But if a few squares become the whole bar, back away from the chocolate slowly!

CHOOSE THE BEST QUALITY MEATS

Paleo and low-carb diets often include meat. Sometimes, *lots* of meat. Unfortunately, most commercial beef, poultry, and even fish come from antibiotic-injected animals subjected to horrific living conditions and other atrocities our Paleo ancestors never had to confront.

Skip the feedlot steaks and hormone-injected chicken breasts for the best quality meats you can afford, ideally from farmers who humanely raise their own cows and chickens. Grass-fed meat provides higher amounts of anti-inflammatory omega-3 fatty acids and the fat-burning fatty acid conjugated linoleic acid (CLA). That makes sense when you consider those cows eat their natural diet rather than corn, soy, and other foods that make them fat and shorten their lives.

The same goes for other animal protein—choose pastured poultry and wild-caught fish rather than the farm-raised fish and chicken-on-steroids most grocery stores sell.

CONSIDER PALEO WITH BENEFITS

Okay, so your Paleo ancestors didn't have legumes growing in their backyards and quinoa may be a little too carb-y for a super low-carb diet. I'm all about bending the rules a little bit if it means big dividends for your health. Focus on low–Sugar Impact foods and allow yourself a little leeway to add more nutrients and variety without going off the rails.

STAY HYDRATED

You're probably getting above-average protein on a low-carb or Paleo diet. There's nothing wrong with that, as long as you don't have a pre-existing kidney or liver problem. Just make sure you increase your filtered water intake to help your kidneys process that increased protein.

Besides, even mild dehydration can stall your metabolic machinery, so if you're plateauing, increasing the amount of water you drink might be the needle mover for you. Start with a glass of water when you get up and drink throughout your day. The only time I don't want you drinking is *during* meals, when too much liquid can dilute the stomach enzymes that break down protein.

PALEO AND LOW-CARB MEAL PLAN

Note: For pure Paleo, use the defatted beef protein–based shake.

Cycle 1

DAY 1

BREAKFAST
Sugar Impact Shake (page 65) with low- or medium-SI fruit

LUNCH

Pork and Mushroom Stew with Sweet Potatoes (page 159)

Mixed green salad with *Dijon Vinaigrette* (page 193)

DINNER

Turkey Meatballs with Parmesan and Tomato Sauce (page 126)

Italian-Style Peppers and Onion Sauté (page 169)

OPTIONAL SNACK

Cinnamon Almond Butter (page 104) with apple slices

DAY 2

BREAKFAST

Pumpkin Spice Shake (page 67) with an apple added

LUNCH

Chicken Soup with Parsnips (page 150)

Mixed green salad with *Caper Vinaigrette* (page 192)

DINNER

Jerk-Spiced Chicken Thighs with Roasted Pineapple Chutney (page 123)

Raw Butternut Squash "Pappardelle" with Garlic and Oil (page 181)

Mixed green salad with *Easy Lemon Vinaigrette* (page 193) with roasted beets added

OPTIONAL SNACK

Strawberry Ice Cream (page 202)

DAY 3

BREAKFAST

Tex-Mex Scrambled Eggs with Avocado and Salsa (page 71) with a coconut wrap

LUNCH

Coconut-Vanilla Shake (page 68) with berries

DINNER
Turkey Cutlets with Marsala and Shiitake Mushrooms (page 130)
½ baked sweet potato

OPTIONAL SNACK
Smoky Baba Ghanoush (page 96) with crudités

DAY 4

BREAKFAST
Super Greens Shake (page 66) with a green apple added

LUNCH
Roasted Beet and Arugula Salad with Shallots and Lemon (page 81) topped with a grilled chicken breast

DINNER
Slow-Cooker Tomato-Braised Lamb Shanks (page 105)
Whole Roasted Cauliflower (page 175)
Spiced Sweet Potato "Fries" (page 188)

OPTIONAL SNACK
Lemon-Chili Roasted Almonds (page 95)

DAY 5

BREAKFAST
Goat Cheese and Vegetable Omelet (page 74) with ½ sweet potato

LUNCH
Espresso-Almond Shake (page 67)
Pear slices with goat cheese

DINNER
Beef Bourguignon (page 156)
Mixed green salad with *Dijon Vinaigrette* (page 193) and beets

OPTIONAL SNACK

Cucumber Chips with Guacamole (page 101)

DAY 6

BREAKFAST

Blueberry-Peach Shake (page 70)

LUNCH

Flank Steak and Vegetable Wrap with Chimichurri Sauce (page 81)
Spiced Sweet Potato "Fries" (page 188)

DINNER

Peppered Shrimp with Mango (page 139)
Stir-Fried Bok Choy (page 178)
Lemony Roasted Artichoke Hearts (page 170)

OPTIONAL SNACK

Chipotle Deviled Eggs (page 102)

DAY 7

BREAKFAST

Pumpkin Bread French Toast with Berry Compote (page 72) with a side of nitrate-free
  bacon or chicken breakfast sausage

LUNCH

Cappuccino Protein Shake (page 69) with ½ banana

DINNER

Spaghetti Squash with Capers, Onion, and Bell Pepper (page 185) with an added ¼ cup
  julienned sun-dried tomatoes, topped with a grilled chicken breast
Mixed green salad with *Caper Vinaigrette* (page 192)

OPTIONAL SNACK

Chipotle Kale Chips (page 103)

Cycle 2

DAY 1

BREAKFAST

Sugar Impact Shake (page 65)

LUNCH

Classic Greek Salad with Pan-Grilled Chicken and Feta Cheese (page 91) (skip the feta if intolerant)

DINNER

Pounded Chicken Breasts with Roasted Pepper and Capers (page 120)

Sautéed Kale with Caramelized Onions (page 172)

Mixed green salad with *Caper Vinaigrette* (page 192)

OPTIONAL SNACK

Cinnamon Almond Butter (page 104) with celery

DAY 2

BREAKFAST

Pumpkin Spice Shake (page 67)

LUNCH

Turkey, Spinach, and Strawberry Wrap (page 78)

DINNER

BLT Wedge Salad with Avocado and Dijon Vinaigrette (page 89)

Chicken Soup with Parsnips (page 150)

OPTIONAL SNACK

Smoky Baba Ghanoush (page 96) with crudités

DAY 3

BREAKFAST

Tex-Mex Scrambled Eggs with Avocado and Salsa (page 71) with a coconut wrap

LUNCH

Super Greens Shake (page 66)

DINNER

Beef and Pork Meat Loaf (page 114)
Roasted Butternut Squash with Thyme (page 187)
Mixed green salad with *Basil Vinaigrette* (page 197)

OPTIONAL SNACK

Chipotle Kale Chips (page 103)

DAY 4

BREAKFAST

Espresso-Almond Shake (page 67)

LUNCH

Lamb Souvlaki with Cultured Coconut Milk Tzatziki (page 87)

DINNER

Pepper-Crusted Turkey Paillards over Spinach with Dijon Vinaigrette (page 120)
Onion-Mushroom Soup (page 154)

OPTIONAL SNACK

Vanilla-Coconut "Yogurt" Pudding Pops (page 202)

DAY 5

BREAKFAST

Coconut-Vanilla Shake (page 68)

LUNCH

Goat Cheese Burger Wrap (page 86) (if intolerant, sub cashew cheese for the goat cheese)

Cucumber Chips with Guacamole (page 101)

DINNER

Thai Coconut Steamed Mussels (page 136)

Coconut Curry Butternut Squash Puree (page 180)

Spicy Ginger and Celery Stir-Fry (page 173)

OPTIONAL SNACK

Chipotle Deviled Eggs (page 102)

DAY 6

BREAKFAST

Goat Cheese and Vegetable Omelet (page 74)

LUNCH

Chocolate, Flax, and Avocado Shake (page 69)

DINNER

Strip Steaks with Tomatoes, Olives, and Parsley (page 109)

Marjoram Seared Mushrooms (page 166)

Just Grilled Asparagus (page 165)

OPTIONAL SNACK

Lemon-Chili Roasted Almonds (page 95)

DAY 7

BREAKFAST

Individual Baked Breakfast Frittatas (page 75)

LUNCH

Cappuccino Protein Shake (page 69)

DINNER

Pounded Chicken Breasts with Roasted Peppers and Capers (page 120)
Sautéed Kale with Caramelized Onions (page 172)
Mixed green salad with *Caper Vinaigrette* (page 192)

OPTIONAL SNACK

Cucumber Chips with Guacamole (page 101)

DAY 8

BREAKFAST

Sugar Impact Shake (page 65)

LUNCH

Turkey, Spinach, and Strawberry Wrap (page 78)

DINNER

Spaghetti Squash with Capers, Onion, and Bell Pepper (page 185) with a grilled chicken breast
Mixed green salad with *Caper Vinaigrette* (page 192)

OPTIONAL SNACK

Cinnamon Almond Butter (page 104) with celery

DAY 9

BREAKFAST

Pumpkin Spice Shake (page 67)

LUNCH

Classic Greek Salad with Pan-Grilled Chicken and Feta Cheese (page 91) (skip the feta if intolerant)

DINNER

Onion and Tomato–Smothered Pork Cutlets (page 116)
Creamy Cauliflower Soup (page 154)
Mixed green salad with *Caper Vinaigrette* (page 192)

OPTIONAL SNACK

Chocolate–Almond Butter Protein Popsicles (page 201)

DAY 10

BREAKFAST

Tex-Mex Scrambled Eggs with Avocado and Salsa (page 71) with a coconut wrap

LUNCH

Coconut-Vanilla Shake (page 68)

DINNER

Herbed Salmon Cakes with Tartar Sauce (page 134)

Roasted Onion Gazpacho with Shrimp (page 160)

Shredded Brussels Sprouts with Easy Lemon Vinaigrette (page 166)

OPTIONAL SNACK

Chipotle Kale Chips (page 103)

DAY 11

BREAKFAST

Espresso-Almond Shake (page 67)

LUNCH

Lamb Souvlaki with Cultured Coconut Milk Tzatziki (page 87)

DINNER

Pounded Chicken Breasts with Roasted Peppers and Capers (page 120)

Sautéed Kale with Caramelized Onions (page 172)

Mixed green salad with Caper Vinaigrette (page 192)

OPTIONAL SNACK

Smoky Baba Ghanoush (page 96) with crudités

DAY 12

BREAKFAST
Goat Cheese and Vegetable Omelet (page 74)

LUNCH
Super Greens Shake (page 66)

DINNER
Beef and Pork Meat Loaf (page 114)
Roasted Butternut Squash with Thyme (page 187)
Mixed green salad with *Basil Vinaigrette* (page 197)

OPTIONAL SNACK
Coconut-Avocado Mousse (page 201)

DAY 13

BREAKFAST
Chocolate, Flax, and Avocado Shake (page 69)

LUNCH
Goat Cheese Burger Wrap (page 86) (if intolerant sub cashew cheese for the goat cheese)
Cucumber Chips with Guacamole (page 101)

DINNER
Beef Pepper Steak–Broccolini Stir-Fry (page 115)
Braised Leeks (page 176)
Grilled Endive with Shallot-Bacon Vinaigrette (page 169)

OPTIONAL SNACK
Lemon Cookies (page 203)

DAY 14

BREAKFAST

Individual Baked Breakfast Frittatas (page 75)

LUNCH

Cappuccino Protein Shake (page 69)

DINNER

BLT Wedge Salad with Avocado and Dijon Vinaigrette (page 89)
Chicken Soup with Parsnips (page 150)

OPTIONAL SNACK

Cucumber Chips with Guacamole (page 101)

Cycle 3

DAY 1

BREAKFAST

Sugar Impact Shake (page 65) with low- or medium-SI fruit

LUNCH

Pork and Mushroom Stew with Sweet Potatoes (page 159)
Mixed green salad with *Dijon Vinaigrette* (page 193)

DINNER

Spaghetti Squash with Capers, Onion, and Bell Pepper (page 185) with an added ¼ cup
    julienned sun-dried tomatoes, topped with a grilled chicken breast
Mixed green salad with *Caper Vinaigrette* (page 192)

OPTIONAL SNACK

Cinnamon Almond Butter (page 104) with apple slices

DAY 2

BREAKFAST

Pumpkin Spice Shake (page 67) with an apple added

LUNCH

    Chicken Soup with Parsnips (page 150)

    Mixed green salad with *Caper Vinaigrette* (page 192)

DINNER

    Turkey Cutlets with Marsala and Shiitake Mushrooms (page 130)

    ½ baked sweet potato

OPTIONAL SNACK

    Cucumber Chips with Guacamole (page 101)

DAY 3

BREAKFAST

    Tex-Mex Scrambled Eggs with Avocado and Salsa (page 71) with a coconut wrap

    ½ baked sweet potato

LUNCH

    Super Greens Shake (page 66) with a green apple added

DINNER

    Jerk-Spiced Chicken Thighs with Roasted Pineapple Chutney (page 123)

    Raw Butternut Squash "Pappardelle" with Garlic and Oil (page 181)

    Mixed green salad with *Easy Lemon Vinaigrette* (page 193) and julienned roasted beets

OPTIONAL SNACK

    Lemon-Chili Roasted Almonds (page 95)

DAY 4

BREAKFAST

    Coconut-Vanilla Shake (page 68) with berries

LUNCH

    Flank Steak and Vegetable Wrap with Chimichurri Sauce (page 81)

    Spiced Sweet Potato "Fries" (page 188)

DINNER

Peppered Shrimp with Mango (page 139)
Stir-Fried Bok Choy (page 178)
Lemony Roasted Artichoke Hearts (page 170)

OPTIONAL SNACK

Fresh-Baked Gluten-Free Sesame "Pretzels" (page 94)

DAY 5

BREAKFAST

Pumpkin Bread French Toast with Berry Compote (page 72) with a side of nitrate-free
bacon or chicken breakfast sausage

LUNCH

Espresso-Almond Shake (page 67)
Pear slices with goat cheese

DINNER

Beef Bourguignon (page 156)
Mixed green salad with *Dijon Vinaigrette* (page 193) and beets

OPTIONAL SNACK

Chipotle Deviled Eggs (page 102)

DAY 6

BREAKFAST

Blueberry-Peach Shake (page 70)

LUNCH

Roasted Beet and Arugula Salad with Shallots and Lemon (page 81) topped with a grilled
chicken breast

DINNER

Turkey Meatballs with Parmesan and Tomato Sauce (page 126)
Italian-Style Peppers and Onion Sauté (page 169)

OPTIONAL SNACK

Slow-Roasted Nuts (page 97) with berries

DAY 7

BREAKFAST

Goat Cheese and Vegetable Omelet (page 74)
½ sweet potato

LUNCH

Cappuccino Protein Shake (page 69) with ½ banana

DINNER

Slow-Cooker Tomato-Braised Lamb Shanks (page 105)
Baked potato with grass-fed butter (high-SI test)
Steamed Broccoli with Garlic Oil Drizzle (page 167)

OPTIONAL SNACK

Strawberry Ice Cream (page 202)

16

VEGAN AND VEGETARIAN

I eat meat, but I can understand why people choose not to. I share your concern about the sad state of animal welfare in this country. The abysmal living conditions, inhumane treatment, and rampant use of hormones and antibiotics are cruel and unnecessary. And to top it off, they degrade the quality of the meat! That said, it hardly seems fair that many restaurants and social gatherings make vegans and vegetarians feel like second-class citizens, serving dishes without meat as an afterthought, if at all.

My dilemma is that we evolved eating meat. Humans developed high-functioning, large brains—which use 20% of our energy—directly as a result of including meat in our diet. That's why I only recommend meat from ethically raised animals fed their natural diet. Fish eat algae and plankton, not grain or soy. Cows eat grass, not soy or corn. Countries like New Zealand have rigorous meat standards and only allow grass-fed beef. Unfortunately, America is not there yet.

I don't recommend going vegetarian or vegan for most people. Many times I actually challenge my vegetarian clients to *reintroduce* lean animal protein into their diets. I'm not trying to sabotage their diet or their beliefs; I think most people fare better with some animal-based protein.

I was a vegan and a vegetarian for many years. During that time, I worked out twice as hard but suffered chronic cystic acne, weight loss resistance, and cratered energy. I see all those problems and more with my vegan and vegetarian clients today.

I also know that too many vegans and vegetarians rely on nutrient-bankrupt, soy-based

Frankenfoods and high–Sugar Impact foods. A high-carbohydrate diet—very common among vegans and vegetarians—creates a roller-coaster ride of blood sugar spikes and crashes that set you up for insulin resistance and type 2 diabetes.

Simply put: if you're a vegan or vegetarian for spiritual reasons, I support you and I want to help you do this in the healthiest way possible. If you're doing it because you think it's the healthiest diet, I hope you'll reconsider. And if you're doing it because you're concerned about animal welfare (who isn't?), I want you to consider reintroducing meat from animals raised humanely and fed their natural diet. Vote with your dollars!

Whatever your reason for not eating meat, I admire your dedication. You've got my full support, and you're going to love the delicious, low–Sugar Impact vegan and vegetarian recipes I've provided for you in this book.

You probably already know you have to work a little harder than meat eaters to get enough protein into your diet from the right sources. You can't store protein, so if you're not getting it from food, your body starts breaking down precious muscle tissue. Not good. So make the commitment to ensure that you're getting enough protein every day.

The healthiest vegetarian and vegan diets draw from low-SI foods including colorful vegetables and fruits, and lean, plant-based sources of protein, such as lentils and other legumes, nuts and seeds, and quinoa. Most vegans and vegetarians I know want creative, unique recipes to liven up their routine—and I've provided lots of great options in this cookbook.

With these strategies, you can become a lean, healthy, energetic vegan or vegetarian without going anywhere near a grass-fed steak (assuming I haven't persuaded you otherwise).

START YOUR MORNING WITH A PROTEIN SHAKE

Breakfast might seem like a meatless mecca if you're vegan or vegetarian—muffins, whole-grain cereals, soy crunch bars…But manufacturers know breakfast is all about convenience, and they've cashed in with lots of high-SI choices that masquerade as healthy, grab-and-go goodies. And if your need for speed in the morning means you skip breakfast entirely, you're making an even worse choice.

A protein shake solves both problems: you get a delicious, nutrient-rich, easy-to-make shake that will fuel your energy and fat loss straight through to lunch...far longer than that vegan scone.

MEET YOUR PROTEIN REQUIREMENTS

Animal protein provides the highest ratio of complete amino acids, but with a little planning, you—whether you're a vegan or a vegetarian—can easily meet your protein requirements. Aim for 2 to 3 protein-rich plant foods at every meal. So you might combine:

- ½ cup lentils
- ½ cup quinoa
- 2 tablespoons walnuts

Simple, right?! With combos like that, you'll easily get 17 grams of protein. Homemade veggie burgers, legumes, nuts and nut butters, and non-gluten grains also make excellent plant-based sources of protein.

UPGRADE YOUR FAVORITES

Lateral shifts, or healthier versions of your favorite foods, give you the satisfaction of comfort food, but they have more nutrients and lower Sugar Impact. Here are a few ideas for some awesome swaps:

- Trade nutrient-empty spaghetti noodles for corn-free quinoa pasta or spaghetti squash.
- Trade cow's milk (you probably have anyway) for unsweetened coconut or almond milk.
- Trade chips and salsa for kale chips with hummus or guacamole.
- Trade cheese for cashew cheese (great with low–Sugar Impact alla Checca sauce smeared on portobello mushroom caps).

Once you get the hang of lateral shifts, you can upgrade nearly any food into a nutrient-dense, delicious alternative to potentially highly reactive, high–Sugar Impact foods.

ELIMINATE FOOD INTOLERANCES

Sorry, vegans and vegetarians, but I'm calling you out on this one, since I see so many of you relying on soy as your go-to protein source. Don't get me wrong—I'm really glad you have protein on your radar, but soy isn't your best option. I addressed soy's many issues in *The Virgin Diet*, so here I'll just say that overdoing soy foods, most of them genetically modified, can create food intolerances and the nasty menu of symptoms that go with them.

And it's not just soy. Even though they sometimes fall into the "healthy category," gluten, dairy, and eggs can trigger intolerances when you eat too much of them.

I'm all for barnyard eggs, a limited amount of organic fermented soy, and grass-fed dairy if you can tolerate them. They're excellent protein sources, but they should never become everyday foods, and if you notice any reactions, I hope you'll eliminate and then challenge those foods as I have outlined in *The Virgin Diet*.

ADDRESS NUTRIENT DEFICIENCIES

Studies show vegans and vegetarians can have lower levels of certain nutrients. One found vegetarians often show low levels of vitamins B12 and D, omega-3 fatty acids, calcium, iron, and zinc.

As a vegan or vegetarian, you have to be vigilant about potential deficiencies. Fortunately, the problem becomes easy to fix when you incorporate nutrient-rich foods like nuts and seeds, which make good sources of zinc and calcium.

Beyond food, I strongly suggest you take a comprehensive multivitamin/mineral supplement every day to fill in nutrient gaps. An essential fatty acids formula can provide omega-3s, which are crucial to balance the omega-6-heavy diet most of us eat. If you can't do fish oil, look for a vegan (algae-derived) DHA supplement. And be sure to incorporate alpha-linolenic acid (ALA)–rich foods like flaxseeds, chia seeds, and walnuts.

MAKE AN OIL CHANGE

Vegetable oils sure sound healthy, don't they? Yet canola and other predominantly omega-6 oils can contribute to inflammation and upset the omega-6/omega-3 balance essential for reducing the risk of serious health conditions.

A vegan or vegetarian diet can also leave you deficient in healthy fats. The solution is easy and delicious: incorporate more nutrient-rich avocado, olives and olive oil, coconut, and nuts and seeds into your diet.

My favorite high-heat cooking oils are coconut oil and Malaysian red palm fruit oil. Use extra-virgin olive oil for drizzling onto salads and veggies.

VEGAN AND VEGETARIAN MEAL PLAN

Some recipes contain dairy—please note the modifications for vegans.

Cycle 1

DAY 1

BREAKFAST
Sugar Impact Shake (page 65) with fruit

LUNCH
Portobello Pizzas (page 143) served on *Sautéed Kale with Caramelized Onions* (page 172)

DINNER
Tuscan White Beans with Roasted Grape Tomatoes and Parmesan (page 179) served on a bed of brown rice
Mixed green salad with *Caper Vinaigrette* (page 192)

OPTIONAL SNACK
Garlic Hummus with Lentil Chips (page 100)

DAY 2

BREAKFAST
Old-Fashioned Oatmeal with Cinnamon, Blueberries, and Raspberries (page 73) topped with 2 tablespoons chopped walnuts

LUNCH
Super Greens Shake (page 66) with berries

DINNER

Quinoa Pasta alla Checca (page 144) with an added ¼ cup chickpeas

Mixed green salad with *Basil Vinaigrette* (page 197)

OPTIONAL SNACK

Grilled Nectarine Salsa (page 99) with lentil chips

DAY 3

BREAKFAST

Blueberry-Peach Shake (page 70)

LUNCH

Easy Vegetarian White Chili (page 144)

Mixed green salad with 1 tablespoon pepitas and *Easy Lemon Vinaigrette* (page 193)

DINNER

Spicy Black Bean Burgers with Goat Cheese and Wilted Tomato Salsa (page 146)

Spiced Sweet Potato "Fries" (page 188)

OPTIONAL SNACK

Smoky Baba Ghanoush (page 96) with rice chips

DAY 4

BREAKFAST

Sugar Impact Shake (page 65) with fruit

LUNCH

Cup of *Yellow Split Pea Soup* (page 151)

Asian Confetti Quinoa Salad with Almonds (page 85)

DINNER

Mushroom, Cashew, Spinach, and Lentil Skillet (page 142) served over brown rice

Mixed green salad with *Dijon Vinaigrette* (page 193)

OPTIONAL SNACK

Cinnamon Almond Butter (page 104) with apple slices

DAY 5

BREAKFAST
Coconut-Vanilla Shake (page 68) with fruit

LUNCH
Roasted Beet and Arugula Salad with Shallots and Lemon (page 81)
Beans and Greens Stew (page 155)

DINNER
Coconut Curry Butternut Squash Puree (page 180)
Red Lentil Dal (page 182)

OPTIONAL SNACK
Lime and Jalapeño Hummus (page 95) with rice chips

DAY 6

BREAKFAST
Coconut-Vanilla Shake (page 68) with fruit

LUNCH
Indian-Style Lentil Soup (page 159)
Mixed green salad with *Basil Vinaigrette* (page 197) and 2 tablespoons nut and seed mixture of your choice

DINNER
Chickpeas with Sautéed Greens (page 183)
Red Quinoa with Slow-Roasted Almonds and Caramelized Shallots (page 183)

OPTIONAL SNACK
White and Red Bean Salsa with White Onion, Tomato, and Cilantro (page 93) with rice chips

DAY 7

BREAKFAST
Blueberry-Peach Shake (page 70)

LUNCH

Winter Vegetable Minestrone (page 162) with an added ⅓ cup cannellini beans, served with rice chips

DINNER

Wild Rice and Vegetable Pilaf (page 189)

Chickpeas with Sautéed Greens (page 183)

OPTIONAL SNACK

Spicy Black Bean Dip with Celery (page 101) with rice chips

Cycle 2

DAY 1

BREAKFAST

Super Greens Shake (page 66)

LUNCH

Cup of *Yellow Split Pea Soup* (page 151)

Asian Confetti Quinoa Salad with Almonds (page 85)

DINNER

Coconut Curry Butternut Squash Puree (page 180)

Red Lentil Dal (page 182)

OPTIONAL SNACK

Lemon-Chili Roasted Almonds (page 95)

DAY 2

BREAKFAST

Pumpkin Spice Shake (page 67)

LUNCH

Easy Vegetarian White Chili (page 144)

Mixed green salad with 1 tablespoon pepitas and *Easy Lemon Vinaigrette* (page 193)

DINNER
  Spicy Black Bean Burgers with Goat Cheese and Wilted Tomato Salsa (page 146)
  Warm Wax Bean and Green Bean Salad (page 174)

OPTIONAL SNACK
  Chipotle Kale Chips (page 103)

DAY 3

BREAKFAST
  Chocolate, Flax, and Avocado Shake (page 69)

LUNCH
  Beans and Greens Stew (page 155)
  Wild Rice and Vegetable Pilaf (page 189)

DINNER
  Spicy Black Bean Burgers with Goat Cheese and Wilted Tomato Salsa (page 146)
  Warm Wax Bean and Green Bean Salad (page 174)

OPTIONAL SNACK
  Spicy Black Bean Dip with Celery (page 101)

DAY 4

BREAKFAST
  Coconut-Vanilla Shake (page 68)

LUNCH
  Lemony Roasted Artichoke Hearts (page 170) and *Lima Beans with Lemon and Spinach* (page 186) served on a bed of quinoa
  Mixed green salad with *Easy Lemon Vinaigrette* (page 193)

DINNER
  Raw Butternut Squash "Pappardelle" with Garlic and Oil (page 181)—double portion with *Marjoram Seared Mushrooms* (page 166)
  Mixed green salad with 2 tablespoons nut and seed mixture of your choice

OPTIONAL SNACK

Fresh-Baked Gluten-Free Sesame "Pretzels" (page 94)

DAY 5

BREAKFAST

Pumpkin Spice Shake (page 67)

LUNCH

Winter Vegetable Minestrone (page 162) with an added ⅓ cup cannellini beans and ½ cup cooked quinoa

Mixed green salad with *Basil Vinaigrette* (page 197)

DINNER

Chickpeas with Sautéed Greens (page 183)

Red Quinoa with Slow-Roasted Almonds and Caramelized Shallots (page 183)

OPTIONAL SNACK

Lime and Jalapeño Hummus (page 95) with crudités

DAY 6

BREAKFAST

Super Greens Shake (page 66)

LUNCH

Indian-Style Lentil Soup (page 159)

Mixed green salad with *Basil Vinaigrette* (page 197) with an added 2 tablespoons nut and seed mixture of your choice

DINNER

Tuscan White Beans with Roasted Grape Tomatoes and Parmesan (page 179) served on a bed of quinoa

Roasted Zucchini and Bell Pepper Medley (page 171)

OPTIONAL SNACK
> *Cucumber Chips with Guacamole* (page 101)

DAY 7

BREAKFAST
> *Cappuccino Protein Shake* (page 69)

LUNCH
> *Roasted Butternut Squash with Thyme* (page 187) topped with *Roasted Spiced Chickpeas* (page 98)
> *Sautéed Kale with Caramelized Onions* (page 172)

DINNER
> *Wild Rice and Vegetable Pilaf* (page 189)
> *Chickpeas with Sautéed Greens* (page 183)

OPTIONAL SNACK
> *Smoky Baba Ghanoush* (page 96) with crudités

DAY 8

BREAKFAST
> *Coconut-Vanilla Shake* (page 68)

LUNCH
> *Easy Vegetarian White Chili* (page 144)
> Mixed green salad with 1 tablespoon pepitas and *Easy Lemon Vinaigrette* (page 193)

DINNER
> *Coconut Curry Butternut Squash Puree* (page 180)
> *Red Lentil Dal* (page 182)

OPTIONAL SNACK
> *Roasted Spiced Chickpeas* (page 98)

DAY 9

BREAKFAST
Chocolate, Flax, and Avocado Shake (page 69)

LUNCH
Indian-Style Lentil Soup (page 159)

Mixed green salad with *Basil Vinaigrette* (page 197) and an added 2 tablespoons nut and seed mixture of your choice

DINNER
Mushroom, Cashew, Spinach, and Lentil Skillet (page 142)

Mixed green salad with *Dijon Vinaigrette* (page 193)

OPTIONAL SNACK
Chipotle Kale Chips (page 103)

DAY 10

BREAKFAST
Super Greens Shake (page 66)

LUNCH
Cup of *Yellow Split Pea Soup* (page 151)

Asian Confetti Quinoa Salad with Almonds (page 85)

DINNER
Beans and Greens Stew (page 155)

Wild Rice and Vegetable Pilaf (page 189)

OPTIONAL SNACK
Spicy Black Bean Dip with Celery (page 101)

DAY 11

BREAKFAST
Cappuccino Protein Shake (page 69)

LUNCH

Lemony Roasted Artichoke Hearts (page 170) and *Lima Beans with Lemon and Spinach* (page 186) served on a bed of quinoa

Mixed green salad with *Easy Lemon Vinaigrette* (page 193)

DINNER

Roasted Butternut Squash with Thyme (page 187) topped with *Roasted Spiced Chickpeas* (page 98)

Sautéed Kale with Caramelized Onions (page 172)

OPTIONAL SNACK

Lemon-Chili Roasted Almonds (page 95)

DAY 12

BREAKFAST

Espresso-Almond Shake (page 67)

LUNCH

Creamy Cauliflower Soup (page 154)

Quinoa with Celery and Mushrooms (page 187) with ½ cup lentils

DINNER

Raw Butternut Squash "Pappardelle" with Garlic and Oil (page 181)—double portion with *Marjoram Seared Mushrooms* (page 166)

Mixed green salad with 2 tablespoons nut and seed mixture of your choice

OPTIONAL SNACK

White and Red Bean Salsa with White Onion, Tomato, and Cilantro (page 93) with romaine or butter lettuce leaves

DAY 13

BREAKFAST

Sugar Impact Shake (page 65)

LUNCH

Indian-Style Lentil Soup (page 159)

Mixed green salad with *Basil Vinaigrette* (page 197) and an added 2 tablespoons nut and seed mixture of your choice

DINNER

Tuscan White Beans with Roasted Grape Tomatoes and Parmesan (page 179) served on a bed of quinoa

Mixed green salad with *Caper Vinaigrette* (page 192)

OPTIONAL SNACK

Fresh-Baked Gluten-Free Sesame "Pretzels" (page 94)

DAY 14

BREAKFAST

Cappuccino Protein Shake (page 69)

LUNCH

Winter Vegetable Minestrone (page 162) with an added ⅓ cup cannellini beans and ½ cup cooked quinoa

Mixed green salad with *Basil Vinaigrette* (page 197)

DINNER

Mushroom, Cashew, Spinach, and Lentil Skillet (page 142)

Mixed green salad with *Dijon Vinaigrette* (page 193)

OPTIONAL SNACK

Roasted Spiced Chickpeas (page 98)

<u>Cycle 3</u>

DAY 1

BREAKFAST

Sugar Impact Shake (page 65) with fruit

LUNCH

Cup of *Yellow Split Pea Soup* (page 151)

Asian Confetti Quinoa Salad with Almonds (page 85)

DINNER

Tuscan White Beans with Roasted Grape Tomatoes and Parmesan (page 179) served on a bed of brown rice

Mixed green salad with *Caper Vinaigrette* (page 192)

OPTIONAL SNACK

White and Red Bean Salsa with White Onion, Tomato, and Cilantro (page 93) with rice chips

DAY 2

BREAKFAST

Blueberry-Peach Shake (page 70)

LUNCH

Indian-Style Lentil Soup (page 159)

Mixed green salad with *Basil Vinaigrette* (page 197)

Rice chips

DINNER

Mushroom, Cashew, Spinach, and Lentil Skillet (page 142) served over brown rice

Mixed green salad with *Dijon Vinaigrette* (page 193)

OPTIONAL SNACK

Smoky Baba Ghanoush (page 96) with rice chips

DAY 3

BREAKFAST

Old-Fashioned Oatmeal with Cinnamon, Blueberries, and Raspberries (page 73) topped with 2 tablespoons chopped walnuts

LUNCH

Super Greens Shake (page 66) with berries

DINNER

Chickpeas with Sautéed Greens (page 183)

Red Quinoa with Slow-Roasted Almonds and Caramelized Shallots (page 183)

OPTIONAL SNACK

Spicy Black Bean Dip with Celery (page 101) with rice chips

DAY 4

BREAKFAST

Sugar Impact Shake (page 65) with fruit

LUNCH

Winter Vegetable Minestrone (page 162) with an added ⅓ cup cannellini beans, served with rice chips

DINNER

Quinoa Pasta alla Checca (page 144) with an added ¼ cup chickpeas

Mixed green salad with *Basil Vinaigrette* (page 197)

OPTIONAL SNACK

Grilled Nectarine Salsa (page 99) with lentil chips

DAY 5

BREAKFAST

Coconut-Vanilla Shake (page 68) with fruit

LUNCH

Spicy Black Bean Burgers with Goat Cheese and Wilted Tomato Salsa (page 146) in a rice tortilla, served with crudités

DINNER

Coconut Curry Butternut Squash Puree (page 180)

Red Lentil Dal (page 182)

OPTIONAL SNACK

Cinnamon Almond Butter (page 104) with apple slices

DAY 6

BREAKFAST

Coconut-Vanilla Shake (page 68) with fruit

LUNCH

Roasted Beet and Arugula Salad with Shallots and Lemon (page 81)
Beans and Greens Stew (page 155)

DINNER

Wild Rice and Vegetable Pilaf (page 189)
Chickpeas with Sautéed Greens (page 183)

OPTIONAL SNACK

Lime and Jalapeño Hummus (page 95) with rice chips

DAY 7

BREAKFAST

Blueberry-Peach Shake (page 70)

LUNCH

Portobello Pizzas (page 143) served on *Sautéed Kale with Caramelized Onions* (page 172)

DINNER

Spicy Black Bean Burgers with Goat Cheese and Wilted Tomato Salsa (page 146)
Baked potato (high-SI trial)

OPTIONAL SNACK

Garlic Hummus with Lentil Chips (page 100)

YOU'RE A SUGAR IMPACT PLAYER

What a trip it's been! It went by in a flash, didn't it? And surprise—you lost weight fast, stopped aging in its tracks, and feel better than you have in years. I'm so tempted to say I told you so! Keep in mind the good feelings aren't going to end just because you've graduated. The Sugar Impact trifecta of looking, feeling, and *being* great is just beginning.

I hope you'll never again look at food without thinking about its Sugar Impact: how will it affect your blood sugar, your energy, your waistline? You're empowered now to make educated choices, and if you can't choose low SI, you know how to work the Scales so you don't go flying off the rails. The Cycle 3 guidelines are clear—stick with them and the high-SI choices you can handle, and you'll look and feel fabulous for the rest of your fat-burning life.

Continue to eat by the Sugar Impact Plate and the Sugar Impact Clock, and make the Sugar Impact Shake (page 65) your go-to breakfast. Keep all the delicious low- and medium-SI recipes in this book in regular rotation, too. They'll also help you stay on track in your lower-SI life—with a revved metabolism, free of symptoms, and looking nowhere near your age. Create your own path forward, to taste. Because now you actually *will* taste all the fabulous, subtle, nuanced flavors the dishes in this book have to offer.

Your lower-SI lifestyle is yours to run with now. Don't be shy about sharing what you've discovered—there are many people who are where you were and who would really benefit from the inspiration of your example. Spread the word!

ACKNOWLEDGMENTS

A cookbook like this can only originate with an expert culinary team. Thank you, Jonathan Heindemause, for beautifully photographing these dishes. Chefs Marge Perry and David Bonom helped translate my low–Sugar Impact philosophy into easy-to-follow recipes, and Julie Grimes provided impeccable nutrition analysis along the way. Suzanne Griffith, you totally rocked the cookbook recipes and blogs.

I have a top-tier publishing team that helped this cookbook reach my loyal readers. A special thanks here to associate publisher Brian McLendon, who did a terrific job handling marketing. Matthew Ballast, my executive director of publicity, ensured this cookbook would become a success from the beginning.

I couldn't have done this without my editorial staff, including Karen Murgolo, editorial director of Grand Central Life & Style; Jamie Raab, president and publisher of Grand Central Publishing, who oversaw the whole imprint; and editor in chief Deb Futter. Elizabeth Connor provided amazing attention to detail with the cover design. Morgan Hedden, editorial assistant, became invaluable orchestrating behind-the-scenes happenings. And what would I do without the fabulous Sarah Pelz, executive editor at Grand Central Life & Style?

Ellyne Lonergan, my scriptwriter for PBS, helped me clarify my message to a much broader audience. Celeste Fine, my literary agent, showed unwavering support throughout every step of this process. Nicole Dunn, thank you for being my PR rock star. With a meticulous photogenic eye for detail, photographer Lesley Bohm helped me feel comfortable in front of the camera when I'm anything but.

This cookbook took shape working with my mentors, who challenged me to see a bigger vision. Better yet, they gave me the tools and support to go after that vision. So thank you, Brendon Burchard, Ali Brown, Joe Polish, Lisa Sasevich, Victoria Labalme, Mike Koenigs, Jon Walker, Dan Sullivan, and Babs Smith.

JJ Virgin & Associates continues to grow, and I have an A-list team that ensures the daily wheels turn smoothly with no stone unturned. Travis Houston heads up my online launches to reach a wider audience, while his wife, Joy, provides valuable support with our online programs. Traci Knoppe has loyally remained with my team for years and oversees tech support. Ben Clark, our incredible designer, makes us look good online and in the real world.

Susan Tafralis helped with product development, but she wears numerous other hats. She's literally the glue that holds my business together and has been for over 14 years now, having run every part of my business. Where would I be without her? As our company grew, Kim Ward stepped in to help with those ever-increasing duties.

My top-notch nutrition coaches Patsy Wallace and Jason Boehm oversee the coaches and community. Kathy White, Jennifer Vega, and Chelsea Early help support the community forums so that every question gets answered. Jason also helps with blogs and research.

Michael Ross, thanks for your keen eye for detail. Mary Ann Guillory, thank you for making sure those orders go out every day and ensuring that everyone gets paid.

Social media helps my message reach a much bigger audience, and I have Mary Agnes Antonopoulous, her husband, Tommy, and her amazing team to thank for that. Mary Agnes does double duty as my copywriter, and Kathy White helps provide community and social media support.

As my president and COO, Camper Bull, always says, customer service is the face of this company. We get a lot of questions here, so thank you, Brandy Burke, for being a great team leader and juggling numerous projects. Nadiya Gillani, Rose Curran, Sigourney Rodriguez, and Melanie Humphrey all ensure every person gets the help and support they need. Gina Callaway is my e-mail list pro. The adorable Lacy Kirkland skillfully helps manage my affiliates and provides team support.

Overseeing this entire process, Camper also helped me launch the company to an entirely new level.

Thank you to Peter Hoppenfeld and Darryl Scheetz for your always excellent legal support. Liana Chauli, your eye for details helps keep me looking great with your impeccable wardrobe advice. Harshini Wijesuriya, thank you for your personal assistant support.

Gratitude, too, for my peers in our Mindshare Collaborative group, including Pattie Ptak, Leslie Scirratt, and Audrey Hagen, for helping me shape my vision into reality.

And I am thrilled to have the vision and support of Johnathan Lizotte, CEO of Designs for Health, to help me offer the best product line to my community.

Everything I do, I do for my family; they belong at the top of any acknowledgment list (even if I mention them last). Bryce, thank you for being kind, brilliant, talented, and supportive. Grant, you are a walking miracle who continues to inspire people with your story every day. And John Virgin, thank you for being an incredible dad and stepping in to help me out while I get my message to the world.

RESOURCES

ONLINE

If you're looking for more recipes to use on the Sugar Impact Diet, and more support during your journey, be sure to check out these additional resources online at http://sugarimpact .com/resources. There are meal plans for every situation under the sun and guides and tools to help you breeze to the finish line.

Use The Virgin Diet/Sugar Impact Diet Conversion Guide to incorporate the *Virgin Diet Cookbook* and you'll have no shortage of delicious low-SI options—it will help you use the *Virgin Diet Cookbook* with the Sugar Impact Diet with ease.

Additional Meal Plans:

- Athletes
- Budget
- Family
- Intensify
- On the Go
- Party
- The Virgin Diet
- Dining Out

Sugar Impact Diet Tools and Support:

- Cycle blueprints
- Food journal
- Full Sugar Impact Scales—by category
- Shopping lists for all meal plans
- Sneaky Sugar Inventory
- Speed-Healing Techniques
- Sugar Impact Plate and Categories—Cycle 2 and low/medium Sugar Impact (SI)

- Sugar Impact Quiz
- Sugar Impact Scale—for Cycle 2 only
- Sugar-Attack Survival Strategies
- Sugar-Withdrawal Strategies
- The Virgin Diet/Sugar Impact Diet Conversion Guide
- Water schedule

MEDITATION AND MIND-SET TRAINING

Sculptations is a brain-entrainment technology designed to shift your thought patterns around sugar cravings. Using our proprietary process of MindSculpting, you immediately begin to reset your negative thought patterns, rewire your habits and behaviors, and recode a new level of thinking that supports you and your success. In as little as 5 minutes, you'll be able to release the hold your sugar cravings have on you and accelerate the sculpting of new mind-sets that support a healthier and more vibrant lifestyle. The scientifically engineered audio tracks are designed to synchronize your conscious desires and your subconscious beliefs (called creating "neural harmony") to empower you to achieve greater health with lightning speed and accuracy. For more information and to download two free Sculptations to help you with your sugar cravings and reach your ideal weight, go to www.sculptations.com/jjvirgin.

JJ'S FAVORITE FOODS AND DRINKS

Andean Dream Quinoa Pasta

www.andeandream.com/OtherProducts.html

Pasta without the high-glycemic load. Andean Dream Quinoa Pasta is the only quinoa pasta I know that doesn't contain corn. Gluten-free and organic, Andean Dream Quinoa Pasta comes in traditional spaghetti as well as noodles, macaroni, and fusilli for all your gluten-free pasta needs.

Bob's Red Mill

www.bobsredmill.com

You've likely seen Bob's Red Mill in your health food store. This company has been around nearly forever (well, since 1978) and provides a wide variety of gluten-free oats and flours as well as golden flaxseeds, chia seeds, and coconut flour. Bob's Red Mill remains the trusted leader in gluten-free flours, seeds, and other foods because they provide consistently superior products.

Hampton Creek Foods Just Mayo

https://hamptoncreekfoods.com/justmayo

Finally, a healthy, egg-free mayo! Made from non-GMO, expeller-pressed canola oil, lemon juice, and white vinegar, this is the perfect condiment to smear on Paleo wraps or anywhere else you want the creamy, delicious taste of mayo without the junk most commercial brands contain. Just Mayo is available at Whole Foods Markets.

Heintzman Farms Golden Flax

www.heintzmanfarms.com

Flaxseeds are one of my favorite foods because these tiny seeds are loaded with protein, fiber, lignans, and omega-3 fatty acids. If you follow my recipe, you know I like to throw flaxseeds into my protein smoothie.

I've been using Heintzman Farms Gold Flax for years—I love when my order of fresh, whole, GMO-free Dakota Flax Gold flaxseeds arrives. Their kit includes three 1-pound bags of seeds and a mini electric grinder so that you can grind the flaxseeds yourself. Toss them into your smoothie or use them anytime you need a fiber and nutrient boost.

Hint Water

www.drinkhint.com

Hint Water evolved when San Francisco native Kara Goldin couldn't find a delicious, refreshing drink for herself or her kids. What she wanted was simple: no sweeteners, sugars, fancy but useless additives, or ingredients you can't pronounce. Just plain, delicious pure springwater with a splash of natural flavor. Sounds easy, right? It wasn't, which is why she created Hint Water. When people tell me they don't like water or are trying to break their soda habit, I always recommend Hint Water in amazing flavors like raspberry-lime and strawberry-kiwi. Who says water has to be boring?

Hydrolyzyme by Designs for Health

www.jjvirginstore.com

Nearly everyone struggling with gas, bloating, and other gastrointestinal issues after drinking a pea protein shake can benefit from taking Hydrolyzyme from Designs for Health. That's because Hydrolyzyme is a proprietary blend of protease enzymes that helps support efficient digestion and absorption of protein supplements consumed as a shake or liquid meal, since liquid protein supplements pass through the stomach more quickly than solid meals.

Benefits of Hydrolyzyme include efficiently breaking down 99% of protein, significantly reducing gastrointestinal discomfort, and helping your body absorb and utilize that protein quickly and efficiently.

Julian Bakery Paleo Wraps

www.julianbakery.com/bread-product/paleo-wraps-1-pack-7-wraps-gluten-free-raw
-vegan-low-carb

When you want the portability and ease of bread without gluten or carbs, Paleo Wraps are your answer: gluten-free, soy-free, GMO-free, raw, vegan, and low-carb. Made from coconut meat and unrefined virgin coconut oil, these are my go-to wraps for everything from hummus to sliced turkey with avocado.

Kerrygold Pure Irish Butter

http://kerrygoldusa.com/products/butter

Sometimes you want the creaminess of pure butter. Kerrygold Pure Irish Butter is miles above regular butter because it comes from grass-fed cows whose milk is higher in nutrients like fat-burning conjugated linolenic acid, yielding the sweetest, richest butter in the world.

KeVita Probiotic Drink

http://kevita.com

We could all use more healthy gut bacteria, but eating fermented foods can sometimes be a challenge, especially when you're busy or on the road. That's why I love KeVita Probiotic Drink. Every sip of this fabulous-tasting beverage provides four strains of live probiotic. KeVita Probiotic Drink comes in delicious flavors like Coconut, Mango Coconut, and Pomegranate. Certified organic, very low in sugar, nondairy, non-GMO, gluten-free, and vegan: what's not to love?

Kite Hill Nondairy Cheeses

www.kite-hill.com

Finally, a nondairy cheese that tastes decadently delicious. Crafted by artisanal cheesemakers, Kite Hill nondairy cheeses fit into your eating plan whether you're vegan, vegetarian, Paleo, or dairy-sensitive. They currently offer three diverse cheeses, with more sure to come: Cassucio, with a soft, fresh, supple, and silky texture; Costanoa, semisoft and dusted with a piquant blend of paprika and fennel pollen; and White Alder, a soft ripened cheese with a delicate white rind, pungent aroma, and velvety texture. Kite Hill nondairy cheeses are sold exclusively at Whole Foods Markets.

SKINNYFat

http://jjvirgin.com/skinnyfat

SKINNYFat Oil Blends bring the health benefits of some of the healthiest oils in the world—including organic virgin coconut oil, medium-chain triglycerides (MCTs), and organic extra-virgin olive oil—into your kitchen, making it easy to avoid highly processed, genetically modified oils, such as corn, canola, and soybean. And because MCTs are used as immediate energy it is nearly impossible to store SKINNYFat as body fat, which makes SKINNYFat perfect for anyone wanting to lose weight, control hunger, boost brain power, and naturally increase their energy. Both flavor varieties, SKINNYFat and SKINNYFat Olive, are so delicious and easy to use that you may just forget they're good for you—but your body won't. Try them in your favorite recipes, including salad dressings, sauces, soups, smoothies, dips, marinades, yogurt, and even ice cream!

Upgraded Cacao Butter

www.jjvirgin.com/bulletproof

If you're a chocolate lover, give your coffee a decadent upgrade or make healthy hot chocolate with this rich, delicious cacao butter. Upgraded Cacao Butter is a superfood made from organic raw cacao butter, sourced from the best cacao beans, processed to minimize toxins, and carefully stored to prevent contamination from heavy metals and fungi.

Upgraded Coffee

www.jjvirgin.com/bulletproof

For years, I avoided coffee because it made me a wired mess. Then I discovered Upgraded Coffee. Perfectly roasted beans with a bold, well-balanced flavor make Upgraded Coffee unlike any other coffee you've tried. Best of all, Upgraded Coffee contains no nasty toxins. Whether you opt for drinking it black or making Bulletproof Coffee with grass-fed butter or ghee, Upgraded Coffee will give you a morning jolt without the jittery aftermath. Also available in decaf.

Upgraded Ghee

www.jjvirgin.com/bulletproof

Ghee is clarified butter, meaning butter with the milk solids removed, so it's ideal for anyone with dairy intolerances. Upgraded ghee comes from grass-fed cows, tastes great, and doesn't contain nasty toxins or other pollutants. Perfect for cooking, adding to your Bulletproof Coffee, or anywhere you normally use butter and want a healthy fat source. Strictly limited edition (currently, they have a shortage on butter from grass-fed cows!), so grab it if they have it in stock.

Upgraded MCT Oil

www.jjvirgin.com/bulletproof

Six times stronger than coconut oil, Upgraded MCT oil converts into energy faster than other oils when you need a fast energy source without stimulants like caffeine. Odorless and flavorless, Upgraded MCT oil blends easily into your coffee (combine with grass-fed butter or ghee to make Bulletproof Coffee), gives you an immune boost, and helps your body better absorb nutrients.

Dark and Raw Chocolate

ChocolaTree

http://chocolatree.com

Your one-stop shop for all things chocolate, including a 78% cacao Raw Love Bar and Velvet Chocolate Coconut Oil/Butter. Lower sugar and higher fiber means you can enjoy many of ChocolaTree's foods guilt-free. ChocolaTree also has a wide selection of Sugar Impact Diet–friendly non-chocolate foods, including nut butters and kale chips.

Soma Chocolatemaker

www.somachocolate.com

Making small batches from premium-grade cacao, this Canadian chocolatier creates some of the richest, healthiest chocolate on the planet. It's absolutely worth seeking out. Soma Arcana 100% is a premium, delicious 100% cacao dark chocolate created with four types of flavor-grade cacao beans and without any sugar, emulsifiers, or flavorings. Just pure, healthy dark chocolate that kicks up flavor in shakes or blended with almond butter.

Coconut

Coconut Secret Coconut Aminos

www.coconutsecret.com/aminos2.html

Skip the soy sauce in your next stir-fry and reach for Coconut Secret Coconut Aminos, a 100% organic, raw, gluten- and soy-free sauce that kicks up your sushi, dressings, marinades, and sautés with a burst of flavor and healthy amino acids. When coconut trees are tapped, the blossoms exude a nutrient-rich sap that creates these aminos. In addition to an impressive amino acid profile, Coconut Secret Coconut Aminos provide rich amounts of B vitamins, vitamin C, and minerals.

Coconut Kefir Starter Mix

Yogurt fans, check out coconut kefir. Its many benefits include probiotics for a healthy gut and better digestion. Kefir also boosts your immune system and is antiaging. If you're curious, give So Delicious coconut kefir a try. I think you'll love it. If you want to make your own kefir (it's fun and super easy, I promise!), get the kefir starter from my brilliant pal Donna Gates at Body Ecology (www.bodyecology.com).

So Delicious Coconut Milk

www.turtlemountain.com/products

You can replace cow's milk with So Delicious unsweetened coconut milk beverage, either as an ingredient in your protein smoothies or as a beverage in its own right. One cup contains just 50 calories and only 1 gram of sugar. It also offers medium-chain fatty acids, a healthy fat that your body easily burns for energy rather than storing it. They also have a line of culinary milks that are perfect to add creaminess to sauces and soups.

If coconut milk isn't your thing, try So Delicious unsweetened almond milk and my new favorite, cashew milk. So Delicious also provides a delicious selection of no-sugar-added coconut milk ice cream and cultured coconut milk. One bite of these delicious treats and you'll wonder why you ever fell for cow's milk. And this is my go-to resource for culinary coconut milks.

Fiber Blends

JJ Virgin's Extra Fiber

www.jjvirginstore.com

My favorite way to meet your 50-gram daily fiber quota, JJ Virgin's Extra Fiber contains 12 different types of soluble and insoluble fiber naturally derived from fruits, vegetables, roots, seeds, and tree extracts, with added friendly bacteria and prebiotics. Antioxidant rich and free of phytates, lectins, gluten, and other harsh ingredients found in some fiber products, JJ Virgin's Diet Extra Fiber is unsweetened and mixes easily into shakes and other liquids.

SunFiber

www.sunfiber.com

Sunfiber promotes intestinal and colon health, aids in the transit of food through the intestines, and assists weight control by providing a satiety effect. Sunfiber promotes the absorption of essential minerals and helps the body combat increased blood glucose levels by controlling the glycemic index of foods.

Grass-Fed Beef

U.S. Wellness Meats

www.grasslandbeef.com

One of my favorite companies from which to buy healthy, sustainable grass-fed beef, wild game, poultry, and wild seafood, delivered right to my door. I love that their website is a one-stop shop for pet foods, raw organic ice cream, and healthy snacks like beef pemmican, a grass-fed jerky.

Carolina Beef and Bison

http://carolinabison.com

Another of my top suppliers for grass-fed beef and bison, and they deliver, too! Founded by author, lecturer, and whole-health practitioner Dr. Frank J. King Jr. in 1985, Carolina Bison is located in the lush Blue Ridge Mountains of Western North Carolina. They raise their cows and bison on top-quality grasses and pure mountain springwater to yield the same pristine meats our Paleolithic ancestors once ate. When I order from Carolina Beef and Bison, I know I'm getting the highest-quality, nutrient-rich, grass-fed, free-range meats with no steroids, antibiotics, or any other nasty stuff found in conventionally raised meats.

Wild Things Seafood

www.wildthingsseafood.com/collections/jjvirgin

Another great resource for grass-fed beef and lamb and pastured pork and chicken is www.WildThingsSeafood.com. Don't let the name fool you, the owner Jeff Moore sources the best clean lean protein.

Protein Powders

JJ Virgin's All-in-One Shake

www.jjvirginstore.com

JJ Virgin's All-in-One Shake lives up to its name. Blended with either plant-based or grass-fed beef protein (yes, defatted beef protein from Swedish grass-fed cows; it has a high biological value similar to egg protein, but without eggs' potential reactivity), this premium powder contains optimal amounts of vitamins, minerals, enzymes, probiotics, whole food complexes (antioxidants), and fiber with no added sugar. Start every morning with JJ Virgin's All-in-One Shake and you'll stay full, focused, and burning fat for hours. Available in chocolate, vanilla, or my favorite, chai.

Designs for Health

www.designsforhealth.com

PaleoMeal DF. A great-tasting, nutrient-rich, very-low-sugar pea-based protein powder. Every serving of PaleoMeal DF combines 17 grams of pea protein isolate with 5 grams of fiber, vitamins, minerals, and conditionally essential nutrients that help support weight control, gastrointestinal health, detoxification, immune issues, heavy metals, and muscle gain. Casein-free, lactose-free, and gluten-free and available in vanilla or berry flavor.

PaleoCleanse. PaleoCleanse is a comprehensive functional food powder ideal for detoxification. Very low in sugar, it combines pea protein isolate with vitamins, minerals, antioxidants, and conditionally essential nutrients to provide comprehensive nutrient support to aid phase 1 and phase 2 detoxification. Blends easily, in a delicious berry-vanilla flavor, with a great mouthfeel.

Natural Sugar Substitutes

Virgin Sprinkles

www.jjvirginstore.com

Finally, a good-for-you sugar substitute that also tastes good. Virgin Sprinkles contain a blend of glycine, erythritol, and stevia—all natural, beneficial sweeteners—that you can use just like sugar and mix easily into your favorite food or beverage. Best of all, Virgin Sprinkles create no weird aftertaste, stomach upset, or other side effects like other natural sugar alternatives.

Natvia

www.natvia.com

A unique blend of 100% natural stevia and erythritol, Natvia is a great-tasting sweetener that bakes and cooks just like sugar. Natvia blends easily in your favorite food or beverage and makes the perfect sweetener for people with diabetes and sugar sensitivities. Available in canisters or perfect on-the-go stick packets.

Norbu Sweetener

http://norbusweetener.com

A 100% natural sweetener with zero calories that's sugar-free and non-GMO, Norbu combines the clean sweet taste of monk fruit with erythritol. Safe for people with diabetes and sugar sensitivities, Norbu is formulated for baking and blends well into your favorite food or beverage. Norbu comes in a powder or convenient on-the-go tablets.

Stevia

www.stevia.com

Known as the "sweet leaf," this no-calorie herbal sweetener comes in packets, liquid form, and shaker bottles. Look for pure stevia, not one of those commercial brands loaded with sugar alcohols and other ingredients. Whole Foods 365 brand makes an organic pure stevia that I highly recommend.

The Ultimate Sweetener Xylitol

http://theultimatelife.net/CatSweet.htm

Xylitol still has some calories, sweetens like sugar, doesn't raise blood sugar levels like sugar does, and provides benefits from cavity prevention and reducing candida to improving bone health. Unfortunately, most xylitol these days comes from corn, a highly reactive food that creates food intolerances. The Ultimate Sweetener from The Ultimate Life uses 100% birch trees for their xylitol. Unlike some other brands, The Ultimate Sweetener contains no artificial sweeteners, sugars, potential food intolerance triggers, or other additives. Just pure birch tree–derived xylitol. Available from Amazon.com or at your local health food store.

Flavor Enhancing Sides and Seasonings

Navitas Naturals

www.navitasnaturals.com

They aren't kidding when they call themselves "The Super Food Company": Navitas Naturals is a family-owned company that provides a wide array of organic, non-GMO, nutrient-rich raw cacao, flax, cashew, coconut, and other delicious foods. Among their "must-trys" are raw cacao nibs and powder as well as chia seed powder.

Pete's Paleo Bacon

http://petespaleo.com

Bacon lovers, rejoice! Pete's Paleo Bacon is my absolute favorite bacon, because unlike most commercial brands, it contains no sugar, nitrates, or nitrites. Dry cured with salt, herbs, and spices, Pete's bacon is cold smoked for 2 days for perfect flavor and texture. Sold in a slab by the pound so you can slice it as thick or thin as you'd like.

Also check out their 30-Day Gut Healing Kit, which includes bone broth sourced from humanely raised animals. Each kit includes bone broth in 10 easy-to-store, resealable containers as well as 30 coconut cream chai–flavored gelatin gummies, 30 berry & mint– or green tea & ginger–flavored gelatin gummies, and 15 soup "packs" consisting of dehydrated veggies (just add broth to make an instant meal).

Real Good Salt

http://get.realgoodsalt.com/thevirgindiet

Real Good Salt is nutrient-rich Aztec sea salt from La Laguna de Cuyutlá (the same place where the Aztecs got their salt over 500 years ago). Traditional *salineros* (salt farmers) continue to harvest this salt using an organic, 100% renewable process (evaporated naturally by the sun) to protect the environment and wildlife. With your purchase, you are supporting this "small salt economy" of *salineros*, their families, and their way of salt harvesting. I wouldn't use any other salt with my food.

Diet Bars and Drinks

JJ Virgin's All-in-One Bars

www.jjvirginstore.com

When you want a healthy, delicious snack or mini meal, reach for JJ Virgin's All-in-One Bars. GMO-free and made with fresh ingredients like organic cashew butter and chia seeds with no fractionated oils or other preservatives, All-in-One Bars provide a sweet, satisfying, chewy, low-sugar treat. Each bar packs healthy fat, 8 grams of protein, and 6 grams of fiber to curb hunger and cravings. Available in Cinnamon Cashew Crunch, Dark Chocolate Cherry, and my new favorite, Toasted Coconut Cacao.

JJ Virgin's Green Balance

www.jjvirginstore.com

This unique fiber and green powder blend provides serious nutrition in a delicious lightly stevia-sweetened orange-cranberry flavor. Every serving of JJ Virgin's Green Balance combines 5 grams of high-quality fiber with alkalizing grass juices, the prebiotic inulin, vegetables, fruits, and berries. The blend of natural soluble and insoluble fiber comes from fruits, vegetables, roots, seeds, and tree extracts with added friendly bacteria and prebiotics. Antioxidant-rich JJ Virgin's Green Balance mimics whole, nutrient-rich, high-fiber plant foods and makes an ideal way to meet your fruit and veggies quota.

Whole Foods 365 brand

Far from being a generic brand, Whole Foods 365 and 365O brands provide high-quality, natural, GMO-free, organic frozen fruit, teas, nonirradiated spices, and much more, all priced to compete against grocery store brands. When I'm not making my own, I choose 365 Organic Smooth Almond Butter, which doesn't have added sugar, trans fat, or other junk found in many commercial nut butters. Also worth mentioning is Whole Foods 365 Natural Stevia Extract Powder. You get pure stevia without the maltodextrin, dextrose, nebulous natural flavors, and other additives in some commercial brands.

Wild Seafood

Wild Things Seafood

www.wildthingsseafood.com/collections/jjvirgin

Wild Things Seafood is a provider of premium "Caught to Be Frozen" chef-ready restaurant-quality seafood, premium grass-fed beef and lamb, pasture-raised chicken, and other clean, lean, and organic protein. Wild Things has created an exclusive Clean and Lean Marketplace stocked with only JJ Virgin–approved seafood and meat. I have negotiated special discounted prices to support my mission to provide healthy, clean, *and* affordable food for clients, readers, and friends.

Vital Choice

www.vitalchoice.com

Buying fish can be confusing. Vital Choice makes it easy because I know they sell only the highest-quality wild and organic seafood. I especially love their Alaskan salmon, which—like all their fish—is cleaned and flash-frozen within hours of harvest (the fish is delivered on dry ice). I also encourage you to venture beyond their fabulous seafood selection. Vital Choice sells other organic and wild foods, including nuts, berries, teas, and my favorite, dark chocolate.

BOOKS

Mira and Jayson Calton, *Rich Food, Poor Food: The Ultimate Grocery Purchasing System*
William Davis, MD, *Wheat Belly*
Mark Hyman, MD, *The Blood Sugar Solution*
David Gillespie, *Sweet Poison*
Richard Johnson, MD, *The Sugar Fix*; *The Fat Switch*
Robert Lustig, MD, *Fat Chance*; *Sugar: The Bitter Truth* (Video: http://www.youtube.com/watch?v =dBnniua6-oM)
Dr. Joseph Mercola, *The No-Grain Diet*; *Sweet Deception*
Michael Moss, *Salt Sugar Fat*
Pamela Peeke, MD, *The Hunger Fix: The Three-Stage Detox and Recovery Plan for Overeating and Food Addiction*
David Perlmutter, MD, *Grain Brain*
Gary Taubes, *Why We Get Fat*
JJ Virgin, *The Virgin Diet*; *The Virgin Diet Cookbook; JJ Virgin's Sugar Impact Diet*
John Yudkin, *Pure, White, and Deadly*

COACHING AND COMMUNITY

Virgin Diet and Sugar Impact Diet Coaches

The Sugar Impact and Virgin Diet One-on-One Coaching

www.jjvirgin.com/coaches

Nearly everyone who excelled at something had a coach somewhere along the way. Customize your food and nutrient plan with one of my rock-star health coaches, whom I've personally trained based on my philosophy. Whatever your needs, preferences, budget, or other restrictions, they can develop a plan that works specifically for you to achieve and maintain your goals. They can also provide support and troubleshoot potential issues that arise along your journey. We offer several one-on-one packages.

Sugar Solution Online Program and Group Challenges

http://virgindiet.com, http://sugarimpact.com

Take your commitment to the next level and do a deep dive into the program. You'll engage in the community forum, find an accountability partner, and get support from Sugar Impact coaches to help ensure your success.

EXERCISE RESOURCES

Exercise Equipment

X-iser Burst Trainer

http://jjvirgin.com/xiserjj

Trash your treadmill…sprint on the X-iser! The days of 30- to 60-minute workouts on oversize machines are over. The sprint training revolution is here. The science behind sprinting combined with the technology of the X-iser gives you a full cardio workout in just a few minutes a day. No… it is not just another stepper! The X-iser is specifically designed to allow people of any age and fitness level a way to sprint train. No other stepping device can provide the same level of benefit.

4x4 Burst Training Videos

JJ's Fit Club

www.jjsfitclub.com

A full-body workout in just 15 minutes, three times a week, in your own home. My 4x4 Workout combines high-intensity burst training with resistance exercise to blast fat, jumpstart metabolism, and keep you lean and sexy. Dump the expensive gym memberships and lame excuses and get moving with my free 4x4 Workout!

FINDING A QUALIFIED PRACTITIONER

Over the years, I've had the good fortune to work with many wonderful practitioners. I've included the top organizations to query to find a practitioner near you.

Age Management Medicine Group (AMMG)

www.agemed.org/Home.aspx

I like this organization because it provides proactive, preventive protocols to help you optimize your health, restore endocrine balance, delay the symptoms of aging, and prevent premature disability and death. The result is a higher quality of life, an enhanced sense of well-being, and a longer life. To find an AMMG-certified practitioner, visit www.agemed.org /Supporters/ProductandServicesDirectory.aspx.

American Academy of Anti-Aging Medicine (A4M)

www.a4m.com

A4M represents 24,000 of the smartest cutting-edge physicians and scientists from 110 countries. They use advanced technology that detects, prevents, and treats aging-related disease. And they're always looking for ways to slow and optimize aging. To keep up with their breakthroughs and antiaging issues in general, as well as find an A4M-certified practitioner, click on Directory on the home page.

American Association of Naturopathic Physicians

www.naturopathic.org

I respect naturopathic medicine because it's based on the belief that the human body has an innate healing ability. Naturopathic doctors (NDs) teach you to use diet, exercise, lifestyle changes, and cutting-edge natural therapies to enhance your body's ability to ward off and combat disease. NDs craft comprehensive treatment plans that blend the best of modern medical science and traditional natural medical approaches to both treat disease and restore health. You can find an ND near you from the home page of this site.

American College for Advancement in Medicine (ACAM)

www.acamnet.org

This nonprofit organization educates doctors and other health care professionals on the safe and effective application of integrative medicine. ACAM's health care model focuses on total wellness and preventing illness. As an ACAM member, you can connect with more than 1,500 physicians in 30 countries who take an integrative approach to patient care. ACAM also empowers you with information about integrative medicine treatment options. You can find an ACAM practitioner directly from the home page of this site.

The Institute for Functional Medicine (IFM)

www.functionalmedicine.org

IFM focuses on functional medicine as the standard of care. Functional medicine is a patient-centered, optimal-health approach that views each person as biochemically unique. To find a functional medicine practitioner, visit www.functionalmedicine.org/practitioner_search.aspx.

National Association of Nutrition Professionals (NANP)

www.nanp.org

This nonprofit organization advocates on behalf of holistically trained food and nutrition professionals. NANP members are nutrition professionals working in a variety of settings who are recognized for their knowledge and expertise in whole-foods nutrition and the safe, effective use of dietary supplements. NANP members include MDs, RNs, chiropractors, acupuncturists, and natural-foods chefs. To find a NANP practitioner, visit www.nanp.org/find-a-professional.

GLUTEN-FREE RESOURCES

GF Harvest: www.glutenfreeoats.com
Amazon: www.amazon.com

GlutenFree.com: www.glutenfree.com

The Gluten-Free Mall: www.glutenfreemall.com

GMO INFORMATION

Institute for Responsible Technology

www.responsibletechnology.org/buy-non-gmo

Expert Jeffrey Smith's site is loaded with great information, including your complete guide on how to avoid genetically modified foods.

KITCHEN EQUIPMENT

Blendtec Blenders

www.blendtec.com

Blendtec designs dependable, affordable, professional-grade blenders that can tackle your toughest jobs from shakes to soups with ease. Their Signature Series offers simple, intuitive touchpad icons, a completely sealed surface for easy cleanup, five preprogrammed blending cycles, and a manual five-speed control with a sleek, modern design. Available at Costco, Bed Bath & Beyond, and other fine retailers.

Food Dehydrator

A food dehydrator is your ultimate kitchen workhorse appliance. I use mine to make jerky without the nitrates and other junk found in commercial jerky. Natto, pemmican, and yogurt are other ideal foods to create in a dehydrator. More than any other food, I use my dehydrator for nuts. Soaking and drying nuts makes nutrients more available and reduces phytic acid and other nutrient inhibitors. Plus, it makes the nuts taste way better. You can find a good-quality hydrator, such as the Nesco FD-60 Snackmaster Express 4-Tray Food Dehydrator, on Amazon.com for less than $50.

Magic Bullet and Nutribullet

www.buythebullet.com, www.nutribullet.com

The Magic Bullet is a portable, space-saving device that makes a great alternative to blenders and food processors. It also travels well and is your perfect device to whip up my All-in-One shake. Honestly, I never travel without it!

The NutriBullet is a revved-up version of the Magic Bullet. The NutriBullet has a higher loading capacity (24 ounces versus the Magic Bullet's 18 ounces) and a higher-watt motor (600 watts versus the Magic Bullet's 250 watts), making it ideal for your toughest grinding jobs—including nut butters.

CONVERTING TO METRICS

VOLUME MEASUREMENT CONVERSIONS	
US	*Metric*
¼ teaspoon	1.25 milliliters (ml)
½ teaspoon	2.5 ml
¾ teaspoon	3.75 ml
1 teaspoon	5 ml
1 tablespoon	15 ml
¼ cup	62.5 ml
½ cup	125 ml
¾ cup	187.5 ml
1 cup	250 ml

WEIGHT CONVERSION MEASUREMENTS	
US	*Metric*
1 ounce	28.4 grams (g)
8 ounces	227.5 g
16 ounces (1 pound)	455 g

COOKING TEMPERATURE CONVERSIONS	
Celsius/Centigrade	F = (C x 1.8) + 32
Fahrenheit	C = (F−32) x 0.5555

Zero degrees Celsius and 100°C are arbitrarily placed as the melting and boiling points of water, while Fahrenheit establishes 0°F as the stabilized temperature when equal amounts of ice, water, and salt are mixed. So, for example, if you are baking at 350°F and want to know that temperature in Celsius, the following calculation will provide it: C = (350–32) × 0.5555 = 176.66°C.

REFERENCES

Introduction: Drop 7 Sugars, Lose 10 Pounds, Just 2 Weeks

J. Bailor, "57 Sneaky Sugars to Avoid," *Huffington Post* blog, November 20, 2013. http://www.huffingtonpost.com/jonathan-bailor/sugars-avoid_b_4222642.html

R.K. Johnson et al., "Dietary Sugars Intake and Cardiovascular Health: A Scientific Statement from the American Heart Association," *Circulation* 120, no. 11 (2009): 1011–20.

United States Department of Agriculture, "Sugar and Sweeteners Yearbook Tables," accessed May 23, 2014. www.ers.usda.gov/data-products/sugar-and-sweeteners-yearbook-tables.aspx#.U393esbSOdL

J. Wachob, "14 Mind-Blowing Facts About Sugar (Infographic)," *Mind Body Green*, April 16, 2012, accessed May 23, 2014. www.mindbodygreen.com/0-4543/14-MindBlowing-Facts-About-Sugar-Infographic.html

PART I. UNDERSTANDING SUGAR IMPACT

Chapter 1. Not All Sugar Is Created Equal

S. Basu et al., "The Relationship of Sugar to Population-Level Diabetes Prevalence: An Econometric Analysis of Repeated Cross-Sectional Data," *PLoS One* 8, no. 2 (Epub 2013).

J. Boyer and R.H. Liu, "Apple Phytochemicals and Their Health Benefits," *Nutrition Journal* 3, no. 5 (2004).

J.F. Hollis et al., "Weight Loss During the Intensive Intervention Phase of the Weight-Loss Maintenance Trial," *American Journal of Preventive Medicine* 35, no. 2 (2008): 118–26.

K. Keskitalo et al., "Same Genetic Components Underlie Different Measures of Sweet Taste Preference," *American Journal of Clinical Nutrition* 86, no. 6 (2007): 1663–9.

M. Lenoir et al., "Intense Sweetness Surpasses Cocaine Reward," *PLoS One* 2, no. 8 (2007): e698.

R. Schachter, "The Shocking Statistical Truth About Sugar," *Wake Up World*, accessed May 23, 2014. http://wakeup-world.com/2012/10/26/the-shocking-statistical-truth-about-sugar/

Chapter 2. The Sugar Impact Plate

M.B. Abou-Donia et al., "Splenda Alters Gut Microflora and Increases Intestinal p-Glycoprotein and Cytochrome p-450 in Male Rats," *Journal of Toxicology and Environmental Health, Part A* 71, no. 21 (2008): 1415–29.

K. Mahdy Ali et al., "Cardiovascular Disease Risk Reduction by Raising HDL Cholesterol—Current Therapies and Future Opportunities," *British Journal of Pharmacology* 167, no. 6 (2012): 1177–94.

A. Ascherio et al., "Trans-Fatty Acids Intake and Risk of Myocardial Infarction," *Circulation* 89, no. 1 (1994): 94–101.

C.S. Berkey et al., "Milk, Dairy Fat, Dietary Calcium, and Weight Gain: A Longitudinal Study of Adolescents," *Archives of Pediatric and Adolescent Medicine* 159, no. 6 (2005): 543–50.

G.A. Bray, "Soft Drink Consumption and Obesity: It Is All About Fructose," *Current Opinion in Lipidology* 21, no. 1 (2010): 51–57.

E.A. Brinton et al., "A Low-Fat Diet Decreases High Density Lipoprotein (HDL) Cholesterol Levels by Decreasing HDL Apolipoprotein Transport Rates," *Journal of Clinical Investigation* 85, no. 1 (1990): 144–51.

L. Calabresi et al., "An Omega-3 Polyunsaturated Fatty Acid Concentrate Increases Plasma High-Density Lipoprotein 2 Cholesterol and Paraoxonase Levels in Patients with Familial Combined Hyperlipidemia," *Metabolism* 53, no. 2 (2004): 153–58.

W.J. Chen et al., "The Antioxidant Activities of Natural Sweeteners, Mogrosides, from Fruits of *Siraitia grosvenori*," *International Journal of Food Sciences and Nutrition* 58, no. 7 (2007): 548–56.

R. Curi et al., "Effect of *Stevia rebaudiana* on Glucose Tolerance in Normal Adult Humans," *Brazilian Journal of Medical and Biological Research* 19, no. 6 (1986): 771–74.

R. Di et al., "Anti-Inflammatory Activities of Mogrosides from *Momordica grosvenori* in Murine Macrophages and a Murine Ear Edema Model," *Journal of Agricultural and Food Chemistry* 59, no. 13 (2011): 7474–81.

G. Fagherazzi et al., "Consumption of Artificially and Sugar-Sweetened Beverages and Incident Type 2 Diabetes in the Etude Epidemiologique aupres des Femmes de la Mutuelle Generale de l'Education Nationale-European Prospective Investigation into Cancer and Nutrition Cohort," *American Journal of Clinical Nutrition* 97, no. 3 (2013): 517–23.

E. Green and C. Murphy, "Altered Processing of Sweet Taste in the Brain of Diet Soda Drinkers," *Physiology & Behavior* 107, no. 4 (2012): 560–67.

J.A. Greenberg and A. Geliebter, "Coffee, Hunger, and Peptide YY," *Journal of the American College of Nutrition* 31, no. 3 (2012): 160–66.

The Nutrition School at the Harvard School of Public Health, "Vegetables and Fruits: Get Plenty Every Day," accessed February 19, 2014. www.hsph.harvard.edu/nutritionsource/vegetables-full-story/

M. Hibi et al., "Nighttime Snacking Reduces Whole Body Fat Oxidation and Increases LDL Cholesterol in Healthy Young Women," *American Journal of Physiology: Regulatory, Integrative, and Comparative Physiology* 304, no. 2 (2013): R94–R101.

J. Hiebowicz et al., "Effect of Cinnamon on Postprandial Blood Glucose, Gastric Emptying, and Satiety in Healthy Subjects," *American Journal of Clinical Nutrition* 85, no. 6 (2007): 1552–56.

J. Hiebowicz et al., "Effects of 1 and 3 g Cinnamon on Gastric Emptying, Satiety, and Postprandial Blood Glucose, Insulin, Glucose-Dependent Insulinotropic Polypeptide, Glucagon-Like Peptide 1, and Ghrelin Concentrations in Healthy Subjects," *American Journal of Clinical Nutrition* 89, no. 3 (2009): 815–21.

A. Hsu et al., "Promoter De-methylation of Cyclin D2 by Sulforaphane in Prostate Cancer Cells," *Clinical Epigenetics* 3, no. 1 (2011): 3.

M. Hyman, "Eggs Don't Cause Heart Attacks—Sugar Does," *Dr. Mark Hyman* (blog), February 13, 2014, accessed May 23, 2014. http://drhyman.com/blog/2014/02/07/eggs-dont-cause-heart-attacks-sugar/

M. Ishikawa et al., "Effects of Oral Administration of Erythritol on Patients with Diabetes," *Regulatory Toxicology and Pharmacology* 24, no. 2, Pt. 2 (1996): S303–8.

R.J. Johnson et al., "Sugar, Uric Acid, and the Etiology of Diabetes and Obesity," *Diabetes* 62, no. 10 (2013): 3307–15.

C.S. Johnston and C.A. Gaas, "Vinegar: Medicinal Uses and Antiglycemic Effect," *Medscape General Medicine* 8, no. 2 (2006): 61.

C.S. Johnston et al., "Vinegar Improves Insulin Sensitivity to a High-Carbohydrate Meal in Subjects with Insulin Resistance or Type 2 Diabetes," *Diabetes Care* 27, no. 1 (2004): 281–82.

T. Just et al., "Cephalic Phase Insulin Release in Healthy Humans After Taste Stimulation?," *Appetite* 51, no. 3 (2008): 622–27.

M.B. Katan et al., "Trans Fatty Acids and Their Effects on Lipoproteins in Humans," *Annual Review of Nutrition* 15 (1995): 473–93.

J. Kawanabe et al., "Noncariogenicity of Erythritol as a Substrate," *Caries Research* 26, no. 5 (1992): 358–62.

A. Keyes et al., "The Diet and 15-Year Death Rate in the Seven Countries Study," *American Journal of Epidemiology* 124, no. 6 (1986): 903–15.

S.E. Lakhan and A. Kirchgessner, "The Emerging Role of Dietary Fructose in Obesity and Cognitive Decline," *Nutrition Journal* 12 (2013): 114.

W.J. Lee et al., "Alpha-Lipoic Acid Increases Insulin Sensitivity by Activating AMPK in Skeletal Muscle," *Biochemical and Biophysical Research Communication* 332, no. 3 (2005): 885–91.

Y. Liang et al., "The Effect of Artificial Sweetener on Insulin Secretion. 1. The Effect of Acesulfame K on Insulin Secretion in the Rat (Studies in vivo)," *Hormone and Metabolic Research* 19, no. 6 (1987): 233–38.

H. Lynch et al., "Xylitol and Dental Caries: An Overview for Clinicians," *Journal of the California Dental Association* 31, no. 3 (2003): 205–9.

K.K. Mäkinen, "Long-Term Tolerance of Healthy Human Subjects to High Amounts of Xylitol and Fructose: General and Biochemical Findings," Internationale Zeitschrift für Vitamin- und Ernährungsforschung, *Beiheft* 15 (1976): 92–104.

K.K. Mäkinen, "Similarity of the Effects of Erythritol and Xylitol on Some Risk Factors of Dental Caries," *Caries Research* 39, no. 3 (2005): 207–15.

Y. Matsuda et al., "Coffee and Caffeine Improve Insulin Sensitivity and Glucose Tolerance in C57BL/6J Mice Fed a High-Fat Diet," *Bioscience, Biotechnology, and Biochemistry* 75, no. 12 (2011): 2309–15.

C.M. Matthews, "Exploring the Obesity Epidemic," *Proceedings (Baylor University Medical Center)* 25, no. 2 (2012): 276–77.

P.T. Mattila et al., "Increased Bone Volume and Bone Mineral Content in Xylitol-Fed Aged Rats," *Gerontology* 47, no. 6 (2001): 300–305.

D. Mozaffarian et al., "Trans Fatty Acids and Cardiovascular Disease," *New England Journal of Medicine* 354, no. 15 (2006): 1601–13.

M.Y. Pepino et al., "Sucralose Affects Glycemic and Hormonal Responses to an Oral Glucose Load," *Diabetes Care* 36, no. 9 (2013): 2530–35.

M. Sisson, "The Definitive Guide to Resistant Starch," *Mark's Daily Apple*, March 26, 2014, accessed May 23, 2014. www.marksdailyapple.com/the-definitive-guide-to-resistant-starch/#axzz2y9u8NTdh

J. Udani et al., "Blocking Carbohydrate Absorption and Weight Loss: A Clinical Trial Using Phase 2 Brand Proprietary Fractionated White Bean Extract," *Alternative Medicine Review: A Journal of Clinical Therapeutic* 9, no. 1 (2004): 63–69.

A. Uittamo et al., "Xylitol Inhibits Carcinogenic Acetaldehyde Production by Candida Species," *International Journal of Cancer* 129, no. 8 (2011): 2038–41.

University of Washington Study, 2002, reported in *Integrated and Alternative Medicine Clinical Highlights* 4, no. 1, 16.

W.C. Willett et al., "Intake of Trans Fatty Acids and Risk of Coronary Heart Disease Among Women," *Lancet* 6, no. 341 (1993): 581–85.

Q. Yang, "Gain Weight by 'Going Diet'? Artificial Sweeteners and the Neurobiology of Sugar Cravings," *Yale Journal of Biology and Medicine* 83, no. 2 (2010): 101–8.

Q. Yang et al., "Added Sugar Intake and Cardiovascular Diseases Mortality Among US Adults," *JAMA (Journal of the American Medical Association) Internal Medicine* 74, no. 4 (2014): 516–24.

J. Zabner et al., "The Osmolyte Xylitol Reduces the Salt Concentration of Airway Surface Liquid and May Enhance Bacterial Killing," *Procedure of the National Academy of Sciences of the United States of America* 97, no. 21 (2000): 11614–19.

PART II. SUGAR IMPACT DIET RECIPES

J.A. Babraj et al., "Extremely Short Duration High Intensity Interval Training Substantially Improves Insulin Action in Young Healthy Males," *BMC Endocrine Disorders* 9, no. 3 (2009): DOI: 10.1186/1472-6823-9-3.

K. Casazza et al., "Myths, Presumptions, and Facts About Obesity," *New England Journal of Medicine* 368, no. 5 (2013): 446–54.

W.J. Craig, "Nutrition Concerns and Health Effects of Vegetarian Diets," *Nutrition in Clinical Practice: Official Publication of the American Society for Parenteral and Enteral Nutrition* 25, no. 6 (2010): 613–20.

E. A. Dennis et al., "Water Consumption Increases Weight Loss During a Hypocaloric Diet Intervention in Middle-Aged and Older Adults," *Obesity (Silver Spring)* 18, no. 2 (2010): 300–7.

E. Donga et al., "A Single Night of Partial Sleep Deprivation Induces Insulin Resistance in Multiple Metabolic Pathways in Healthy Subjects," *Journal of Clinical Endocrinology and Metabolism* 95, no. 6 (2010): 2963–68.

M.C. Gannon et al., "An Increase in Dietary Protein Improves the Blood Glucose Response in Persons with Type 2 Diabetes," *American Journal of Clinical Nutrition* 78, no. 4 (2003): 734–41.

J. Han et al., "Modulating Gut Microbiota as an Anti-Diabetic Mechanism of Berberine," *Medical Science Monitor: International Medical Journal of Experimental and Clinical Research* 17, no. 7 (2011): RA164–67.

S.B. Heymsfield et al., "Weight Management Using a Meal Replacement Strategy: Meta and Pooling Analysis from Six Studies," *International Journal of Obesity and Related Metabolic Disorders: Journal of the International Association for the Study of Obesity* 27, no. 5 (2003): 537–49.

A.H. Hite et al., "Low-Carbohydrate Diet Review: Shifting the Paradigm," *Nutrition in Clinical Practice: Official Publication of the American Society for Parenteral and Enteral Nutrition* 26, no. 3 (2011): 300–8.

C.W. Kendall et al., "Health Benefits of Nuts in Prevention and Management of Diabetes," *Asia Pacific Journal of Clinical Nutrition* 1, no. 19 (2010): 110–16.

A.C. Logan and T.M. Beauline, "The Treatment of Small Intestinal Bacterial Overgrowth with Enteric-Coated Peppermint Oil: A Case Report," *Alternative Medicine Review: A Journal of Clinical Therapeutic* 7, no. 5 (2002): 410–17.

L.M. Nackers et al., "The Association Between Rate of Initial Weight Loss and Long-Term Success in Obesity Treatment: Does Slow and Steady Win the Race?," *International Journal of Behavioral Medicine* 17, no. 3 (2010): 161–67.

E.M. Quigley and R. Quera, "Small Intestinal Bacterial Overgrowth: Roles of Antibiotics, Prebiotics, and Probiotics," *Gastroenterology* 130, no. 2, Suppl. 1 (2006): S78–90.

J.L. Slavin, "Dietary Fiber and Body Weight," *Nutrition* 21, no. 3 (2005): 411–18.

K. Spiegel et al., "Sleep Loss: A Novel Risk Factor for Insulin Resistance and Type 2 Diabetes," *Journal of Applied Physiology* 99, no. 5 (2005): 2008–19.

X. Wittebole et al., "A Historical Overview of Bacteriophage Therapy as an Alternative to Antibiotics for the Treatment of Bacterial Pathogens," *Virulence* 5, no. 1 (2014): 226–35.

PART III. THE SUGAR IMPACT DIET MEAL PLANS

Chapter 13: Diabetes and Insulin Resistance

J.A. Babraj et al., "Extremely Short Duration High Intensity Interval Training Substantially Improves Insulin Action in Young Healthy Males." *BMC Endocrine Disorders* 9, no. 3 (2009). DOI: 10.1186/1472-6823-9-3.

I. Chiodini et al., "Cortisol Secretion in Patients with Type 2 Diabetes: Relationship with Chronic Complications," *Diabetes Care* 30, no. 1 (2007): 83–88.

M.C. Gannon et al., "An Increase in Dietary Protein Improves the Blood Glucose Response in Persons with Type 2 Diabetes," *American Journal of Clinical Nutrition* 78, no. 4 (2003): 734–41.

C.W. Kendall et al., "Health Benefits of Nuts in Prevention and Management of Diabetes," *Asia Pacific Journal of Clinical Nutrition* 19, no. 1 (2010): 110–16.

J.P. Little et al., "Low-Volume High-Intensity Interval Training Reduces Hyperglycemia and Increases Muscle Mitochondrial Capacity in Patients with Type 2 Diabetes," *Journal of Applied Physiology* 111, no. 6 (2011): 1554–60. DOI: 10.1152/japplphysiol.00921.2011. Epub 2011 Aug. 25.

K. Spiegel et al., "Sleep Loss: A Novel Risk Factor for Insulin Resistance and Type 2 Diabetes," *Journal of Applied Physiology* 99, no. 5 (2005): 2008–19.

C.C. Sung et al., "Role of Vitamin D in Insulin Resistance," *Journal of Biomedicine and Biotechnology* 2012 (2012). Article ID 634195. DOI: 10.1155/2012/634195. Epub 2012 Sep. 3.

Chapter 14: Gastrointestinal Healing

R.A. Gianella et al., "Jejunal Brush Border Injury and Impaired Sugar and Amino Acid Uptake in the Blind Loop Syndrome," *Gastroenterology* 67 (1974): 965–74.

J. Han et al., "Modulating Gut Microbiota as an Anti-Diabetic Mechanism of Berberine," *Medical Science Monitor* 17, no. 7 (2011): RA164–67.

A.C. Logan et al., "The Treatment of Small Intestinal Bacterial Overgrowth with Enteric-Coated Peppermint Oil: A Case Report," *Alternative Medicine Review* 7, no. 5 (2002): 410–17.

M. Pimentel et al., "Eradication of Small Intestinal Bacterial Overgrowth Reduces Symptoms of Irritable Bowel Syndrome," *American Journal of Gastroenterology* 95, no. 12 (2000): 3503–36.

P.M. Quigley et al., "Small Intestinal Bacterial Overgrowth: Roles of Antibiotics, Prebiotics, and Probiotics," *Gastroenterology* 130, no. 2, Suppl 1 (2006): S78–90.

www.ncbi.nlm.nih.gov/pmc/articles/PMC2890937/

www.blogtalkradio.com/drloradio/2011/05/04/digestive-health-with-dr-allison-siebecker

Chapter 15: Paleo and Low Carb

A.H. Hite et al., "Low-Carbohydrate Diet Review: Shifting the Paradigm," *Nutrition in Clinical Practice* 26, no. 3 (2011): 300–8. DOI: 10.1177/0884533611405791.

J.L. Slavin, "Dietary Fiber and Body Weight," *Nutrition* 21, no. 3 (2005): 411–18.

Chapter 16: Vegan and Vegetarian

W.J. Craig, "Nutrition Concerns and Health Effects of Vegetarian Diets," *Nutrition in Clinical Practice* 25, no. 6 (2010): 613–20. DOI: 10.1177/0884533610385707.

INDEX

ABOUT THE AUTHOR

JJ Virgin, CNS, CHFS, is a highly regarded fitness and nutrition expert, public speaker, and media personality. Her most recent book, *JJ Virgin's Sugar Impact Diet*, made her a three-time *New York Times* bestselling author. Her book *The Virgin Diet: Drop 7 Foods, Lose 7 Pounds, Just 7 Days* has appeared on numerous bestselling nonfiction lists, including the *New York Times*, *USA Today*, the *Chicago Tribune*, and the *Wall Street Journal*. Her second book, *The Virgin Diet Cookbook: 150 Easy and Delicious Recipes to Lose Weight and Feel Better Fast*, is also a *New York Times* bestseller.

Internationally recognized as an expert in helping people overcome "weight-loss resistance" (a term she uses to describe the condition of people who do everything right according to current dieting strategies but still can't lose weight), JJ has helped hundreds of thousands of people achieve fast fat loss by addressing food allergies, food sensitivities, and other food intolerances. Clients feel better in days and achieve fast, lasting fat loss when they drop the 7 highly reactive foods she has identified.

JJ's recent media appearances include PBS, *Access Hollywood*, *Rachael Ray*, *The Dr. Oz Show*, *The Doctors*, and the *Today Show*. She is a frequent blogger for Livestrong.com, MindBodyGreen.com, the *Huffington Post*, and *Prevention* magazine. JJ has been interviewed in numerous publications, including *Fox News Magazine*, *Women's World*, *Health*, *LA Weekly*, *Cosmopolitan*, *InStyle* magazine, and the *Los Angeles Times*.

High-performance athletes, CEOs, and A-list celebrities seek out JJ to deliver the results they need and expect. She has worked with Nicole Eggert, Tracie Thoms, and Tamara Johnson-George, and she helped Brandon Routh get in top physical form for *Superman Returns*.

For two years, JJ was the nutrition expert on the top-rated *Dr. Phil* show, and she spent two seasons as cohost of TLC's *Freaky Eaters*. She has two public television pledge shows, *Drop 7 Foods, Feel Better Fast!*, based on the Virgin Diet principles, and *The Sugar Impact*

Secret, based on the Sugar Impact Diet. She is also the bestselling author of *Six Weeks to Sleeveless and Sexy* and creator of the 4x4 Workout series.

JJ is a lifelong learner and has completed 40 graduate and doctoral courses in the areas of exercise science, nutrition, functional medicine, and psychology. She is a board-certified nutrition specialist through the American College of Nutrition, board certified in holistic nutrition, and a certified health and fitness specialist through the American College of Sports Medicine.

Most important, JJ is the mom of two amazing teenage boys. One of them survived a near fatal auto accident, and JJ used her knowledge, expertise, and peer network to take him from comatose to thriving. Every day, JJ wakes up with gratitude to be able to spend another day with her children and to help more people live fuller lives by achieving better health.

For more information, please visit JJ at jjvirgin.com.